Coffee and Caffeine Consumption for Human Health

Coffee and Caffeine Consumption for Human Health

Special Issue Editor

Juan Del Coso

MDPI • Basel • Beijing • Wuhan • Barcelona • Belgrade • Manchester • Tokyo • Cluj • Tianjin

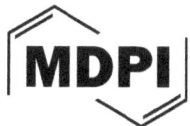

Special Issue Editor
Juan Del Coso
Rey Juan Carlos University
Spain

Editorial Office
MDPI
St. Alban-Anlage 66
4052 Basel, Switzerland

This is a reprint of articles from the Special Issue published online in the open access journal *Nutrients* (ISSN 2072-6643) (available at: https://www.mdpi.com/journal/nutrients/special_issues/Coffee_Caffeine_Health).

For citation purposes, cite each article independently as indicated on the article page online and as indicated below:

LastName, A.A.; LastName, B.B.; LastName, C.C. Article Title. *Journal Name* **Year**, *Article Number*, Page Range.

ISBN 978-3-03928-628-7 (Pbk)
ISBN 978-3-03928-629-4 (PDF)

Cover image courtesy of pixabay.com.

© 2020 by the authors. Articles in this book are Open Access and distributed under the Creative Commons Attribution (CC BY) license, which allows users to download, copy and build upon published articles, as long as the author and publisher are properly credited, which ensures maximum dissemination and a wider impact of our publications.
The book as a whole is distributed by MDPI under the terms and conditions of the Creative Commons license CC BY-NC-ND.

Contents

About the Special Issue Editor ix

Juan Del Coso, Juan José Salinero and Beatriz Lara
Effects of Caffeine and Coffee on Human Functioning
Reprinted from: *Nutrients* **2020**, *12*, 125, doi:10.3390/nu12010125 1

Juan José Salinero, Beatriz Lara, Ester Jiménez-Ormeño, Blanca Romero-Moraleda, Verónica Giráldez-Costas, Gabriel Baltazar-Martins and Juan Del Coso
More Research Is Necessary to Establish the Ergogenic Effect of Caffeine in Female Athletes
Reprinted from: *Nutrients* **2019**, *11*, 1600, doi:10.3390/nu11071600 7

Millán Aguilar-Navarro, Gloria Muñoz, Juan José Salinero, Jesús Muñoz-Guerra, María Fernández-Álvarez, María del Mar Plata and Juan Del Coso
Urine Caffeine Concentration in Doping Control Samples from 2004 to 2015
Reprinted from: *Nutrients* **2019**, *11*, 286, doi:10.3390/nu11020286 11

Alejandro F. San Juan, Álvaro López-Samanes, Pablo Jodra, Pedro L. Valenzuela, Javier Rueda, Pablo Veiga-Herreros, Alberto Pérez-López and Raúl Domínguez
Caffeine Supplementation Improves Anaerobic Performance and Neuromuscular Efficiency and Fatigue in Olympic-Level Boxers
Reprinted from: *Nutrients* **2019**, *11*, 2120, doi:10.3390/nu11092120 23

Domingo Jesús Ramos-Campo, Andrés Pérez, Vicente Ávila-Gandía, Silvia Pérez-Piñero and Jacobo Ángel Rubio-Arias
Impact of Caffeine Intake on 800-m Running Performance and Sleep Quality in Trained Runners
Reprinted from: *Nutrients* **2019**, *11*, 2040, doi:10.3390/nu11092040 39

Sandro Venier, Jozo Grgic and Pavle Mikulic
Caffeinated Gel Ingestion Enhances Jump Performance, Muscle Strength, and Power in Trained Men
Reprinted from: *Nutrients* **2019**, *11*, 937, doi:10.3390/nu11040937 49

Michal Wilk, Aleksandra Filip, Michal Krzysztofik, Adam Maszczyk and Adam Zajac
The Acute Effect of Various Doses of Caffeine on Power Output and Velocity during the Bench Press Exercise among Athletes Habitually Using Caffeine
Reprinted from: *Nutrients* **2019**, *11*, 1465, doi:10.3390/nu11071465 63

Blanca Romero-Moraleda, Juan Del Coso, Jorge Gutiérrez-Hellín and Beatriz Lara
The Effect of Caffeine on the Velocity of Half-Squat Exercise during the Menstrual Cycle: A Randomized Controlled Trial
Reprinted from: *Nutrients* **2019**, *11*, 2662, doi:10.3390/nu11112662 75

Michal Wilk, Michal Krzysztofik, Aleksandra Filip, Adam Zajac and Juan Del Coso
The Effects of High Doses of Caffeine on Maximal Strength and Muscular Endurance in Athletes Habituated to Caffeine
Reprinted from: *Nutrients* **2019**, *11*, 1912, doi:10.3390/nu11081912 85

Michal Wilk, Michal Krzysztofik, Aleksandra Filip, Adam Zajac and Juan Del Coso
Correction: Wilk et al. "The Effects of High Doses of Caffeine on Maximal Strength and Muscular Endurance in Athletes Habituated to Caffeine" Nutrients, 2019, 11(8), 1912
Reprinted from: *Nutrients* **2019**, *11*, 2660, doi:10.3390/nu11112660 99

Hamdi Chtourou, Khaled Trabelsi, Achraf Ammar, Roy Jesse Shephard and Nicola Luigi Bragazzi
Acute Effects of an "Energy Drink" on Short-Term Maximal Performance, Reaction Times, Psychological and Physiological Parameters: Insights from a Randomized Double-Blind, Placebo-Controlled, Counterbalanced Crossover Trial
Reprinted from: *Nutrients* **2019**, *11*, 992, doi:10.3390/nu11050992 101

Juan Del Coso, Beatriz Lara, Carlos Ruiz-Moreno and Juan José Salinero
Challenging the Myth of Non-Response to the Ergogenic Effects of Caffeine Ingestion on Exercise Performance
Reprinted from: *Nutrients* **2019**, *11*, 732, doi:10.3390/nu11040732 115

Paulo Estevão Franco-Alvarenga, Cayque Brietzke, Raul Canestri, Márcio Fagundes Goethel, Bruno Ferreira Viana and Flávio Oliveira Pires
Caffeine Increased Muscle Endurance Performance Despite Reduced Cortical Activation and Unchanged Neuromuscular Efficiency and Corticomuscular Coherence
Reprinted from: *Nutrients* **2019**, *11*, 2471, doi:10.3390/nu11102471 123

Akbar Shabir, Andy Hooton, George Spencer, Mitch Storey, Olivia Ensor, Laura Sandford, Jason Tallis, Bryan Saunders and Matthew F. Higgins
The Influence of Caffeine Expectancies on Simulated Soccer Performance in Recreational Individuals
Reprinted from: *Nutrients* **2019**, *11*, 2289, doi:10.3390/nu11102289 137

Juan Mielgo-Ayuso, Diego Marques-Jiménez, Ignacio Refoyo, Juan Del Coso, Patxi León-Guereño and Julio Calleja-González
Effect of Caffeine Supplementation on Sports Performance Based on Differences Between Sexes: A Systematic Review
Reprinted from: *Nutrients* **2019**, *11*, 2313, doi:10.3390/nu11102313 159

Juan Mielgo-Ayuso, Julio Calleja-Gonzalez, Juan Del Coso, Aritz Urdampilleta, Patxi León-Guereño and Diego Fernández-Lázaro
Caffeine Supplementation and Physical Performance, Muscle Damage and Perception of Fatigue in Soccer Players: A Systematic Review
Reprinted from: *Nutrients* **2019**, *11*, 440, doi:10.3390/nu11020440 177

Satoshi Tsuda, Tatsuya Hayashi and Tatsuro Egawa
The Effects of Caffeine on Metabolomic Responses to Muscle Contraction in Rat Skeletal Muscle
Reprinted from: *Nutrients* **2019**, *11*, 1819, doi:10.3390/nu11081819 193

Antonella Samoggia and Bettina Riedel
Consumers' Perceptions of Coffee Health Benefits and Motives for Coffee Consumption and Purchasing
Reprinted from: *Nutrients* **2019**, *11*, 653, doi:10.3390/nu11030653 207

Regina Wierzejska, Mirosław Jarosz and Barbara Wojda
Caffeine Intake During Pregnancy and Neonatal Anthropometric Parameters
Reprinted from: *Nutrients* **2019**, *11*, 806, doi:10.3390/nu11040806 229

Hyeong Jun Kim, Min Sun Choi, Shaheed Ur Rehman, Young Seok Ji, Jun Sang Yu, Katsunori Nakamura and Hye Hyun Yoo
Determination of Urinary Caffeine Metabolites as Biomarkers for Drug Metabolic Enzyme Activities
Reprinted from: *Nutrients* **2019**, *11*, 1947, doi:10.3390/nu11081947 239

Ki-Young Ryu and Jaesook Roh
The Effects of High Peripubertal Caffeine Exposure on the Adrenal Gland in Immature Male and Female Rats
Reprinted from: *Nutrients* **2019**, *11*, 951, doi:10.3390/nu11050951 255

Marina Sartini, Nicola Luigi Bragazzi, Anna Maria Spagnolo, Elisa Schinca, Gianluca Ottria, Chiara Dupont and Maria Luisa Cristina
Coffee Consumption and Risk of Colorectal Cancer: A Systematic Review and Meta-Analysis of Prospective Studies
Reprinted from: *Nutrients* **2019**, *11*, 694, doi:10.3390/nu11030694 267

About the Special Issue Editor

Juan Del Coso is the Director of the Exercise and Training Laboratory at Rey Juan Carlos University and he lectures on athletics and sports performance assessment. During the last 15 years, he has been working in the field of exercise physiology, devoted to developing new strategies to increase sports performance. After he obtained a bachelor's degree in Sport Sciences (2002, Castilla La Mancha University), he started to investigate the benefits of merging rehydration, carbohydrate intake, and caffeine intake on endurance performance and this was the topic of his Ph.D. dissertation in sports performance (2007, Castilla La Mancha University). He obtained two post-doc fellowships at the Institute for Exercise and Environmental Medicine at Texas Health Presbyterian Hospital Dallas and UT Southwestern Medical Center (2007) and in the Spanish Anti-Doping Agency (2008). Then, he became the Director of the Exercise Physiology Laboratory at Camilo José Cela University (2010), where he spent 9 years building a research group focused on studying sports nutrition, genetics, and doping behaviors. He has just started a new step in his career at Rey Juan Carlos University where he will collaborate to expand the knowledge on evidence-based, safe, and legal approaches to enhance sport performance.

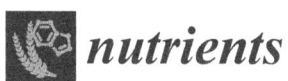

Editorial

Effects of Caffeine and Coffee on Human Functioning

Juan Del Coso [1,*], Juan José Salinero [2] and Beatriz Lara [2]

1. Centre for Sport Studies, Rey Juan Carlos University, Fuenlabrada, 28943 Madrid, Spain
2. Exercise Physiology Laboratory, Camilo José Cela University, 28692 Madrid, Spain; jjsaalinero@ucjc.edu (J.J.S.); blara@ucjc.edu (B.L.)
* Correspondence: juan.delcoso@urjc.es; Tel.: +34-918444694

Received: 17 December 2019; Accepted: 20 December 2019; Published: 2 January 2020

As expected, 2019 has been a prolific year in terms of new evidence regarding the effects of coffee and caffeine consumption on diverse aspects of human functioning. A search in PubMed for published studies in 2019 on the effects of caffeine or coffee on humans, following the Preferred Reporting Items for Systematic Review and Meta-Analyses (PRISMA) guidelines [1], showed a total of 202 manuscripts that contained "coffee" (n = 65, which represents 32.2% of the total) or "caffeine" (n = 137, which represents 67.8% of the total) in the title of the manuscript (Figure 1). In the group of studies that investigated the effect of coffee intake, 58 (89.2%) were related to the use of this beverage to modify one or more health outcomes, five (7.7%) were related to the use of coffee to improve human performance and two (3.1%) assessed regular intake of coffee. In the group of studies that investigated the effect of caffeine intake (in most cases measured as the sum of all the sources containing caffeine such as coffee, tea, chocolate, energy drinks, etc.), 79 (57.7%) were associated with the use of caffeine with health variables, 52 (38.0%) were associated with the use of caffeine with ergogenic purposes, six (4.4%) were associated with regular caffeine intake. Briefly, this analysis shows the elevated amount of new information published each year regarding the utility of coffee and caffeine to produce a change in human functioning while reveals that most of the indications of coffee and caffeine are associated with producing a benefit on health or with enhancing human performance.

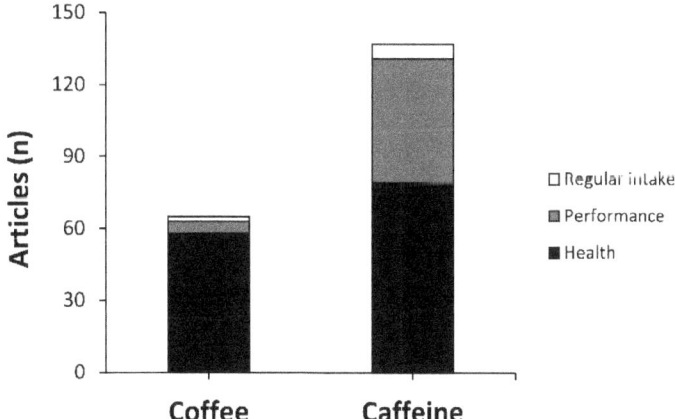

Figure 1. Number of articles published in 2019 that investigated the effects of coffee or caffeine on humans.

This special edition in Nutrients has brought together a variety of investigation that imitates the pattern of published manuscripts commented above. This issue entitled "Coffee and Caffeine

Consumption for Human Health" gathered 20 manuscripts; two (10.0%) were associated with coffee intake and 18 (90%) were associated with caffeine intake. In the manuscripts associated with the use of coffee, one original investigation was geared to study the perceptions of consumers regarding the health benefits that they might obtain with the regular consumption of this beverage [2]. Interestingly, 75.2% of the study sample perceived coffee as negative for their health, while the investigation determined that coffee users that seek potential health benefits of coffee are more likely to be male, young, and working. The other investigation associated with coffee intake was a systematic review and meta-analysis of prospective studies on the effect of this beverage on the risk of colorectal cancer [3]. In this study, a total of 26 investigations were analyzed while the main finding was a weak but significant protective effect of habitual coffee intake on the risk of suffering colon cancer. In addition, the regular intake of decaffeinated coffee exerted a protective effect against colorectal cancer, suggesting that part of the positive effect of coffee to reduce the risk of suffering colorectal cancer is independent of caffeine. Both investigations reflect the beliefs and patterns of our society because evidence shows that the regular intake of coffee can have a positive impact on several health outcomes [4]. Nevertheless, consumers are still cautious about drinking coffee because of the negative image of coffee-(particularly caffeinated coffee), which is not based on the latest scientific evidence [2]. More efforts should be made to translate to our society the new pieces of evidence that support the positive effect of regular coffee consumption on health, in addition to the caution that should be taken in terms of dose, interactions with other substances, and prevalence of side-effects (e.g., stimulant-like effects).

The remaining 18 studies of this issue investigated the effect of caffeine. There was a particular focus on the ergogenic effect of caffeine as 14 (77.8% of the investigations with caffeine in this special issue) investigations were related to this topic. The amount of caffeine ingested on a regular basis was associated with two (11.1%), and the remaining two (11.1%) determined the effect of caffeine on health variables. In the investigations that studied caffeine's ergogenicity, several shared a common message because they reflect that the acute intake of caffeine (from ~1 to ~6 mg/kg of body mass) was effective to improve different aspects of physical and sport performance [5–9], along with enhancement in reaction times and psychological parameters [6]. In addition, several investigations responded to an Editorial [10] that fostered investigations to assess the effect of acute caffeine intake in female athletes because most of the current knowledge about the caffeine's ergogenicity is based on investigations carried out with only-male study samples. As an answer to this call, Mielgo-Ayuso et al. [11] presented an analysis, based on a systematic review, indicating that acute caffeine intake exhibited a similar ergogenic benefit for aerobic performance in men and women athletes. However, the ergogenic effect of caffeine was inferior in women than in men in strength- and power-based tests, even when the same dose of caffeine was being administered. This significant, although low in magnitude, effect of caffeine to increase muscle power and force in women was confirmed by Romero-Moraleda [12], but these authors suggested that caffeine's ergogenicity was similar across the menstrual cycle (by investigating placebo-caffeine comparisons in the early follicular, late follicular and mid-luteal phases). All these investigations have contributed to explaining the effect of caffeine on human performance, which is present in several exercise situations and with several dosages, although further investigations should be carried out to explain the individual differences in the magnitude of the ergogenic effect of caffeine [13].

The clear evidence provided by this special issue confirming the ergogenic effect of caffeine might be behind the slight increase in the use of caffeine in sports since its removal from the list of banned substances in 2004 [14]. By analyzing the concentration of caffeine in post-competition urine samples, it has been found that about three out of four athletes consume caffeine or caffeine-containing products to increase performance [14]. Interestingly, the investigation by Shabir et al. [15], who used a double-dissociation experimental design where caffeine and a placebo were administered in situations in which participants were informed or misinformed of the substance that they had ingested, determined that part of the ergogenic effect of caffeine on human performance is explained by the psychological impact of the expectancy of ergogenicity that caffeine produces in athletes. Thus, believing to have ingested caffeine, or feeling the stimulation that it produces, might be an important part of the actual ergogenic effect of caffeine [16]. In this regard, caffeine ergogenicity can be obtained by the synergistic action of the pharmacological effect of this substance on the central nervous system [8] and in other peripheral tissues [17], together with the psychological effect of this potent stimulant [15].

Nevertheless, habituation to caffeine through the regular intake of this substance might be an important modifier for the obtaining of caffeine ergogenicity. The ingestion of 6 mg/kg of caffeine did not improve the time employed to complete an 800 m competition in athletes habituated to caffeine while it negatively affected sleep quality [18]. Similarly, low-to-moderate doses of caffeine (from 3 to 9 mg/kg), were found to be ergogenic in other situations with individuals who do not consume caffeine or are low caffeine consumers [19,20] and seemed ineffective in increasing muscle performance in athletes habituated to caffeine intake [21]. These two investigations [18,21] indicate that the use of moderate doses of caffeine might not be ergogenic in individuals habituated to caffeine, likely due to the progressive tolerance to the ergogenic effect of this substance when it is ingested chronically [22]. For athletes habituated to caffeine, the use of high doses (up to 11 mg/kg) might exert a positive effect on maximal strength values, but may negatively affect muscle endurance while increasing the prevalence of caffeine-induced drawbacks [23]. All this information taken together suggests that athletes who are consuming caffeine in a habitual manner should refrain from caffeine intake for several days to remove/reduce tolerance to the ergogenic effect of this substance. For athletes habituated to caffeine who seek caffeine's ergogenicity, the dishabituation to caffeine is recommended instead of using doses of caffeine higher than the daily habitual intake.

Other contributions to science published in this issue suggest the possibility of using the measurement of urinary caffeine metabolites as a routine clinical examination for evaluating drug metabolic phenotypes [24], the harmful effects of the administration of high doses of caffeine on the adrenal glands of immature rats [25], and the safety of a mean caffeine intake <200 mg/day to avoid any effect on neonatal weight, length, or head, and chest circumference [26].

The diversity of the articles published in this special issue highlights the extent of the effects of coffee and caffeine on human functioning while it underpins the positive nature of most of these effects. More work is necessary to completely understand the complex mechanisms behind each effect of caffeine on body tissues, although this issue has greatly contributed to unveil how coffee and caffeine might be used to improve human functioning.

Author Contributions: J.D.C., J.J.S., and B.L. wrote the Editorial. All authors have read and agreed to the published version of the manuscript.

Funding: This research received no external funding.

Conflicts of Interest: The authors declare no conflict of interest.

References

1. Moher, D.; Liberati, A.; Tetzlaff, J.; Altman, D.G. PRISMA Group Preferred Reporting Items for Systematic Reviews and Meta-Analyses: The PRISMA Statement. *PLoS Med.* **2009**, *6*, e1000097. [CrossRef] [PubMed]
2. Samoggia, A.; Riedel, B. Consumers' Perceptions of Coffee Health Benefits and Motives for Coffee Consumption and Purchasing. *Nutrients* **2019**, *11*, 653. [CrossRef] [PubMed]
3. Sartini, M.; Bragazzi, N.; Spagnolo, A.; Schinca, E.; Ottria, G.; Dupont, C.; Cristina, M. Coffee Consumption and Risk of Colorectal Cancer: A Systematic Review and Meta-Analysis of Prospective Studies. *Nutrients* **2019**, *11*, 694. [CrossRef] [PubMed]
4. De Mejia, E.G.; Ramirez-Mares, M.V. Impact of caffeine and coffee on our health. *Trends Endocrinol. Metab.* **2014**, *25*, 489–492. [CrossRef] [PubMed]
5. Venier, S.; Grgic, J.; Mikulic, P. Caffeinated Gel Ingestion Enhances Jump Performance, Muscle Strength, and Power in Trained Men. *Nutrients* **2019**, *11*, 937. [CrossRef] [PubMed]

6. Chtourou, H.; Trabelsi, K.; Ammar, A.; Shephard, R.J.; Bragazzi, N.L. Acute Effects of an "Energy Drink"; on Short-Term Maximal Performance, Reaction Times, Psychological and Physiological Parameters: Insights from a Randomized Double-Blind, Placebo-Controlled, Counterbalanced Crossover Trial. *Nutrients* **2019**, *11*, 992. [CrossRef]
7. San Juan, A.F.; López-Samanes, Á.; Jodra, P.; Valenzuela, P.L.; Rueda, J.; Veiga-Herreros, P.; Pérez-López, A.; Domínguez, R. Caffeine Supplementation Improves Anaerobic Performance and Neuromuscular Efficiency and Fatigue in Olympic-Level Boxers. *Nutrients* **2019**, *11*, 2120. [CrossRef]
8. Franco-Alvarenga, P.E.; Brietzke, C.; Canestri, R.; Goethel, M.F.; Viana, B.F.; Pires, F.O. Caffeine Increased Muscle Endurance Performance Despite Reduced Cortical Activation and Unchanged Neuromuscular Efficiency and Corticomuscular Coherence. *Nutrients* **2019**, *11*, 2471. [CrossRef]
9. Mielgo-Ayuso, J.; Calleja-Gonzalez, J.; Del Coso, J.; Urdampilleta, A.; León-Guereño, P.; Fernández-Lázaro, D. Caffeine Supplementation and Physical Performance, Muscle Damage and Perception of Fatigue in Soccer Players: A Systematic Review. *Nutrients* **2019**, *11*, 440. [CrossRef]
10. Salinero, J.J.; Lara, B.; Jiménez-Ormeño, E.; Romero-Moraleda, B.; Giráldez-Costas, V.; Baltazar-Martins, G.; Del Coso, J. More Research Is Necessary to Establish the Ergogenic Effect of Caffeine in Female Athletes. *Nutrients* **2019**, *11*, 1600. [CrossRef]
11. Mielgo-Ayuso, J.; Marques-Jiménez, D.; Refoyo, I.; Del Coso, J.; León-Guereño, P.; Calleja-González, J. Effect of Caffeine Supplementation on Sports Performance Based on Differences Between Sexes: A Systematic Review. *Nutrients* **2019**, *11*, 2313. [CrossRef]
12. Romero-Moraleda, B.; Del Coso, J.; Gutiérrez-Hellín, J.; Lara, B. The Effect of Caffeine on the Velocity of Half-Squat Exercise during the Menstrual Cycle: A Randomized Controlled Trial. *Nutrients* **2019**, *11*, 2662. [CrossRef]
13. Del Coso, J.; Lara, B.; Ruiz-Moreno, C.; Salinero, J.J. Challenging the Myth of Non-Response to the Ergogenic Effects of Caffeine Ingestion on Exercise Performance. *Nutrients* **2019**, *11*, 732. [CrossRef] [PubMed]
14. Aguilar-Navarro, M.; Muñoz, G.; Salinero, J.J.; Muñoz-Guerra, J.; Fernández-Álvarez, M.; Plata, M.D.M.; Del Coso, J. Urine Caffeine Concentration in Doping Control Samples from 2004 to 2015. *Nutrients* **2019**, *11*, 286. [CrossRef] [PubMed]
15. Shabir, A.; Hooton, A.; Spencer, G.; Storey, M.; Ensor, O.; Sandford, L.; Tallis, J.; Higgins, M.F.; Higgins, M.F. The Influence of Caffeine Expectancies on Simulated Soccer Performance in Recreational Individuals. *Nutrients* **2019**, *11*, 2289. [CrossRef]
16. Hurst, P.; Schipof-Godart, L.; Hettinga, F.; Roelands, B.; Beedie, C. Improved 1000-m Running Performance and Pacing Strategy With Caffeine and Placebo: A Balanced Placebo Design Study. *Int. J. Sports Physiol. Perform.* **2019**, in press. [CrossRef]
17. Tsuda, S.; Hayashi, T.; Egawa, T. The Effects of Caffeine on Metabolomic Responses to Muscle Contraction in Rat Skeletal Muscle. *Nutrients* **2019**, *11*, 1819. [CrossRef] [PubMed]
18. Ramos-Campo, D.J.; Pérez, A.; Ávila-Gandía, V.; Pérez-Piñero, S.; Rubio-Arias, J.Á. Impact of Caffeine Intake on 800-m Running Performance and Sleep Quality in Trained Runners. *Nutrients* **2019**, *11*, 2040. [CrossRef]
19. Del Coso, J.; Salinero, J.J.; González-Millán, C.; Abián-Vicén, J.; Pérez-González, B. Dose response effects of a caffeine-containing energy drink on muscle performance: A repeated measures design. *J. Int. Soc. Sports Nutr.* **2012**, *9*, 21. [CrossRef]
20. Grgic, J.; Mikulic, P.; Schoenfeld, B.J.; Bishop, D.J.; Pedisic, Z. The Influence of Caffeine Supplementation on Resistance Exercise: A Review. *Sports Med.* **2019**, *49*, 17–30. [CrossRef]
21. Wilk, M.; Filip, A.; Krzysztofik, M.; Maszczyk, A.; Zajac, A. The Acute Effect of Various Doses of Caffeine on Power Output and Velocity during the Bench Press Exercise among Athletes Habitually Using Caffeine. *Nutrients* **2019**, *11*, 1465. [CrossRef] [PubMed]
22. Lara, B.; Ruiz-Moreno, C.; Salinero, J.J.; Del Coso, J. Time course of tolerance to the performance benefits of caffeine. *PLoS ONE* **2019**, *14*, e0210275. [CrossRef] [PubMed]
23. Wilk, M.; Krzysztofik, M.; Filip, A.; Zajac, A.; Del Coso, J. Correction: Wilk et al. "The Effects of High Doses of Caffeine on Maximal Strength and Muscular Endurance in Athletes Habituated to Caffeine" Nutrients, 2019, 11(8), 1912. *Nutrients* **2019**, *11*, 2660. [CrossRef] [PubMed]
24. Kim, H.J.; Choi, M.S.; Rehman, S.U.; Ji, Y.S.; Yu, J.S.; Nakamura, K.; Yoo, H.H. Determination of Urinary Caffeine Metabolites as Biomarkers for Drug Metabolic Enzyme Activities. *Nutrients* **2019**, *11*, 1947. [CrossRef] [PubMed]

25. Ryu, K.-Y.; Roh, J. The Effects of High Peripubertal Caffeine Exposure on the Adrenal Gland in Immature Male and Female Rats. *Nutrients* **2019**, *11*, 951. [CrossRef] [PubMed]
26. Wierzejska, R.; Jarosz, M.; Wojda, B. Caffeine Intake During Pregnancy and Neonatal Anthropometric Parameters. *Nutrients* **2019**, *11*, 806. [CrossRef]

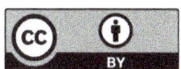

© 2020 by the authors. Licensee MDPI, Basel, Switzerland. This article is an open access article distributed under the terms and conditions of the Creative Commons Attribution (CC BY) license (http://creativecommons.org/licenses/by/4.0/).

Editorial

More Research Is Necessary to Establish the Ergogenic Effect of Caffeine in Female Athletes

Juan José Salinero, Beatriz Lara, Ester Jiménez-Ormeño, Blanca Romero-Moraleda, Verónica Giráldez-Costas, Gabriel Baltazar-Martins and Juan Del Coso *

Exercise Physiology Laboratory, Camilo José Cela University, 28692 Madrid, Spain
* Correspondence: jdelcoso@ucjc.edu; Tel.: +34-9185-3131

Received: 9 July 2019; Accepted: 12 July 2019; Published: 15 July 2019

Dear Editor-in-Chief,

Today, there is a significant gap in research on the ergogenicity of caffeine, and on sports nutrition in general: the benefits/drawbacks for a given substance are typically assumed for the whole population of athletes when most of the evidence is supported by investigations with only male samples. As a result of this assumption, acute pre-exercise ingestion of 3–9 mg/kg of caffeine is considered an effective strategy to increase sports performance [1], while data on urine caffeine concentration indicates that the use of caffeine in sport is similar in both sexes [2]. A few recent investigations using women as study samples, have also found that caffeine increases sports performance [3–6]. However, evidence regarding the overall ergogenicity of caffeine in women is much scarcer than in men, and it seems unsafe to conclude that the ergogenic effect of a moderate dose of caffeine is of similar magnitude in men and women.

A search for published studies on the effects of caffeine on physical performance in PubMed and Scopus, following with the Preferred Reporting Items for Systematic Review and Meta-Analyses (PRISMA) guidelines [7], showed a total of 362 original investigations that have compared caffeine to a placebo/control situation, with the measurement of at least one physical performance variable (Figure 1).

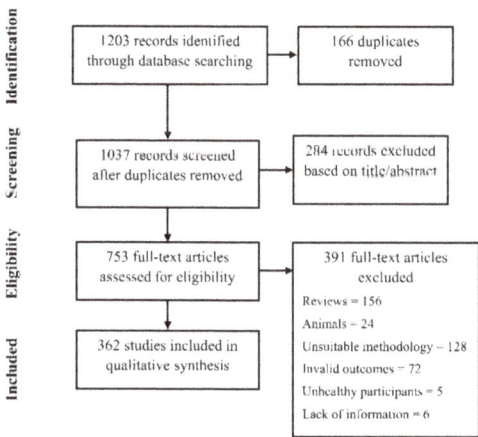

Figure 1. Selection of studies.

After filters were applied to remove duplicates or publications with unsuitable methodology, the search illustrated that a total of 5321 individuals have been tested to assess caffeine ergogenicity, since the seminal investigation by Costill et al. [8]. From this sample, 703 participants were women, which represents only 13.2% of the total sample.

Although investigations on this topic have a higher tendency to include women, especially since 2013, women still represent only 16.3% of individuals participating in research carried out in 2018 (Figure 2). In addition, there is no investigation that has measured caffeine ergogenicity in women with doses below 1 mg/kg or above 9 mg/kg, and the number of women in investigations about caffeine effects on speed and muscle power is very low (Table 1).

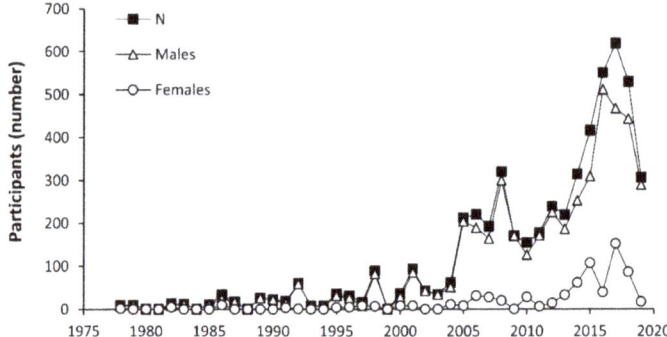

Figure 2. Evolution of the number of participants (n = total, males and females) in investigations aimed at determining the ergogenic effects of caffeine.

Table 1. Number (frequency) of male and female participants in investigations aimed at determining the ergogenic effects of caffeine depending on dose, type of exercise, and participant's level.

		Males	Females
Caffeine dose	< 1 mg/kg	10 (100.0%)	0 (0.0%)
	1.0–2.9 mg/kg	608 (90.2%)	66 (9.8%)
	3.0–5.9 mg/kg	2295 (85.2%)	400 (14.8%)
	6.0–9.0 mg/kg	1590 (87.0%)	237 (13.0%)
	>9 mg/kg	115 (100.0%)	0 (0.0%)
Type of exercise	Speed	128 (89.5%)	15 (10.5%)
	Strength	527 (83.1%)	107 (16.9%)
	Power	98 (83.8%)	19 (16.2%)
	Anaerobic-like	587 (88.0%)	80 (12.0%)
	Endurance-like	2019 (89.0%)	249 (11.0%)
	Team-sport	241 (70.9%)	99 (29.1%)
	Other	1018 (88.4%)	134 (11.6%)
Athlete' level	Trained	2777 (87.8%)	385 (12.2%)
	Active	1421 (85.7%)	237 (14.3%)
	Untrained	420 (83.8%)	81 (16.2%)

Interestingly, there are no investigations measuring the ergogenic effect of caffeine during the different phases of the menstrual cycle, despite the interactions between caffeine and female sex hormones [9]. In fact, it has been found that the effect of caffeine on increasing blood pressure is higher in the follicular than in the luteal phase in female adolescents [10]. All this information indicates that it is still too early to establish that women experience the same ergogenic response to caffeine as men, and further research is needed to describe the optimal conditions of caffeine use in sport and exercise for women. With this Editorial, we want to encourage authors to provide objective information about the dose-effect of caffeine on female athletes' physical performance. We also want to embolden research focused to determine the magnitude of the ergogenic effect of caffeine during the different phases of the menstrual cycle. The Nutrients' Special Issue on "Coffee and Caffeine Consumption for

Human Health" is open to receive investigations on these topics that hold to "bridge the gap" on the ergogenicity of caffeine in female athletes.

Author Contributions: Conceptualization, J.D.C.; methodology, J.J.S., B.L., E.J.-O., B.R.-M., V.G.-C., and G.B.-M.; formal analysis, J.J.S., and J.D.C.; writing—original draft preparation, J.D.C.; writing—review and editing, J.J.S., B.L., E.J.-O., B.R.-M., V.G.-C., and G.B.-M; supervision, J.D.C.

Funding: This research received no external funding.

Acknowledgments: We want to acknowledge all the authors that are investigating the effects of acute caffeine intake in several aspects of physical performance.

Conflicts of Interest: The authors declare no conflict of interest.

References

1. Baltazar-Martins, J.G.; Brito de Souza, D.; Aguilar, M.; Grgic, J.; Del Coso, J. Infographic. The road to the ergogenic effect of caffeine on exercise performance. *Br. J. Sports Med.* **2019**. [CrossRef] [PubMed]
2. Aguilar-Navarro, M.; Muñoz, G.; Salinero, J.J.; Muñoz-Guerra, J.; Fernández-Álvarez, M.; Plata, M.D.M.; Del Coso, J. Urine Caffeine Concentration in Doping Control Samples from 2004 to 2015. *Nutrients* **2019**, *11*, 286. [CrossRef] [PubMed]
3. Lara, B.; Gonzalez-Millán, C.; Salinero, J.J.; Abian-Vicen, J.; Areces, F.; Barbero-Alvarez, J.C.; Muñoz, V.; Portillo, L.J.; Gonzalez-Rave, J.M.; Del Coso, J. Caffeine-containing energy drink improves physical performance in female soccer players. *Amino Acids* **2014**, *46*, 1385–1392. [CrossRef] [PubMed]
4. Del Coso, J.; Portillo, J.; Muñoz, G.; Abián-Vicén, J.; Gonzalez-Millán, C.; Muñoz-Guerra, J. Caffeine-containing energy drink improves sprint performance during an international rugby sevens competition. *Amino Acids* **2013**, *44*, 1511–1519. [CrossRef] [PubMed]
5. Pérez-López, A.; Salinero, J.J.; Abian-Vicen, J.; Valadés, D.; Lara, B.; Hernandez, C.; Areces, F.; González, C.; Del Coso, J. Caffeinated energy drinks improve volleyball performance in elite female players. *Med. Sci. Sports Exerc.* **2015**, *47*, 850–856. [CrossRef] [PubMed]
6. Skinner, T.L.; Desbrow, B.; Arapova, J.; Schaumberg, M.A.; Osborne, J.; Grant, G.D.; Anoopkumar-Dukie, S.; Leveritt, M.D. Women Experience the Same Ergogenic Response to Caffeine as Men. *Med. Sci. Sports Exerc.* **2019**, *51*, 1195–1202. [CrossRef] [PubMed]
7. Moher, D.; Liberati, A.; Tetzlaff, J.; Altman, D.G. Preferred Reporting Items for Systematic Reviews and Meta-Analyses: The PRISMA Statement. *PLoS Med.* **2009**, *6*, e1000097. [CrossRef] [PubMed]
8. Costill, D.L.; Dalsky, G.P.; Fink, W.J. Effects of caffeine ingestion on metabolism and exercise performance. *Med. Sci. Sports* **1978**, *10*, 155–158. [PubMed]
9. Arnaud, M.J. Pharmacokinetics and Metabolism of Natural Methylxanthines in Animal and Man. *Handb. Exp. Pharmacol.* **2011**, 33–91. [CrossRef]
10. Temple, J.L.; Ziegler, A.M. Gender Differences in Subjective and Physiological Responses to Caffeine and the Role of Steroid Hormones. *J. Caffeine Res.* **2011**, *1*, 41–48. [CrossRef] [PubMed]

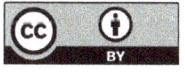

© 2019 by the authors. Licensee MDPI, Basel, Switzerland. This article is an open access article distributed under the terms and conditions of the Creative Commons Attribution (CC BY) license (http://creativecommons.org/licenses/by/4.0/).

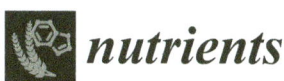

Article

Urine Caffeine Concentration in Doping Control Samples from 2004 to 2015

Millán Aguilar-Navarro [1,2], Gloria Muñoz [3], Juan José Salinero [1], Jesús Muñoz-Guerra [4], María Fernández-Álvarez [3], María del Mar Plata [4] and Juan Del Coso [1,*]

[1] Exercise Physiology Laboratory, Camilo José Cela University, 28692 Madrid, Spain; millan.aguilar@ufv.es (M.A.-N.); jjsalinero@ucjc.edu (J.J.S.)
[2] Faculty of Education, Francisco de Vitoria University, 28223 Madrid, Spain
[3] Doping Control Laboratory, Spanish Agency for Health Protection in Sport, 28040 Madrid, Spain; gloria.munoz@aepsad.god.es (G.M.); maria.fernandez@aepsad.god.es (M.F.-Á.)
[4] Department for Doping Control, Spanish Agency for Health Protection in Sport, 28016 Madrid, Spain; jesus.munoz@aepsad.god.es (J.M.-G.); maria.plata@aepsad.god.es (M.d.M.P.)
* Correspondence: jdelcoso@ucjc.edu; Tel.: +34-918-153-131

Received: 28 November 2018; Accepted: 23 January 2019; Published: 29 January 2019

Abstract: The ergogenic effect of caffeine is well-established, but the extent of its consumption in sport is unknown at the present. The use of caffeine was considered "prohibited" until 2004, but this stimulant was moved from the List of Prohibited Substances to the Monitoring Program of the World Anti-Doping Agency to control its use by monitoring urinary caffeine concentration after competition. However, there is no updated information about the change in the use of caffeine as the result of its inclusion in the Monitoring Program. The aim of this study was to describe the changes in urine caffeine concentration from 2004 to 2015. A total of 7488 urine samples obtained in official competitions held in Spain and corresponding to athletes competing in Olympic sports (2788 in 2004, 2543 in 2008, and 2157 in 2015) were analyzed for urine caffeine concentration. The percentage of samples with detectable caffeine (i.e., >0.1 µg/mL) increased from ~70.1%, in 2004–2008 to 75.7% in 2015. The median urine caffeine concentration in 2015 (0.85 µg/mL) was higher when compared to the median value obtained in 2004 (0.70 µg/mL; $p < 0.05$) and in 2008 (0.70 µg/mL; $p < 0.05$). The urine caffeine concentration significantly increased from 2004 to 2015 in aquatics, athletics, boxing, judo, football, weightlifting, and rowing ($p < 0.05$). However, the sports with the highest urine caffeine concentration in 2015 were cycling, athletics, and rowing. In summary, the concentration of caffeine in the urine samples obtained after competition in Olympic sports in Spain increased from 2004 to 2015, particularly in some disciplines. These data indicate that the use of caffeine has slightly increased since its removal from the list of banned substances, but urine caffeine concentrations suggest that the use of caffeine is moderate in most sport specialties. Athletes of individual sports or athletes of sports with an aerobic-like nature are more prone to using caffeine in competition.

Keywords: pharmacokinetics; energy drink; exercise; elite athlete; performance

---

1. Introduction

Caffeine (1,3,7-trimethylxanthine) is a stimulant naturally present in a variety of foods and drinks, although it is also artificially included in dietary and sports supplements, over-the-counter medications, and beverages. In the sport setting, caffeine is widely utilized because it might have the capacity to enhance endurance performance [1,2], anaerobic-based performance [3], and strength/power-oriented performance [4,5] in exercise and sports of different nature [6–8]. There is strong evidence supporting that caffeine, when ingested prior to exercise, and at a dosage of 3–6 mg per kg of body mass, could benefit sports performance as it has been recently recognized by the International Olympic Committee in its consensus statement on dietary supplements [9]. However, the ergogenicity of caffeine might be affected by the scenario of use and may vary widely among individuals because of several factors that include genetic variants, the microbiome and habituation to caffeine [10]. Specifically, it has been recently found that AA homozygotes for a single nucleotide polymorphism in the CYP1A2 gene (rs762551, also known as −163C>A) might obtain greater ergogenic benefits from acute caffeine intake (2–6 mg/kg) than C-allele carriers [11–13], although this is not always the case [14–17]. In addition, previous investigations have suggested that the ergogenic effect of acute caffeine ingestion (3–5 mg/kg) might be reduced by habitual caffeine intake [18,19], suggesting a progressive tolerance to the ergogenic effects of this substance when this substance is ingested chronically. However, other investigations have shown that naïve/low caffeine consumers benefited from the acute intake of 3–6 mg/kg of caffeine to a similar extent to habitual caffeine consumers [20,21], and, to date, there is not a clear consensus about time course of tolerance to the performance benefits of caffeine. Although the reasons to explain tolerance to caffeine require further investigation, it seems clear that the physiological responses to acute caffeine intake have a great inter-individual variability [22].

The use of caffeine in sports can also have several drawbacks, such as increased ratings of nervousness and insomnia [23] that might limit its efficacy to enhance performance. In this respect, the "more is better" philosophy (i.e., >9 mg/kg), when applied to caffeine, may result in a higher prevalence of side effects [24,25] that outweigh the potential performance benefits of this stimulant. Likely due to these and other drawbacks, caffeine was considered a banned substance in sport by the medical commission of the International Olympic Committee and other anti-doping authorities between 1984 and 2004, and its use was prohibited only in competition. A 12 µg/mL threshold for urine caffeine concentration was set in 1987 to limit the use of high doses of caffeine and athletes that surpassed this threshold were penalized for doping misconduct. The World Anti-Doping Agency (WADA) decided to remove caffeine from the list of banned substances with effect from January 1, 2004, and since then, athletes have been able to consume caffeine-containing products freely. However, WADA included caffeine in its Monitoring Program; a program designed to monitor and detect patterns of misuse in substances not included in the prohibited list, but with the possibility of being harmful in sport [26]. Since 2004, WADA has monitored the proportion of urine samples with a caffeine concentration of over 6 µg/mL in order to monitor the use of high doses that could be harmful for athletes, although the data are not public. Interestingly, the concentration of caffeine in the urine samples used for doping control remained similar between 1993–2002 (i.e., when caffeine was in the list of banned substances) [27] and 2004–2008 (i.e., when caffeine was removed from the list of banned substances) [28,29]. These data suggest that the use of caffeine was not substantially modified with the removal of caffeine from the list of banned substances, likely because the "12-µg/mL-threshold" was not an effective deterrent to prevent the use of caffeine to increase physical performance. However, since 2008, there is no investigation that have studied the trends in the use of caffeine sports despite the evidence that support the ergogenicity of caffeine has greatly increased in the last years [1,2,5,30,31]. Thus, the aim of this study was to describe the changes in urine caffeine concentrations in Olympic sports using samples obtained in 2004, 2008, and 2015. The ultimate goal of this study was to use the evolution in urinary caffeine concentration to infer changes in the use of caffeine in sport.

2. Materials and Methods

For this study, we measured the urine caffeine concentration in all samples submitted to the Madrid Doping Control Laboratory (Spain) in 2004, 2008, and 2015 as part of the WADA Monitoring Program. The samples measured corresponded to specimens gathered after national and international competitions held in Spain, since urine specimens collected out-of-competition are not routinely analyzed for caffeine detection. The current study presents an analysis of the 7488 urine samples that corresponded to athletes competing in Olympic sports (2788 in 2004, 2543 in 2008, and 2157 in 2015). In 2004, 25.4% of the samples pertained to women athletes, 26.0% in 2008 and 24.2% in 2015. To obtain representative data on each sport discipline, a threshold of >25 samples per year was established to include any Olympic sport in the analysis. Information about the athlete's sex (included on the anti-doping form) was integrated into a database for the analysis. The investigation used anonymized data obtained for the doping control and thus did not require ethical approval. Participants' rights and confidentiality were protected during the whole study, and the data were only used for the purposes included in this investigation. The study conformed to the Declaration of Helsinki.

2.1. Urine Analysis

All samples were obtained following the Guidelines for Urine Sample Collection described by WADA [32]. Upon collection, the samples were sent to the Doping Control Laboratory by special refrigerated transport and arrived at the laboratory with an anonymized format (alpha-numeric code). After arrival, a portion of the sample was used to measure urine caffeine concentration and the remaining amount was destined to other anti-doping purposes. Specifically, a portion (5 mL) of each urine sample was poured into a 15-mL screw-capped glass tube. Then, 50 µL of internal standard (diphenylamine 100 µg/mL) was added to the sample. After that, 100 µL of sodium hydroxide 10 mol/L and 0.5 g of sodium sulphate were added to increase the transfer of analytes from the aqueous to the organic phase. Alkaline extraction was performed by adding 5 mL of methyl tert-butyl ether and centrifuging the sample at 60 rpm for 20 min. After that, the sample was frozen in a cryogenic bath, and the organic phase (upper phase and not frozen) was transferred to a clean vial. The extract was concentrated with nitrogen, and 2 µL of the remaining extract was injected into the system for caffeine quantification.

The methodology to quantify urine caffeine concentration was based on gas chromatography–mass spectrometry (GC-MS), and was validated according to ISO17025. The measurement of each batch of urine samples was preceded by a calibration process, using a solution with an established caffeine concentration (6 µg/mL). GC-MS analysis was performed using a 6890N Gas Chromatograph (Agilent Technologies, Santa Clara, CA, USA) coupled to a 5973N Mass Selective Detector (Agilent Technologies). All the chromatograms in the samples analyzed in 2004 and in 2008 were obtained in the scan mode range. At this time, the GC was equipped with a fused silica capillary column OV-1 (J & W Scientific Inc., Folsom, CA, USA). In 2015, the chromatograms were obtained in the single ion monitoring (SIM) mode and the GC was equipped with a capillary column Ultra-1 (J & W Scientific Inc., Folsom, CA, USA). In all analyses the carrier gas was helium, and they were carried out at a constant pressure of 15 psi. To facilitate separation, the initial column temperature was set at 90 °C and the final column temperature was set at 300 °C. The temperature on the injector port was set at 275 °C.

2.2. Validation Procedure

The between-days reproducibility was evaluated using 20 measurements of the calibration solution obtained over two months. The between-days coefficient of variation (at 6 µg/mL) was 7%. Accuracy was calculated in terms of the recovery factor (experimental value/theoretical value, expressed as a percentage). The value obtained was 105%, and no tendencies were observed. Combined uncertainty was estimated taking into account the contributions of accuracy and reproducibility and the value obtained was 11%. The limit of detection (LOD) was 0.1 µg/mL.

2.3. Statistical Analysis

All samples with a urinary caffeine concentration below the LOD were considered to be specimens without any caffeine content. The remaining samples were categorized into intervals of 1.0 µg/mL, with a maximal caffeine concentration of 13.0 µg/mL. Most of the samples had a urinary caffeine concentration between 0.0 and 13.0 µg/mL, but 32 samples had a urinary caffeine concentration of >13.0 µg/mL (14 in 2004, 11 in 2008, and 7 in 2015). These samples were included in the statistical analysis, but they were not included in the graphical presentation of the data per 1.0 µg/mL-categories. The samples were grouped by sport discipline, by year of collection, and by athlete's sex. Normality for each year of collection was tested with the Kolmogorov-Smirnov test.

Data are presented as median ± and interquartile range (25% and 75% percentile) for quantitative variables (urine caffeine concentration), while qualitative variables (distribution) are presented as percentages. Urine caffeine concentration had a non-normal distribution and thus, non-parametric statistics were later employed. The comparison of the urine caffeine concentration among the three years (2004 vs. 2008 vs. 2015) was tested with the Kruskal-Wallis test. The changes in the evolution of the urine caffeine concentration within each sport were also identified with the Kruskal-Wallis test. The differences in distribution of samples among ranges of urine caffeine concentration were tested with crosstab and Chi Square tests, including adjusted standardized residuals. The comparison among sport specialties was only performed for the samples obtained in 2015 because a previous publication provided this comparison for 2004–2008 [29]. Finally, the differences between sexes were analyzed with the U-Mann Whitney test. The data were analyzed with the statistical package SPSS v 21.0 (SPSS Inc., Chicago, IL, USA). The significance level for all these statistical analyses was set at $p < 0.05$.

3. Results

The median urine caffeine concentration in 2015 (0.9; 0.1–2.4 µg/mL) was higher when compared to the median value obtained in 2004 (0.7; 0.0–2.4 µg/mL; $p < 0.05$) and 2008 (0.70; 0.1–2.1 µg/mL; $p < 0.05$; Figure 1). The maximal value of caffeine concentration was 21.1, 19.2 and 18.6 µg/mL for 2004, 2008, and 2015, respectively.

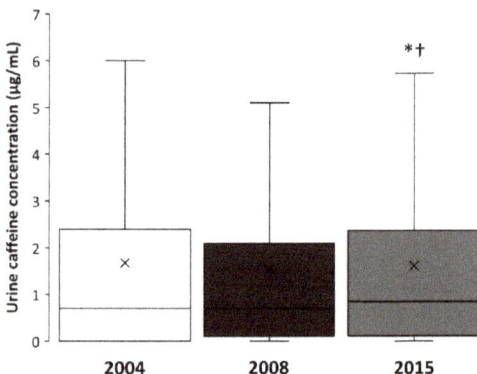

Figure 1. Box-and-whisker plot for caffeine concentration in the urine samples of Olympic sports collected in 2004, 2008, and 2015. The cross depicts the mean value while the lower, middle and upper lines of the box represent the 25%, 50% and 75% percentile. Whiskers represent 1.5 × interquartile range. Outlier data have been removed to facilitate the comprehension of the figure. (*) Different from 2004 at $p < 0.05$; (†) Different from 2008 at $p < 0.05$.

Figure 2 depicts the distribution of urine samples in each year of analysis according to their urine caffeine concentration, using 1 µg/mL intervals. The distribution of the samples was slightly different among these years because in 2015, the percentage of samples below the limit of detection was lower than expected ($p < 0.05$) while the percentage of samples between 2 and 4 µg/mL was higher than expected ($p < 0.05$). The percentage of samples with detectable caffeine (i.e., > 0.1 µg/mL) was 70.3%, 69.8%, and 75.7% in 2004, 2008, and 2015, respectively. The proportion of samples with urine caffeine concentrations of >12 µg/mL was 0.79%, 0.87%, and 0.60% in 2004, 2008, and 2015, respectively.

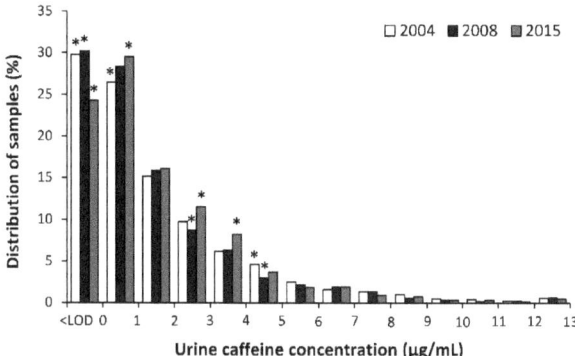

Figure 2. Distribution of urine samples according to the concentration of caffeine in 2004, 2008, and 2015. (*) Different from the expected value. LOD: limit of detection.

Figure 3 depicts box-and-whisker plots for the changes in urine caffeine concentrations in 2004, 2008, and 2015 in men and women. The median values obtained in 2015 were different from 2004 and 2008 in men (upper panel) and women (lower panel), respectively ($p < 0.05$), while the median values were always higher in men than in women ($p < 0.05$).

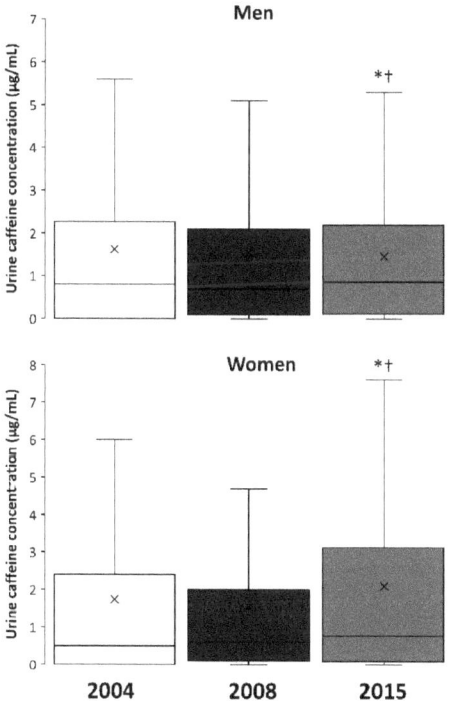

Figure 3. Box-and-whisker plot for caffeine concentrations in the urine samples from men and women collected in 2004, 2008, and 2015. The cross depicts the mean value while the lower, middle and upper lines of the box represent the 25%, 50%, and 75% percentile. Whiskers represent 1.5 × interquartile range. Outlier data have been removed to facilitate the comprehension of the figure. (*) Different from 2004 at $p < 0.05$; (†) Different from 2008 at $p < 0.05$.

Figure 4 depicts urine caffeine concentration in Olympic sports in 2015 using box-and-whisker plots. The sports with the highest concentration of caffeine in urine were cycling, rowing, triathlon, athletics, weightlifting, and volleyball (all with median values >1.0 µg/mL); the sports with the lowest urine caffeine concentration were shooting, fencing, hockey, basketball, and golf (all with median values <0.5 µg/mL). Golf presented urine caffeine concentrations lower than cycling, athletics, rowing, triathlon, handball, and football ($p < 0.05$). Table 1 contains information on the changes in the median urine caffeine concentrations in Olympics sports for the years 2004, 2008, and 2015. Specifically, the values obtained in 2015 were significantly higher than those obtained in 2004 and 2008 in aquatics, athletics, boxing, judo, and football. In golf and skiing, the data from 2015 were higher only when compared to 2008, while in rowing and weightlifting, the values in 2015 were only different to 2004.

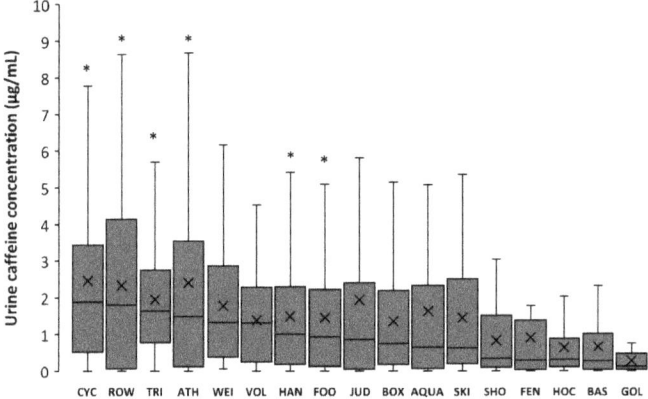

Figure 4. Box-and-whisker plot for caffeine concentrations in the urine samples of Olympic sports collected in 2015. The cross depicts the mean value while the lower, middle, and upper lines of the box represent the 25%, 50%, and 75% percentile. Whiskers represent 1.5 × interquartile range. Outlier data have been removed to facilitate the comprehension of the figure. CYC = Cycling; ROW = Rowing; TRI = Triathlon; ATH = Athletics; WEI = Weightlifting; VOL = Volleyball; HAN = Handball; FOO = Football; JUD = Judo; BOX = Boxing; AQUA = Aquatics; SKI = Skiing; SHO = Shooting; FEN = Fencing; HOC = Hockey; BAS = Basketball; GOL = Golf. (*) Different from GOL at $p < 0.05$.

Table 1. Urine caffeine concentrations (µg/mL) in Olympic sports in 2004, 2008, and 2015. Data are medians (25% and 75% percentile) for each sport.

Sport	2004	2008	2015	p Value
Aquatics	0.1 (0.0–0.8)	0.1 (0.0–1.2)	0.7 (0.1–2.3) *†	<0.01
Athletics	0.7 (0.0–2.6)	0.8 (0.1–2.4)	1.5 (0.1–3.6) *†	<0.01
Basketball	0.2 (0.0–0.9)	0.4 (0.0–1.2)	0.3 (0.1–1.0)	0.13
Boxing	0.5 (0.0–0.9)	0.0 (0.0–0.8)	0.8 (0.2–2.2) *†	<0.01
Cycling	2.0 (0.5–4.0)	1.7 (0.5–3.6)	1.9 (0.5–3.4)	0.30
Fencing	0.5 (0.0–0.9)	0.1 (0.0–0.8)	0.3 (0.1–1.4)	0.19
Football	0.7 (0.0–2.0)	0.5 (0.1–1.6)	0.9 (0.1–2.2) *†	<0.01
Golf	0.0 (0.2–0.4)	0.0 (0.0–0.0) *	0.1 (0.0–0.5) †	<0.01
Handball	1.0 (0.2–2.7)	0.9 (0.1–2.1)	1.0 (0.2–2.3)	0.40
Hockey	0.4 (0.0–1.6)	0.9 (0.2–2.2)	0.3 (0.3–0.9)	0.60
Judo	0.2 (0.0–0.8)	0.2 (0.0–0.5)	0.9 (0.1–2.4) *†	<0.01
Rowing	0.4 (0.1–1.6)	2.7 (0.1–5.0) *	1.8 (0.1–4.1) *	<0.01
Shooting	0.4 (0.0–2.0)	0.1 (0.0–1.7)	0.3 (0.1–1.5)	0.24
Skiing	0.2 (0.0–1.0)	0.3 (0.1–0.9)	0.6 (0.2–2.5) †	0.03
Triathlon	1.2 (0.3–4.2)	3.0 (1.5–6.2) *	1.6 (0.8–2.8)	<0.01
Volleyball	0.9 (0.1–2.0)	1.5 (0.2–2.6)	1.3 (0.3–2.2)	0.45
Weightlifting	0.2 (0.0–1.2)	0.6 (0.0–1.8)	1.3 (0.4–2.9) *†	0.01

(*) Different from 2004 at $p < 0.05$. (†) Different from 2008 at $p < 0.05$.

4. Discussion

The purpose of this investigation was to describe the changes in urine caffeine concentration of samples obtained in competition of Olympic sports for the years 2004, 2008, and 2015. The final goal was to determine the evolution in the use of caffeine in sports, especially one decade after it was removed from the banned list. For this purpose, we measured caffeine concentration in 7488 urine samples received by the WADA-accredited Doping Control Laboratory in Madrid as part of the Monitoring Program. The main outcomes of this investigation indicate the following: (a) in 2015, there was a slight but statistically significant increase in urine caffeine concentration when compared to both 2004 and 2008. This increase is reflected by a lower proportion of athletes with urinary caffeine concentrations below the limit of detection and a higher proportion of athletes with concentrations between 2 and 4 µg/mL; (b) the increase in urine caffeine concentration in 2015 was similarly present in both men and women but it was unequal in all sport disciplines. Sports such as aquatics, athletics, boxing, judo and weightlifting had a progressive increase in urine caffeine concentration from 2004 to 2015, while the concentration in other Olympic sports remained stable throughout this period; (c) in 2015, cycling, athletics, and rowing were the sports with the highest urine caffeine concentration, while shooting, basketball, and golf were the disciplines with the lowest concentrations of urinary caffeine. All this information suggests that the use of caffeine in sports increased from 2008 to 2015, particularly in some individual sports. However, the magnitude of the change in the urine caffeine concentrations obtained in competition does not reflect misuse of this substance in most sport disciplines.

After the removal of caffeine from the list of prohibited substances in 2004, athletes were free to consume caffeine at any amount before, during or even after competitions without the burden of being sanctioned by the anti-doping authorities. In the first five years after this administrative decision, the urinary concentration of caffeine in sport did not significantly change, as was shown by the comparative values of the reports made before [27] and after 2004 [28,29]. The absence of change suggested a high but stable utilization of caffeine by athletes, with most of the samples in the low-to-middle range of urinary caffeine concentrations. However, more than 300 new studies dealing with the effects of caffeine in sports have appeared since 2008, particularly original investigations determining the effects of caffeine on team sports, strength- and power-based sports or those with an intermittent nature. Besides, caffeine-containing products have become more accessible in all types of markets because of the conception of new supplements that incorporate caffeine in their formulation (e.g., pre-work-outs, carbohydrate gels, etc.) or the increase in the popularity of caffeinated drinks. Even so, the use of caffeine in sports competition has not dramatically changed since 2008 although a slight increase in 2015 is suggested by the changes in the distribution of urine caffeine concentration. First, the percentage of samples with a urine caffeine concentration below the limit of detection decreased from 31.2 in 2008 to 24.3% in 2015 (Figure 2), indicating that the proportion of athletes that do not consume caffeine before or during sports competition has slightly shrunk in the last few years. Furthermore, the proportion of athletes with urine caffeine concentrations in the range of 2–4 µg/mL increased in 2015. Thus, it can be suggested that caffeine is a recurrent substance used by ~75% of athletes in competition with a minor but significant evolution towards a higher use in sports in 2015.

Caffeine is a substance present in a multitude of foods and drinks, but the amount of caffeine included in most commercially available products with caffeine has not been shown to have a clear effect on physical performance (a dose of at least 3 mg/kg is usually necessary to increase performance [4,9]). The omnipresence of caffeine in the diet means that this substance can be consumed by some athletes without the intention of increasing physical performance (i.e., social use of caffeine). Although there is no consensus about the urinary caffeine concentration that differentiates the social use of caffeine from the intentional use of caffeine to enhance performance, previous investigations have revealed that lower doses of caffeine that increase performance (i.e., 3–6 mg/kg of body mass) derive in urinary caffeine concentrations of 2–5 µg/mL after simulated and real competitions [33–35] or other forms of exercise [36]. Despite this evidence, WADA only considers relevant, in terms of misuse and abuse of caffeine, those samples with urinary caffeine concentration of above 6 µg/mL [32] despite the fact that this might be indicative of caffeine dosages of >9 mg/kg [37]. In the current data, the proportion of samples above 6 µg of caffeine per mL of urine was 5.9%, 5.4%, and 4.8% for 2004, 2008, and 2015, respectively. By using the cut-off point proposed by WADA, one might assume that caffeine abuse has remained constant and low in the last decade. However, urinary caffeine concentrations between 2 and 6 µg/mL might also be indicative of intentional use of caffeine in sports.

Interestingly, the increase in the concentration of caffeine has not been equally present in all sports. The mean urinary concentration of athletes tested in aquatics, athletics, boxing, judo, and weightlifting increased from 2004 to 2015, suggesting a rise in the use of this substance among these particular sports. Other sports such as basketball, cycling, fencing, handball, hockey, shooting, and volleyball have maintained urine caffeine concentration at relatively stable values, suggestive of a steady-state use of caffeine in the last decade. Despite the uneven evolution or urinary caffeine concentration from 2004 to 2015 among sports, the individual disciplines with an aerobic-based performance continue to be the sports with the highest concentrations of caffeine, while team sports and accuracy sports are the disciplines with the lowest concentrations of caffeine (Figure 4). The higher urinary caffeine concentrations found in aerobic-based sports might be related to the traditional evidence that supported the ergogenic effects of caffeine by using laboratory-based research protocols with endurance-like exercise. However, more recent evidences, obtained in sport-specific situations, have demonstrated that the beneficial effects of pre-competition caffeine intake is extended to sprint- and power-based exercise [5,38], team sports [6,39,40], combat sports [8,41] and sports in which accuracy is a key element for success [42,43]. With these new evidences, it might be expected a higher consumption of caffeine—and a higher urinary caffeine concentration—in these type of sport disciplines in the next years that should be investigated in future research.

The urinary concentration of caffeine has significantly increased in both male and female athletes since 2004 (Figure 2) and median values reached 0.9 (0.1–2.2) and 0.8 (0.1–3.1) µg/mL, respectively, in 2015. Although the median values for men and women are very comparable, the proportion of samples from women athletes at high urinary caffeine concentrations is higher than expected in comparison to the proportion of urine samples from male athletes. For example, ~65.0% of all urine samples with a concentration >10 µg/mL corresponded to female participants, despite urine samples from women representing only about 25.3% of all the samples analyzed. In the opinion of these authors, the higher incidence of women's samples in the highest ranges of urinary concentrations of caffeine could be the result of the unintended intake of larger relative doses of caffeine, in terms of mg per kg of body mass. Caffeine-containing products are equally available in the market for both men and women, but the habitual lower mean body mass of female athletes might mean that the same absolute amount of caffeine ingested (for example, 160 mg of caffeine in a 500 mL can of an energy drink) results in a higher relative dose in mg/kg. This is also supported by the similar urinary pharmacokinetic parameters found for male and female adults [44], which suggests that the higher urinary caffeine excretion in women is related to the ingestion of higher relative doses rather than differences in caffeine metabolism and excretion.

The current analysis presents some limitations that should be discussed to correctly understand the outcomes of the investigation. First, the analysis included data from urine caffeine concentration in three selected years (2004, 2008, and 2015). According to WADA's Monitoring Program specifications, only urine samples with a urinary caffeine concentration above 6.0 µg/mL had to be reported to WADA (and those samples with concentrations below this cut-off remained unreported. Thus, due to the high number of samples analyzed in the Madrid Doping Control Laboratory between 2004 and 2015, we have been only able of obtaining the data of all urine samples, irrespective of their urinary caffeine concentration, in these three specific years. Second, the urine samples included in the analysis were exclusively obtained in national and international competitions held in Spain. Although in these competitions participate athletes of different nationalities, it is expected that a high proportion of the samples analyzed pertained to Spanish athletes. Thus, it is still possible that the evolution of urinary caffeine concentration could have been different in other countries due to social, genetic and lifestyle factors. In addition, the absence of out-of-competition urine samples impeded us to have a control to differentiate the use of caffeine on a day-to-day basis vs. the use before sports competition. Third, absorption, distribution, metabolism, and excretion of caffeine in the human body is affected by a myriad of genetic and environmental factors [45] that could affect the concentration of caffeine in urine in individuals taking the same dose before exercise. Post-competition urinary caffeine levels might be affected by the timing of the urine sample in relation to the caffeine dose [46] or the opportunities to urinate during or after an event. In this regard, the sport disciplines analyzed in this investigation have different regulations, particularly different durations or the presence of several competitions within the same day. Since caffeine is typically consumed before exercise, a longer competition period might allow more time for metabolism and excretion of the substance, affecting those sports with longer competition durations. In addition, caffeine could be ingested more than once in long-lasting events to maintain the effects of the substance on performance. Nevertheless, we believe that the high number of samples analyzed per year minimizes the effect of these factors on the outcomes of the investigation, and the authors believe that the data provided by this research reflect the evolution of the use of caffeine in sports.

5. Conclusions

In summary, the concentration of caffeine in the urine samples obtained after competition in Olympic sports increased from 2004 to 2015, which might indicate a slightly higher use of this substance in both men and women athletes. The analysis by disciplines revealed that some, but not all, sports have shown increases in the concentration of urinary caffeine, suggesting that the popularity of this substance has grown in some sports. Athletes of individual sports or athletes of sports with an aerobic-like nature are more prone to using caffeine in competition. Finally, investigations about the effects of caffeine on female athlete populations should be promoted because women athletes present slightly higher urinary concentrations than men counterparts.

Author Contributions: Conceptualization, M.A.-N., G.M., J.M.-G., and J.D.C.; methodology, M.A.-N., G.M., J.J.S., J.M.-G., M.F.-Á., M.d.M.P., and J.D.C.; formal analysis, M.A., J.J.S., and J.D.C.; writing—original draft preparation, M.A.-N.; writing—review and editing, G.M., J.J.S., J.M.-G., M.F.-Á., M.d.M.P., and J.D.C.; supervision, J.D.C.; project administration, J.D.C.

Funding: This investigation did not receive any funding.

Acknowledgments: The authors of this investigation want to acknowledge the effort of all the laboratory personnel of the Doping Control Laboratory in Madrid that participated in the measurement of the urine samples that made this investigation possible.

Conflicts of Interest: The authors declare no conflict of interest.

References

1. Souza, D.B.; Del Coso, J.; Casonatto, J.; Polito, M.D. Acute effects of caffeine-containing energy drinks on physical performance: A systematic review and meta-analysis. *Eur. J. Nutr.* **2017**, *56*, 13–27. [CrossRef] [PubMed]
2. Southward, K.; Rutherfurd-Markwick, K.J.; Ali, A. The effect of acute caffeine ingestion on endurance performance: A systematic review and meta-analysis. *Sports Med.* **2018**, *48*, 1913–1928. [CrossRef] [PubMed]
3. Grgic, J. Caffeine ingestion enhances wingate performance: A meta-analysis. *Eur. J. Sport Sci.* **2018**, *18*, 219–225. [CrossRef] [PubMed]
4. Del Coso, J.; Salinero, J.J.; Gonzalez-Millan, C.; Abian-Vicen, J.; Perez-Gonzalez, B. Dose response effects of a caffeine-containing energy drink on muscle performance: A repeated measures design. *J. Int. Soc. Sports Nutr.* **2012**, *9*, 21. [CrossRef]
5. Grgic, J.; Trexler, E.T.; Lazinica, B.; Pedisic, Z. Effects of caffeine intake on muscle strength and power: A systematic review and meta-analysis. *J. Inter. Soc. Sports Nutr.* **2018**, *15*, 11. [CrossRef]

6. Puente, C.; Abian-Vicen, J.; Salinero, J.J.; Lara, B.; Areces, F.; Del Coso, J. Caffeine improves basketball performance in experienced basketball players. *Nutrients* **2017**, *9*, 1033. [CrossRef]
7. Del Coso, J.; Estevez, E.; Mora-Rodriguez, R. Caffeine effects on short-term performance during prolonged exercise in the heat. *Med. Sci. Sports Exerc.* **2008**, *40*, 744–751. [CrossRef]
8. Diaz-Lara, F.J.; Del Coso, J.; Garcia, J.M.; Portillo, L.J.; Areces, F.; Abian-Vicen, J. Caffeine improves muscular performance in elite brazilian jiu-jitsu athletes. *Eur. J. Sport Sci.* **2016**, *16*, 1079–1086. [CrossRef]
9. Maughan, R.J.; Burke, L.M.; Dvorak, J.; Larson-Meyer, D.E.; Peeling, P.; Phillips, S.M.; Rawson, E.S.; Walsh, N.P.; Garthe, I.; Geyer, H. IOC consensus statement: Dietary supplements and the high-performance athlete. *Int. J. Sport Nutr. Exerc. Metab.* **2018**, *28*, 104–125. [CrossRef]
10. Pickering, C.; Kiely, J. Are the current guidelines on caffeine use in sport optimal for everyone? Inter-individual variation in caffeine ergogenicity, and a move towards personalised sports nutrition. *Sports Med.* **2018**, *48*, 7–16. [CrossRef] [PubMed]
11. Womack, C.J.; Saunders, M.J.; Bechtel, M.K.; Bolton, D.J.; Martin, M.; Luden, N.D.; Dunham, W.; Hancock, M. The influence of a CYP1A2 polymorphism on the ergogenic effects of caffeine. *J. Int. Soc. Sports Nutr.* **2012**, *9*, 7. [CrossRef] [PubMed]
12. Rahimi, R. The effect of CYP1A2 genotype on the ergogenic properties of caffeine during resistance exercise: A randomized, double-blind, placebo-controlled, crossover study. *Ir. J. Med. Sci.* **2018**. [CrossRef]
13. Guest, N.; Corey, P.; Vescovi, J.; El-Sohemy, A. Caffeine, CYP1A2 genotype, and endurance performance in athletes. *Med. Sci. Sports Exerc.* **2018**, *50*, 1570–1578. [CrossRef] [PubMed]
14. Pataky, M.W.; Womack, C.J.; Saunders, M.J.; Goffe, J.L.; D'Lugos, A.C.; El-Sohemy, A.; Luden, N.D. Caffeine and 3-km cycling performance: Effects of mouth rinsing, genotype, and time of day. *Scand. J. Med. Sci. Sports* **2016**, *26*, 613–619. [CrossRef]
15. Algrain, H.; Thomas, R.; Carrillo, A.; Ryan, E.; Kim, C.; Lettan, R.; Ryan, E. The effects of a polymorphism in the cytochrome p450 CYP1A2 gene on performance enhancement with caffeine in recreational cyclists. *J. Caffeine Res.* **2015**, *6*, 1–6. [CrossRef]
16. Salinero, J.J.; Lara, B.; Ruiz-Vicente, D.; Areces, F.; Puente-Torres, C.; Gallo-Salazar, C.; Pascual, T.; Del Coso, J. CYP1A2 genotype variations do not modify the benefits and drawbacks of caffeine during exercise: A pilot study. *Nutrients* **2017**, *9*, 269. [CrossRef]
17. Puente, C.; Abian-Vicen, J.; Del Coso, J.; Lara, B.; Salinero, J.J. The CYP1A2-163C>A polymorphism does not alter the effects of caffeine on basketball performance. *PLoS ONE* **2018**, *13*, e0195943. [CrossRef]
18. Bell, D.G.; McLellan, T.M. Exercise endurance 1, 3, and 6 h after caffeine ingestion in caffeine users and nonusers. *J. Appl. Physiol.* **2002**, *93*, 1227–1234. [CrossRef]
19. Beaumont, R.; Cordery, P.; Funnell, M.; Mears, S.; James, L.; Watson, P. Chronic ingestion of a low dose of caffeine induces tolerance to the performance benefits of caffeine. *J. Sports Sci.* **2017**, *35*, 1920–1927. [CrossRef]
20. Dodd, S.L.; Brooks, E.; Powers, S.K.; Tulley, R. The effects of caffeine on graded exercise performance in caffeine naive versus habituated subjects. *Eur. J. Appl. Physiol. Occup. Physiol.* **1991**, *62*, 424–429. [CrossRef]
21. Goncalves, L.S.; Painelli, V.S.; Yamaguchi, G.; Oliveira, L.F.; Saunders, B.; da Silva, R.P.; Maciel, E.; Artioli, G.G.; Roschel, H.; Gualano, B. Dispelling the myth that habitual caffeine consumption influences the performance response to acute caffeine supplementation. *J. Appl. Physiol.* **2017**, *123*, 213–220. [CrossRef]
22. Fulton, J.L.; Dinas, P.C.; Carrillo, A.E.; Edsall, J.R.; Ryan, E.J. Impact of genetic variability on physiological responses to caffeine in humans: A systematic review. *Nutrients* **2018**, *10*, 1373. [CrossRef] [PubMed]
23. Salinero, J.J.; Lara, B.; Abian-Vicen, J.; Gonzalez-Millan, C.; Areces, F.; Gallo-Salazar, C.; Ruiz-Vicente, D.; Del Coso, J. The use of energy drinks in sport: Perceived ergogenicity and side effects in male and female athletes. *Br. J. Nutr.* **2014**, *112*, 1494–1502. [CrossRef]
24. Peeling, P.; Binnie, M.J.; Goods, P.S.; Sim, M.; Burke, L.M. Evidence-based supplements for the enhancement of athletic performance. *Int. J. Sport Nutr. Exerc. Metab.* **2018**, *28*, 178–187. [CrossRef] [PubMed]
25. Spriet, L.L. Exercise and sport performance with low doses of caffeine. *Sports Med.* **2014**, *44*, 175–184. [CrossRef]
26. World Anti-Doping Agency. Monitoring program. Available online: https://www.wada-ama.org/en/resources/science-medicine/monitoring-program (accessed on 1 July 2018).
27. Van Thuyne, W.; Roels, K.; Delbeke, F. Distribution of caffeine levels in urine in different sports in relation to doping control. *Int. J. Sports Med.* **2005**, *26*, 714–718. [CrossRef] [PubMed]

28. Van Thuyne, W.; Delbeke, F. Distribution of caffeine levels in urine in different sports in relation to doping control before and after the removal of caffeine from the wada doping list. *Int. J. Sports Med.* **2006**, *27*, 745–750. [CrossRef]
29. Del Coso, J.; Muñoz, G.; Muñoz-Guerra, J. Prevalence of caffeine use in elite athletes following its removal from the world anti-doping agency list of banned substances. *Appl. Physiol. Nutr. Metab.* **2011**, *36*, 555–561. [CrossRef] [PubMed]
30. Lopez-Gonzalez, L.M.; Sanchez-Oliver, A.J.; Mata, F.; Jodra, P.; Antonio, J.; Dominguez, R. Acute caffeine supplementation in combat sports: A systematic review. *J. Int. Soc. Sports Nutr.* **2018**, *15*, 60. [CrossRef] [PubMed]
31. Salinero, J.J.; Lara, B.; Del Coso, J. Effects of acute ingestion of caffeine on team sports performance: A systematic review and meta-analysis. *Res. Sports Med.* **2018**, 1–19. [CrossRef] [PubMed]
32. World Anti-Doping Agency. Guidelines for Urine Sample Collection. Available online: https://www.wada-ama.org/sites/default/files/resources/files/WADA_Guidelines_Urine_Sample_Collection_v5.1_EN.pdf (accessed on 25 June 2018).
33. Del Coso, J.; Munoz-Fernandez, V.E.; Munoz, G.; Fernandez-Elias, V.E.; Ortega, J.F.; Hamouti, N.; Barbero, J.C.; Munoz-Guerra, J. Effects of a caffeine-containing energy drink on simulated soccer performance. *PLoS ONE* **2012**, *7*, e31380. [CrossRef]
34. Del Coso, J.; Portillo, J.; Munoz, G.; Abian-Vicen, J.; Gonzalez-Millan, C.; Munoz-Guerra, J. Caffeine-containing energy drink improves sprint performance during an international rugby sevens competition. *Amino Acids* **2013**, *44*, 1511–1519. [CrossRef] [PubMed]
35. Del Coso, J.; Ramirez, J.A.; Munoz, G.; Portillo, J.; Gonzalez-Millan, C.; Munoz, V.; Barbero-Alvarez, J.C.; Munoz-Guerra, J. Caffeine-containing energy drink improves physical performance of elite rugby players during a simulated match. *Appl. Physiol. Nutr. Metab.* **2013**, *38*, 368–374. [CrossRef] [PubMed]
36. Kovacs, E.M.; Martin, A.M.; Brouns, F. The effect of ad libitum ingestion of a caffeinated carbohydrate-electrolyte solution on urinary caffeine concentration after 4 hours of endurance exercise. *Int. J. Sports Med.* **2002**, *23*, 237–241. [CrossRef] [PubMed]
37. Pasman, W.J.; van Baak, M.A.; Jeukendrup, A.E.; de Haan, A. The effect of different dosages of caffeine on endurance performance time. *Int. J. Sports Med.* **1995**, *16*, 225–230. [CrossRef] [PubMed]
38. Lara, B.; Ruiz-Vicente, D.; Areces, F.; Abian-Vicen, J.; Salinero, J.J.; Gonzalez-Millan, C.; Gallo-Salazar, C.; Del Coso, J. Acute consumption of a caffeinated energy drink enhances aspects of performance in sprint swimmers. *Br. J. Nutr.* **2015**, *114*, 908–914. [CrossRef]
39. Perez-Lopez, A.; Salinero, J.J.; Abian-Vicen, J.; Valades, D.; Lara, B.; Hernandez, C.; Areces, F.; Gonzalez, C.; Del Coso, J. Caffeinated energy drinks improve volleyball performance in elite female players. *Med. Sci. Sports Exerc.* **2015**, *47*, 850–856. [CrossRef]
40. Chia, J.S.; Barrett, L.A.; Chow, J.Y.; Burns, S.F. Effects of caffeine supplementation on performance in ball games. *Sports Med.* **2017**, *47*, 2453–2471. [CrossRef] [PubMed]
41. Coswig, V.S.; Gentil, P.; Irigon, F.; Del Vecchio, F.B. Caffeine ingestion changes time-motion and technical-tactical aspects in simulated boxing matches: A randomized double-blind pla-controlled crossover study. *Eur.J. Sport Sci.* **2018**, *18*, 975–983. [CrossRef] [PubMed]
42. Gallo-Salazar, C.; Areces, F.; Abian Vicen, J.; Lara, B.; Salinero, J.J.; Gonzalez-Millan, C.; Portillo, J.; Munoz, V.; Juarez, D.; Del Coso, J. Enhancing physical performance in elite junior tennis players with a caffeinated energy drink. *Int. J. Sports Physiol. Perform.* **2015**, *10*, 305–310. [CrossRef]
43. Abian, P.; Del Coso, J.; Salinero, J.J.; Gallo-Salazar, C.; Areces, F.; Ruiz-Vicente, D.; Lara, B.; Soriano, L.; Munoz, V.; Abian-Vicen, J. The ingestion of a caffeinated energy drink improves jump performance and activity patterns in elite badminton players. *J. Sports Sci.* **2015**, *33*, 1042–1050. [CrossRef]
44. McLean, C.; Graham, T.E. Effects of exercise and thermal stress on caffeine pharmacokinetics in men and eumenorrheic women. *J. Appl. Physiol.* **2002**, *93*, 1471–1478. [CrossRef]
45. Magkos, F.; Kavouras, S.A. Caffeine use in sports, pharmacokinetics in man, and cellular mechanisms of action. *Crit. Rev. Food Sci. Nutr.* **2005**, *45*, 535–562. [CrossRef]
46. Burke, L.M. Caffeine and sports performance. *Appl. Physiol. Nutr. Metab.* **2008**, *33*, 1319–1334. [CrossRef]

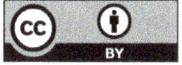

© 2019 by the authors. Licensee MDPI, Basel, Switzerland. This article is an open access article distributed under the terms and conditions of the Creative Commons Attribution (CC BY) license (http://creativecommons.org/licenses/by/4.0/).

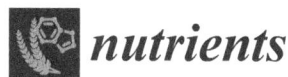

Article

Caffeine Supplementation Improves Anaerobic Performance and Neuromuscular Efficiency and Fatigue in Olympic-Level Boxers

Alejandro F. San Juan [1], Álvaro López-Samanes [2], Pablo Jodra [3], Pedro L. Valenzuela [4], Javier Rueda [1], Pablo Veiga-Herreros [5], Alberto Pérez-López [6,*] and Raúl Domínguez [7]

1. Laboratorio de Biomecánica Deportiva, Departamento de Salud y Rendimiento Humano, Facultad de Ciencias de la Actividad Física y del Deporte, Universidad Politécnica de Madrid, 28040 Madrid, Spain
2. School of Physiotherapy, Faculty of Health Sciences, Francisco de Vitoria University, 28223 Madrid, Spain
3. Faculty of Health Sciences, Alfonso X El Sabio University, 28691 Villanueva de la Cañada (Madrid), Spain
4. Department of Systems Biology, University of Alcalá, 28805 Madrid, Spain
5. Departamento de Nutrición Humana y Dietética, Facultad de Ciencias de la Salud, Universidad Alfonso X El Sabio, 28691 Villanueva de la Cañada (Madrid), Spain
6. Department of Biomedical Sciences, Faculty of Medicine and Health Sciences, University of Alcalá, 28805 Madrid, Spain
7. Facultad de Ciencias de la Salud, Universidad Isabel I, 09003 Burgos, Spain
* Correspondence: alberto_perez-lopez@hotmail.com; Tel.: +34-918-855-4536

Received: 19 August 2019; Accepted: 30 August 2019; Published: 5 September 2019

Abstract: Background: this study examined the effects of caffeine supplementation on anaerobic performance, neuromuscular efficiency and upper and lower extremities fatigue in Olympic-level boxers. Methods: Eight male athletes, members of the Spanish National Olympic Team, were enrolled in the study. In a randomized double-blind, placebo-controlled, counterbalanced, crossover design, the athletes completed 2 test sessions after the intake of caffeine (6 mg·kg^{-1}) or placebo. Sessions involved initial measures of lactate, handgrip and countermovement jump (CMJ) performance, followed by a 30-seconds Wingate test, and then final measures of the previous variables. During the sessions, electromyography (EMG) data were recorded on the gluteus maximus, biceps femoris, vastus lateralis, gastrocnemius lateral head and tibialis anterior. Results: caffeine enhanced peak power (6.27%, $p < 0.01$; Effect Size (ES) = 1.26), mean power (5.21%; $p < 0.01$; ES = 1.29) and reduced the time needed to reach peak power (−9.91%, $p < 0.01$; ES = 0.58) in the Wingate test, improved jump height in the CMJ (+2.4 cm, $p < 0.01$), and improved neuromuscular efficiency at peak power in the vastus lateralis (ES = 1.01) and gluteus maximus (ES = 0.89), and mean power in the vastus lateralis (ES = 0.95) and tibialis anterior (ES = 0.83). Conclusions: in these Olympic-level boxers, caffeine supplementation improved anaerobic performance without affecting EMG activity and fatigue levels in the lower limbs. Further benefits observed were enhanced neuromuscular efficiency in some muscles and improved reaction speed.

Keywords: anaerobic; caffeine; CMJ; ergogenic aids; exercise; nutrition; sport supplement; Wingate; electromyography; efficiency

---

1. Introduction

Caffeine is one of the five nutritional supplements considered ergogenic aids (EA) with good to strong evidence of benefits in specific sports scenarios [1,2], along with other EA such as beetroot juice, sodium bicarbonate, β-alanine, and creatine. All are included in the classification system for nutritional supplements of the Australian Institute of Sports (AIS) based on the demonstrated level of scientific evidence (Level A) [3]. Briefly, the ergogenic effect of caffeine on sports performance can be attributed mainly to: 1) central nervous system stimulation (i.e., blockade of adenosine receptors and release of neurotransmitters such as dopamine, catecholamine and acetylcholine, improving cognitive processes: surveillance, learning, attention and reaction time) [4–6], and 2) enhancement of muscle contraction (i.e., improved calcium output from the sarcoplasmic reticulum to the sarcoplasm after the muscle action potential, and increased recruitment of motor units) [7–9].

There is clear consensus in the literature regarding the effects of caffeine consumption on aerobic performance [10,11]. While fewer studies have focused on sports modalities inducing a predominantly anaerobic metabolism than one mostly dependent on oxidative processes, it is now emerging that caffeine may also have an ergogenic effect on anaerobic efforts [12,13].

The characteristics of combat sports are similar to those of other sports modalities including intermittent dynamics (i.e., high-intensity efforts interspersed with periods of low-intensity activity) [14]. Therefore, at the energy level, combat sports require an important contribution of both aerobic (i.e., oxidative phosphorylation) [15] and anaerobic metabolism (i.e., glycolysis and phosphagen system) during high-intensity actions [16]. Also, combat sports athletes require high levels of isometric handgrip strength [17,18] and muscular endurance in the upper and lower extremities [19]. Competition analysis has revealed that maintenance of power performance during combats is crucial for high-performance in these athletes [20].

As combats sports are characterized by high-intensity power actions and both aerobic and anaerobic energy metabolism systems are required, caffeine could be an EA in these sport modalities. However, the effect of this supplement on combat sport performance or fatigue levels has not yet been addressed in the literature. The present study was therefore designed to examine the effects of caffeine supplementation on anaerobic performance, neuromuscular efficiency and neuromuscular fatigue levels in the upper and lower limbs in Olympic-level boxers. We hypothesized that caffeine supplementation would improve anaerobic performance in a 30-seconds all-out Wingate test, improving muscular efficiency without inducing greater mechanical or neuromuscular fatigue.

2. Materials and Methods

2.1. Participants Selection: Inclusion and Exclusion Criteria

Eight young, healthy male athletes, members of the Spanish National Olympic Team for the Tokyo 2020 Olympic Games (age: 22.0 ± 1.778 years, height: 1.69 ± 0.09 m, body-mass: 65.63 ± 10.79 kg, Body Mass Index (BMI): 22.69 ± 1.31, load Wingate test: 4.91 ± 0.82 kp), were enrolled in the study.

Exclusion criteria were: (1) age younger than 18 years, (2) having consumed any substance that could affect hormone levels or sport performance in the previous 3 months such as nutrition complements or steroids, (3) having consumed narcotic and/or psychotropic agents, drugs or stimulants during the test or supplementation period, and (4) being diagnosed with any cardiovascular, metabolic, neurologic, pulmonary or orthopedic disorder that could limit performance in the different tests.

At the study outset, participants were informed of the study protocol, schedule and nature of the exercises and tests to be performed before signing an informed consent form. The study protocol adhered to the tenets of the Declaration of Helsinki and was approved by the Ethics Committee of the Alfonso X El Sabio University.

2.2. Experimental Design

A randomized double-blind, placebo-controlled, counterbalanced, crossover design was used in this study. The participants completed 2 identical assessment sessions (see Figure 1) in the laboratory at the same time slot (±0.5 hours) to avoid the detrimental effects of performance associated with circadian rhythm [21]. The test sessions started with initial measures of lactate, handgrip and countermovement jump (CMJ) performance, followed by a 30-seconds Wingate test, and then final measures of the previously collected variables (see Figure 1).

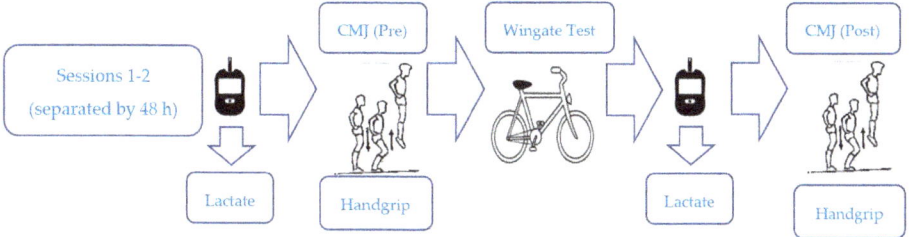

Figure 1. Experimental design. CMJ = countermovement jump test.

The two sessions were separated by 48 hours. Over a period of 48 hours before the start of the first session until the end of the study, subjects were instructed to follow a series of nutrition requirements and refrain from any type of physical exercise.

2.3. Supplementation and Diet Control

The authors packaged and prepared the capsules containing caffeine or placebo (sucrose). The capsules used were no.1 opaque red (Guinama S.L.U, 0044634, La Pobla de Valbona, Spain). For the encapsulation process, we followed the normalized working procedures described for this purpose [22]. The filling equipment used was a manual semiautomatic Carsunorm 2000 system (Miranda de Ebro, Spain).

The subjects arrived at the laboratory 75 minutes before the start of the session, when they were given a capsule containing either a caffeine supplement (6 mg·kg^{-1}) or sucrose (6 mg·kg^{-1}, placebo). Caffeine dosage selection (6 mg·kg^{-1}) was made to promote the higher ergogenic effects producing the minimum side-effects possible [1]. The protocol timing was designed considering that caffeine reaches peak concentrations in blood after 1 hour of intake [23], and the degradation quality control tests its half-life (13.4 minutes) according to previous description [22].

In addition, participants received dietary guidelines to ensure that they all followed a diet with the same content of macronutrients (i.e., 60% of energy intake in the form of carbohydrates, 30% lipids and 10% proteins) in the 48 hours prior to each session. A list of foods rich in caffeine was provided to all participants (e.g., coffee, tea, mate, tea soft drinks, energy drinks, cola drinks, chocolate drinks and chocolate) so that they avoided caffeine intake from 24 hours before the study to the end of the study.

2.4. Wingate Test

A 30-seconds all-out Wingate test was performed on a Monark cycloergometer (Ergomedic 828E, Vansbro, Sweden). Before the test, a warm-up protocol was conducted consisting of 5 minutes pedaling at low intensity (i.e., subjects chose the load and cadence), followed by another 5 minutes pedaling at 60 revolutions per minute (rpm) with a load of 2 kiloponds (Kp). In the last 5 seconds of each minute, the subjects performed a maximum intensity sprint. After three minutes, subjects performed three countermovement jumps (CMJs) at increasing intensity with 10 seconds recovery between jumps. Then, 2 CMJs were executed on the force platform. After two minutes of recovery, the Wingate test began. Subjects pedaled as fast as possible for 30 seconds against a constant load (Kp) calculated according to the 7.5% of each participant body mass [24]. The instructions given to them were: i) reach maximum rpm in the shortest time and ii) try to keep the highest number of rpm until the end of the test. During the test, subjects were encouraged by 4 researchers from the beginning until the end. Power output (W) was analyzed during each second and, later, peak power output (W_{peak}), time (s) to reach W_{peak} (TW_{peak}), mean power output during the 30 seconds sprint (W_{mean}) and minimum power output during the last 10 seconds of the test (W_{min}) were calculated. In addition to W_{mean} during the entire sprint, mean power output was also calculated every 5 seconds of the sprint ($Split_{1-5S}$, $Split_{6-10S}$, $Split_{11-15S}$, $Split_{16-20S}$, $Split_{21-25S}$, $Split_{26-30S}$).

2.5. Electromyographic Assessment

Electromiography (EMG) data were recorded from the following muscles: gluteus maximus (GM), biceps femoris (BF), vastus lateralis (VL), gastrocnemius lateral head (GL), and tibialis anterior (TA) and the mean of the five muscles analyzed (MED). We used a "Trigno Wireless SystemTM Delsys" (Delsys Inc. Massachusetts, MA, USA). Briefly, one active electrode was placed on the bellies of each muscle of the right thigh and leg following the protocol established by the SENIAM Project (Surface ElectroMyoGraphy for the Non-invasive Assessment of Muscles) [25]. These electrodes recorded the surface electrical activity corresponding to the underlying muscle, sampled at a frequency of 1024 Hz. The EMG signal was filtered by a band pass between 20 and 300 Hz, and subsequently the EMG Root Mean Square signal (rms-EMG) was calculated. The rms-EMG variable obtained from each of the 5 muscles was normalized to the maximum value obtained in the corresponding muscle for 1 second. In our study, rms-EMG was used as an estimate of "total myoelectric activity" of the exercising muscle as it has been previously shown that this computation: 1) is an accurate measure of EMG amplitude and 2) is highly correlated with the number of active motor units (fiber recruitment) [26,27].

To facilitate the analysis of results, the 30 seconds of each Wingate test was divided into groups of 5 seconds and we calculated the rms-EMG mean in this time period (e.g., EMG_{0-5s}, EMG_{6-10s}, EMG_{11-15s}). In addition, we calculated the average rms-EMG (EMG_{mean}), the rms-EMG corresponding to the time where W_{peak} was reached (EMG_{Wpeak}), the time (s) to reach the rms-EMG peak record ($TEMG_{peak}$) and the rms-EMG corresponding to the time when W_{min} was reached (EMG_{Wmin}). Data of rms-EMG is expressed as a base index one where the value 1 is equal to 100% (i.e., the value 0.75 is equal to 75 %).

Additionally, to analyze neuromuscular efficiency (NME), we used the ratios between W_{peak} and EMG_{Wpeak} (NME_{Wpeak}) and between W_{mean} and EMG_{Wmean} (NME_{Wmean}). Neuromuscular efficiency (NME) was used as an index of neuromuscular fatigue [28] and was estimated from the ratio of power to non-normalized RMS (raw EMG data in volts). We adapted the methodology described by Hug and Dorel [28], and we propose a ratio of power output to normalized RMS (EMG data in percent of muscle activation). Our rationale was that to determine NME, it is better to relate power to percent of motor units activated than to raw volts, as described in the literature, and more often used as a measure of fatigue [28].

2.6. Blood Lactate

Before the warm-up period and immediately after the Wingate test, 5 µ·l samples of capillary blood from the soft part of the index finger of the left hand were obtained and subjected to blood lactate concentration determination using a Lactate ProTM 2 LT-1710 blood analyzer (Arkray Factory Inc., KDK Corporation, Shiga, Japan).

2.7. Neuromuscular Fatigue

Neuromuscular fatigue in the lower limbs was measured in a CMJ [29] performed on a force platform (Quattro Jump model 9290AD; Kistler Instruments, Winterthur, Switzerland). Before the jump was initiated, participants stood on the platform with legs extended and hands on hips. For the jump, the legs were first flexed to 90° (eccentric action) and then explosively extended in a coordinated manner (concentric action) trying to reach maximum height. During the flight stage, the knees were extended. Contact with the ground was made with the toes first. During the test, subjects were instructed to keep their hands on their hips and avoid any sideways displacements during the flight stage. This same protocol was applied for the CMJs performed before and after the Wingate test.

From each CMJ test, jump height, mean (CMJ_{Wmean}) and peak power produced (CMJ_{Wpeak}) were extracted, as indicators of neuromuscular fatigue [30].

2.8. Handgrip Strength

Isometric handgrip strength (IHS) was measured twice for the dominant hand using a calibrated handgrip dynamometer (Takei 5101, Tokyo, Japan) with 30 seconds of passive recovery between trials. Participants sat with 0 of shoulder flexion and elbow flexion, and the forearm and hand in a neutral position and exerted their maximal strength during 5 seconds [31]. The highest value of the dominant hand was recorded and used for statistical analysis as the maximum voluntary handgrip strength.

2.9. Statistical Analysis

Results for all parameters are presented as mean ± standard deviation (SD). Data analyses were carried out using the commercial software "Statistical Package for Social Sciences" SPSS v21.0 software (SPSS Inc., Chicago, IL, USA). The effects of caffeine supplementation on Wingate test performance, lactate, CMJ and strength grip performance were assessed through a two-way ANOVA test for condition (caffeine versus placebo) and time (pre-versus post-Wingate for CMJ handgrip strength measures, and during each 5 seconds period of the Wingate test). Levene's test revealed the homogeneity of variances of the data and the Shapiro-Wilk's test confirmed their normal distribution. When a significant main effect was detected, pairwise comparisons were assessed using the Holm-Bonferroni test in order to ensure protection against multiple comparisons. Additionally, W_{peak}, TW_{peak}, W_{mean}, W_{min}, EMG_{Wpeak}, $TEMG_{max}$, EMG_{mean} and EMG_{Wmin} and efficiency measures (NME_{Wpeak}, NME_{Wmean} and NME_{Wmin}) were analyzed using the Student's t-test. Pairwise comparisons significance was assessed by calculating Cohen's d Effect Size (ES) [32]. Effect sizes (d) above 0.8, between 0.8 and 0.5, between 0.5 and 0.2 and lower than 0.2 were considered as large, moderate, small, and trivial, respectively [33,34].

3. Results

3.1. Wingate Test

Compared to placebo, caffeine consumption produced a significant and large effect in W_{peak} (10.84 ± 0.49 versus 10.20 ± 0.59; $p < 0.01$; Effect Size (ES) = 1.26) and W_{mean} (8.68 ± 0.34 versus 8.25 ± 0.37; $p < 0.01$; ES = 1.29), a decrease in TW_{peak} (8.00 ± 1.60 versus 8.88 ± 1.64; $p < 0.01$; ES = 0.58), while this improvement after caffeine supplementation in W_{min} it was not significantly different ($p = 0.123$) (see Table 1). Moreover, there was an effect of the time factor ($p < 0.001$), verified in the analysis of power output levels throughout the 6 partial tests, as well as for the supplementation factor ($p = 0.006$). Significant differences were observed in $Split_{6-10s}$ ($p = 0.026$) and $Split_{11-15s}$ ($p = 0.009$), as well as a significant trend $Split_{16-20s}$ ($p = 0.062$) (see Table 2). There was no significant interaction between factors (supplementation-time).

Table 1. Data for power output and root mean square-EMG (rms-EMG) recorded during the Wingate test.

Variable	Experimental Condition	W$_{peak}$-EMG$_{Wpeak}$ M ± SD	p-Value	ES	TW$_{peak}$-TEMG$_{peak}$ M ± SD	p-Value	ES	W$_{mean}$-EMG$_{mean}$ M ± SD	p-Value	ES	W$_{min}$-EMG$_{Wmin}$ M ± SD	p-Value	ES
W$_{output}$	Placebo	10.20 ± 0.59	<0.01 *	1.26	8.88 ± 1.64	0.01 *	0.58	8.25 ± 0.37	0.01 *	1.29	6.19 ± 0.56	0.123	0.75
	Caffeine	10.84 ± 0.49			8.00 ± 1.60			8.68 ± 0.34			6.49 ± 0.22		
EMG$_{VL}$	Placebo	0.78 ± 0.09	0.268	0.71	12.25 ± 9.27	0.270	0.68	0.74 ± 0.11	0.247	0.62	0.41 ± 0.15	0.332	0.47
	Caffeine	0.69 ± 0.17			7.38 ± 5.58			0.66 ± 0.16			0.33 ± 0.21		
EMG$_{BF}$	Placebo	0.67 ± 0.19	0.435	0.29	8.63 ± 3.70	0.292	0.36	0.55 ± 0.14	0.254	0.37	0.26 ± 0.11	0.430	0.37
	Caffeine	0.72 ± 0.18			12.13 ± 8.43			0.60 ± 0.15			0.31 ± 0.17		
EMG$_{GM}$	Placebo	0.68 ± 0.16	0.311	0.73	3.63 ± 3.66	0.022 *	0.91	0.64 ± 0.08	0.728	0.25	0.36 ± 0.31	0.387	0.22
	Caffeine	0.56 ± 0.19			8.00 ± 6.26			0.62 ± 0.09			0.31 ± 0.15		
EMG$_{TA}$	Placebo	0.73 ± 0.21	0.984	0.00	7.75 ± 3.45	0.722	0.16	0.63 ± 0.10	0.298	0.59	0.23 ± 0.12	0.423	0.26
	Caffeine	0.73 ± 0.20			7.13 ± 4.55			0.55 ± 0.18			0.20 ± 0.13		
EMG$_{GL}$	Placebo	0.74 ± 0.15	0.824	0.16	8.00 ± 5.37	0.936	0.05	0.67 ± 0.12	0.935	0.09	0.40 ± 0.11	0.980	0.00
	Caffeine	0.76 ± 0.12			7.75 ± 5.03			0.66 ± 0.13			0.40 ± 0.16		
EMG$_{MED}$	Placebo	0.72 ± 0.07	0.607	0.60				0.65 ± 0.05	0.261	0.44	0.33 ± 0.07	0.343	0.22
	Caffeine	0.69 ± 0.03						0.62 ± 0.09			0.31 ± 0.12		

W$_{peak}$: Peak power (w/kg); EMG-$_{Wpeak}$: rms-EMG at W$_{peak}$; TW$_{peak}$: time (s) to achieve the maximal power; TEMG$_{peak}$: time (s) to achieve the maximal rms-EMG record; W$_{mean}$: Average power (w/kg); EMG$_{mean}$: Average rms-EMG; W$_{min}$: Minimum power (w/kg); EMG$_{Wmin}$: rms-EMG at W$_{min}$; EMG$_{VL}$: rms-EMG recorded on the vastus lateralis; EMG$_{BF}$: rms-EMG recorded on the biceps femoris; EMG$_{GM}$: rms-EMG recorded on the gluteus maximus; EMG$_{GL}$: rms-EMG recorded on the gastrocnemius lateral head; EMG$_{TA}$: rms-EMG recorded on the tibialis anterior; EMG$_{MED}$: Mean rms-EMG recorded on the five muscles analyzed; Data of power output expressed as Watts·kg^{-1}, and rms-EMG data as a base index one. * Significant difference between Placebo and Caffeine condition at $p < 0.05$.

Table 2. Mean and standard deviations (SD) of power output and rms-EMG data during 6 splits in the Wingate Test.

Variable		Split$_{1-5s}$	Split$_{6-10s}$	Split$_{11-15s}$	Split$_{16-20s}$	Split$_{21-25s}$	Split$_{26-30s}$	p-Value Time	p-Value Supplementation	p-Value Time Supplementation
W$_{output}$	Placebo	6.61 ± 0.89 #A	9.98 ± 0.59 #D *	9.63 ± 0.65 #H *	8.80 ± 0.64 #L	7.78 ± 0.36 #O	6.68 ± 0.38	<0.001 #	0.006 *	0.696
	Caffeine	7.05 ± 1.11 #A	0.54 ± 0.56 #D	10.19 ± 0.58 #H	9.18 ± 0.70 #L	8.05 ± 0.56 #O	7.04 ± 0.34			
EMG$_{VL}$	Placebo	0.72 ± 0.10	0.76 ± 0.10	0.79 ± 0.10	0.79 ± 0.14 #M	0.73 ± 0.16	0.67 ± 0.17	0.018 #	0.247	0.985
	Caffeine	0.62 ± 0.19	0.69 ± 0.15	0.72 ± 0.19	0.68 ± 0.16	0.64 ± 0.20	0.58 ± 0.20			
EMG$_{BF}$	Placebo	0.53 ± 0.14 #B	3.75 ± 0.10 #E	0.65 ± 0.16 #I	0.54 ± 0.22 #N	0.43 ± 0.19	0.36 ± 0.16 #P	0.002 #	0.250	0.089
	Caffeine	0.60 ± 0.14	0.71 ± 0.10	0.71 ± 0.16 #I	0.64 ± 0.20 #N	0.52 ± 0.20	0.46 ± 0.19			
EMG$_{GM}$	Placebo	0.73 ± 0.13	0.63 ± 0.12	0.65 ± 0.08	0.65 ± 0.10	0.59 ± 0.05	0.57 ± 0.10	0.094	0.734	0.286
	Caffeine	0.63 ± 0.16	0.59 ± 0.19	0.61 ± 0.15	0.66 ± 0.11	0.66 ± 0.12	0.56 ± 0.11			
EMG$_{TA}$	Placebo	0.61 ± 0.16 #B	0.75 ± 0.16	0.76 ± 0.11 #J	0.65 ± 0.14 #M	0.56 ± 0.11	0.47 ± 0.08 #Q	<0.001 #	0.298	0.033 T
	Caffeine	0.57 ± 0.17	0.70 ± 0.16 #F	0.59 ± 0.22 #K	0.51 ± 0.20	0.45 ± 0.22	0.43 ± 0.24			
EMG$_{GL}$	Placebo	0.77 ± 0.12 #C	0.76 ± 0.09 #G	0.68 ± 0.14	0.65 ± 0.14	0.61 ± 0.16	0.53 ± 0.16	<0.001 #	0.948	0.592
	Caffeine	0.75 ± 0.11 #C	0.75 ± 0.08	0.68 ± 0.18	0.70 ± 0.19 #M	0.61 ± 0.19	0.51 ± 0.17			

EMG$_{VL}$: rms-EMG recorded on the vastus lateralis; EMG$_{BF}$: rms-EMG recorded on the biceps femoris; EMG$_{GM}$: rms-EMG recorded on the gluteus maximus; EMG$_{GL}$: rms-EMG recorded on the gastrocnemius lateral head; EMG$_{TA}$: rms-EMG recorded on the tibialis anterior; Data of power output expressed as Watts·kg^{-1}, and rms-EMG data as a base index one. #: Significant differences in factor time at $p < 0.05$. *: Significant differences between Placebo and Caffeine condition at $p < 0.05$. T: Significant difference in interaction Time-Supplementation at $p < 0.05$. Significance differences between splits: #A: Split$_{1-5s}$, Split$_{6-10s}$, Split$_{11-15s}$ and Split$_{16-20s}$ versus Split$_{1-5s}$. #B: Split$_{6-10s}$ versus Split$_{1-5s}$. #C: Split$_{26-30s}$ versus Split$_{1-5s}$. #D: Split$_{0-5s}$, Split$_{16-20s}$, Split$_{21-25s}$ and Split$_{25-30s}$ versus Split$_{6-10s}$. #E: Split$_{21-25s}$, Split$_{26-30s}$ versus Split$_{6-10s}$. #F: Split$_{16-20s}$, Split$_{21-25s}$, Split$_{26-30s}$ versus Split$_{6-10s}$. #G: Split$_{26-30s}$ versus Split$_{6-10s}$. #H: Split$_{1-5s}$, Split$_{6-10s}$, Split$_{16-20s}$, Split$_{21-25s}$ and Split$_{25-30s}$ versus Split$_{11-15s}$. #I: Split$_{26-30s}$ versus Split$_{11-15s}$. #J: Split$_{26-30s}$ versus Split$_{11-15s}$. #K: Split$_{21-25s}$ versus Split$_{11-15s}$. #L: Split$_{1-5s}$, Split$_{6-10s}$, Split$_{16-20s}$, Split$_{21-25s}$ and Split$_{25-30s}$ versus Split$_{16-20s}$. #M: Split$_{26-30s}$ versus Split$_{16-20s}$. #O: Split$_{6-10s}$, Split$_{16-20s}$, Split$_{21-25s}$ and Split$_{25-30s}$ versus Split$_{21-25s}$. #P: Split$_{6-10s}$, Split$_{11-15s}$ and Split$_{16-20s}$ versus Split$_{26-30s}$. #Q: Split$_{6-10s}$, Split$_{11-15s}$, Split$_{16-20s}$, Split$_{21-25s}$ versus Split$_{26-30s}$.

3.2. Electromyographic Assessment and Neuromuscular Efficiency

In the analysis of rms-EMG, there were no significant differences ($p > 0.05$) between supplementation in EMG_{Wpeak}, EMG_{mean} and EMG_{Wmin} during the Wingate test (see Table 1). Also, we observed a higher $TEMG_{max}$ in the gluteus maximus for the caffeine condition (8.00 ± 6.26 versus 3.63 ± 3.66; $p = 0.022$; ES = 0.91).

On the other hand, there was a time factor effect in EMG_{VL}, EMG_{BF}, EMG_{TA}, EMG_{GL} ($p < 0.05$), in the placebo and caffeine conditions at different Wingate time splits (see Table 2). There were no significant differences for supplementation conditions or the interaction between factors (supplementation-time) ($p > 0.05$), except for EMG_{TA} (time·suplementation: $p = 0.033$).

In the analysis of neuromuscular efficiency there were no significant differences between caffeine and placebo conditions, but a large effect was detected for NME_{Wpeak} in the vastus lateralis (ES = 1.01) and gluteus maximus (ES = 0.89), and NME_{Wmean} for vastus lateralis (ES = 0.95) and tibialis anterior (ES = 0.83). There was also a moderate effect near large values (i.e. ≈ 0.8), in NME_{MED} at W_{peak} (ES = 0.77), and at W_{mean} (ES = 0.74) (see Table 3).

Table 3. Data of neuromuscular efficiency for the different muscles analyzed during the Wingate test.

Variable	Experimental Condition	NME_{Wpeak} M ± SD	p-Value	ES	NME_{Wmean} M ± SD	p-Value	ES
NME_{VL}	Placebo	13.29 ± 1.63	0.115	1.01	11.34 ± 1.98	0.105	0.95
	Caffeine	16.71 ± 4.87			13.99 ± 3.71		
NME_{BF}	Placebo	16.75 ± 5.87	0.785	0.12	16.19 ± 5.00	0.678	0.17
	Caffeine	16.11 ± 5.28			15.39 ± 5.30		
NME_{GM}	Placebo	15.74 ± 4.01	0.187	0.89	13.14 ± 1.75	0.261	0.61
	Caffeine	22.18 ± 10.19			14.27 ± 2.19		
NME_{TA}	Placebo	15.72 ± 7.59	0.957	0.04	13.43 ± 3.06	0.181	0.83
	Caffeine	15.93 ± 4.66			18.11 ± 7.94		
NME_{GL}	Placebo	14.47 ± 3.77	0.947	0.04	12.76 ± 2.88	0.556	0.31
	Caffeine	14.58 ± 2.20			13.82 ± 4.35		
NME_{MED}	Placebo	14.35 ± 1.99	0.184	0.77	12.87 ± 1.41	0.054	0.74
	Caffeine	15.92 ± 2.34			14.36 ± 2.71		

NME_{Wpeak}: ratio between W_{peak} and EMG_{Wpeak}; NME_{Wmean}: ratio between W_{mean} and EMG_{Wmean}; NME_{VL}: neuromuscular efficiency measured on the vastus lateralis; NME_{BF}: neuromuscular efficiency measured on the biceps femoris; NME_{GM}: neuromuscular efficiency measured on the gluteus maximus; NME_{GL}: neuromuscular efficiency measured on the gastrocnemius lateral head; NME_{TA}: neuromuscular efficiency measured on the tibialis anterior; NME_{MED}: neuromuscular efficiency measured as the mean values of the five muscles analyzed; * Significant difference between Placebo and Caffeine condition at $p < 0.05$.

3.3. Blood Lactate

Blood lactate concentrations increased from rest (placebo 1.86 ± 0.55 mmol·L^{-1} versus caffeine 1.53 ± 0.56 mmol·L^{-1}) to exhaustion after the Wingate test (placebo 11.88 ± 1.55 mmol·L^{-1} versus caffeine 15.36 ± 1.57 mmol·L^{-1}), with significant differences in the placebo ($p < 0.001$) and caffeine conditions ($p < 0.001$), but not between conditions ($p > 0.05$) (see Figure 2).

3.4. Neuromuscular Fatigue (CMJ) and Handgrip Strength

Before the Wingate test, caffeine consumption increased jump height (Placebo versus Caffeine, 43.1 ± 3.7 versus 45.4 ± 4.2 cm; $p = 0.006$), but not CMJ_{Wmean} (Placebo versus Caffeine, 28.8 ± 3.0 versus 29.1 ± 4.9 W; $p > 0.05$) or CMJ_{Wpeak} (Placebo versus Caffeine, 51.3 ± 3.4 versus 51.6 ± 5.7 W; $p > 0.05$). The analysis of the CMJs performed before and after the Wingate test revealed a significant decrease in jump height, CMJ_{Wmean} and CMJ_{Wpeak} after caffeine and placebo ingestion (ANOVA time effect, $p = 0.001$). Although compared to placebo, caffeine promoted a less pronounced decrease in jump height, CMJ_{Wmean} and CMJ_{Wpeak} (−2.5%, −1.3% and −2.0%, respectively) only jump height showed a difference between conditions (ANOVA effect, $p = 0.020$). In the analysis of handgrip strength, there were no differences detected for supplementation, time or time·supplementation ($p > 0.05$).

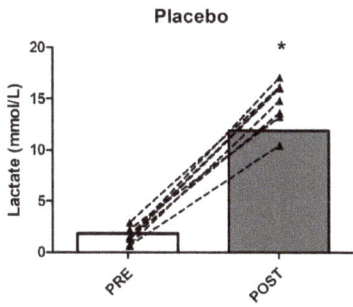 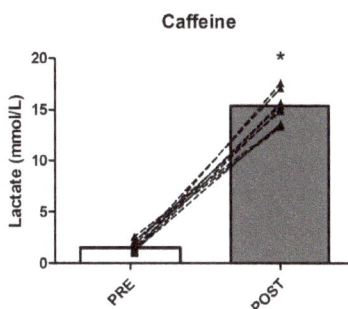

Figure 2. Blood lactate concentrations pre-post Wingate. * $p < 0.05$, significant differences compared to pre-Wingate values (PRE).

4. Discussion

Our results show that the ingestion of caffeine in Olympic-level boxers significantly improves anaerobic performance and has a positive effect on neuromuscular efficiency. Caffeine was also found to reduce lower limbs fatigue levels after an anaerobic test. To our knowledge, this is the first study that has examined the effects of caffeine in Olympic-level boxers.

The main findings of the present study were that caffeine supplementation (6 mg·kg^{-1}) enhanced W$_{peak}$ (6.27%, $p < 0.01$; ES = 1.26) and W$_{mean}$ (5.21%; $p < 0.01$; ES = 1,29) and reduced TW$_{peak}$ (−9.91%, $p < 0.01$; ES = 0.58) in the Wingate test, improved jump height in the CMJ (+2.4 cm, $p < 0.01$) and showed a large effect on neuromuscular efficiency, improving NME$_{Wpeak}$ in the vastus lateralis (ES = 1.01) and gluteus maximus (ES = 0.89) and NME$_{Wmean}$ for the vastus lateralis (ES = 0.95) and tibialis anterior (ES = 0.83). Thereby, these results are in accordance with the 21 meta-analysis review conducted by Grgic et al. [35], who stated that ingestion of caffeine enhanced a large span of exercise performance variables (e.g., muscle endurance and strength, anaerobic power).

Our results with caffeine ingestion seem to improve the most important physical capacities for elite level boxers [36] (e.g., maximal strength and power output, muscle resistance). We observed significant improvements in peak power (6.27%) and mean power (5.21%) in the Wingate test, and in CMJ jump height (5.1%). These findings are consistent with a meta-analysis that have found similar results for peak and mean power [12] and power production [13]. Also, these results are competitively relevant because improvements around 0.6% are enough to make a difference in elite-level sports [37,38].

During the Wingate test, boxers in both conditions, generated the highest power during the second split (6–10 seconds) and then power production decreased progressively until the end of the test. In a Wingate test, W$_{peak}$ is commonly reached during the first 6 seconds of the sprint where free adenosine triphosphate (ATP) and phosphocreatine (PCr) stores are essential energy sources [24,39]. Accordingly, during the 5–10 seconds of the sprint the critical reduction of PCr pools in the muscle promotes adenosine diphosphate (ADP) accumulation which causes the end of the exercise [40]. Given the physiological characteristic of boxing, the delayed time to reach W$_{peak}$ in elite boxers may be explained by an increased capacity to store PCr in their muscles. Further, the caffeine condition showed a higher mean power output in all the splits (differences in splits ranged from +0.27 to +0.56 W·kg^{-1}). These data support the conclusion reached in two caffeine meta-analyses [12,13] where the ergogenic effect of this supplement was attributed to the capacity to improve the production of power by skeletal muscle.

Another main result observed in the present study is the higher neuromuscular efficiency (NME) measured by superficial EMG during the Wingate test in the caffeine condition. To our knowledge, this is the first attempt to asses this question in Olympic level boxers. Mean EMG recordings were similar between both conditions ($p > 0.05$). However, as we described before, the caffeine condition showed a significantly improved power released (i.e., peak power (+0.64 W·kg^{-1}) and time to achieve peak power (−0.88 seconds), and mean power (+0.43 W·kg^{-1})), so the boxers in the caffeine condition developed higher power with the same muscle activation (i.e., greater NME). Moreover, we observed a moderate effect near to large values (i.e., ES > 0.8) for the five muscles measured together NME_{MED} peak (ES = 0.77) and mean (ES = 0.74), and large effect for neuromuscular efficiency (ES > 0.80) for some muscles (i.e., vastus lateralis, gluteus maximus, tibialis anterior). This improved neuromuscular efficiency may be due to the caffeine-enhanced intra- and inter-muscle coordination [41]. Moreover, the vastus lateralis and the gluteus maximus are two of the main muscles involved in pedaling, mostly in the down-stroke phase [42]. Further, in vitro findings observed the increase in calcium release from the sarcoplasmic reticulum after an action potential that could explain these ergogenic effects [43]. In parallel, the significantly longer time (>4 seconds) to achieve EMG peak in the gluteus maximum ($TEMG_{peak\ GM}$) in the caffeine condition, also supports this improved neuromuscular efficiency. Then, during the Wingate test, we observed a greater mean power released in the caffeine condition in each 5 seconds split, with global maintained fiber recruitment (even with a tendency towards lower muscle activation), and with a delay to achieve peak muscle activity in one of the most important muscles in cycling, the gluteus maximum. Therefore, it seems that the higher power production and delayed muscle activity of the gluteus maximum caused by caffeine consumption, facilitated an increased time to produce higher power output (>4 seconds) at the beginning of the test. Also, the higher NME of the tibialis anterior, overall an important up-stroke muscle during the Wingate test, may help to produce this higher power output in the caffeine condition. But further, the NME_{MED} of the five muscles contribute to maintain this greater power production during the 30 seconds of the Wingate test with the same muscle recruitment, resulting in better neuromuscular efficiency. This improved duration during high-power actions was observed by Coswig et al. [44] after caffeine supplementation, ten Judo athletes increased the duration of high-intensity actions and decreased the rest duration during simulated boxing matches. However, Greer, Morales, and Coles [45] studied the effects of caffeine ingestion on Wingate performance and surface EMG in eighteen active males. They observed no differences in neuromuscular efficiency (i.e., same power output and EMG amplitude between conditions). This lack of ergogenic effect may be explained because it could be exclusive to athletes with high levels of performance, as there are other studies with poorly trained subjects where there have been no significant differences between caffeine and placebo conditions [46–49]. More deeply, MacIntosh et al. [50] and Lucia et al. [27] studied this neuromuscular efficiency in cycle ergometry with active healthy subjects and professional elite cyclists, respectively. Both showed that at high power outputs (i.e. ≈ 400 W), higher pedaling cadence produced lower rms-EMG amplitude, and then lower motor unit activation. In the present study, the cycle ergometer was set with the same fixed load for each boxer in both conditions. In the caffeine condition, they produce higher power output with these fixed loads, so caffeine permits a higher pedaling cadence to produce this increased power. Then, this higher cadence may in part explain the better neuromuscular efficiency observed in these elite boxers.

On the other hand, there was a significant EMG fatigue effect in the placebo and caffeine conditions at different Wingate time splits (ANOVA time effect: EMG_{VL}, EMG_{BF}, EMG_{TA}, EMG_{GL}, $p < 0.05$; EMG_{GM} $p = 0.094$). The data revealed in the five muscles mean EMG differences of −13.9% ± 7.0% (range −4% to −24%) from the first Wingate split (0–5 seconds) to the last (26–30 seconds). The rms-EMG used in the present study is an accurate measure of the EMG amplitude and is highly correlated with the number of active motor units (fiber recruitment) [26,27]. Then, fiber recruitment decreased progressively during the Wingate test influenced by higher fatigue levels. The same behavior was described in the Wingate test by Greer, Morales, and Coles [45]. They measured vastus lateralis and gastrocnemius muscles and observed a significantly decreased EMG amplitude during the 30-seconds all-out test, with no differences between caffeine and placebo conditions. In combat sports, Cortez et al. [51] observed the same fatigue effect at the level of the rectus femoris in a dollyo chagi kick (i.e., Taekwondo technique), before and after a strenuous task, and observed that caffeine supplementation reduced this fatigue effect compared to the intake of placebo (≈ −5% Caffeine versus ≈ −20% Placebo).

Caffeine has shown to be effective at improving reaction speed (i.e., reducing the execution time of the bandal tchagui kick) [52], or reaction time in response to a visual stimulus [53], in combat sports. Although, the reaction speed of the upper extremities has not been measured, the shorter time to reach the achieve peak power during the Wingate test (~10%) seems to support this ergogenic effect of caffeine in boxers. This effect of caffeine intake on reaction speed could be mediated by increased neurotransmitter delivery, enhancing motor neuron transmission [54–56], and by increased activity of the sodium-potassium pump, improving the sarcoplasmic availability of calcium [55].

In the present study, caffeine consumption enhanced neuromuscular performance and diminished neuromuscular fatigue, measured with the countermovement jump test, by significantly increasing vertical jump height (+2.3 cm) and attenuating the decrease in vertical jump height after the Wingate test (−2.5%) respectively, and compared to placebo. Fatigue is a very important variable in combat sports such as Olympic boxing, as the competitions include multiple fights on consecutive days, and then the maintenance of power levels between fights is considered a valuable performance variable [20]. Our results agree with those of Cortez et al. [51], who observed higher neuromuscular performance and lower levels of fatigue in a dollyo chagi kick (i.e., Taeckwondo technique) in taekwondo athletes supplemented with caffeine, before and after a strenuous task compared to placebo intake.

Our data showed that an anaerobic effort such as a Wingate Test results in a significant increase in blood lactate concentrations in both conditions (time factor for both placebo and caffeine), but not between conditions ($p > 0.05$). These findings are in agreement with other data published in well-trained men [57], Judo athletes [58], and male wrestlers [20]. However, although we did not find significant differences between conditions, we detected higher lactate concentrations for caffeine supplementation versus placebo. This large amount of lactate production in the caffeine condition may be explained by the observed better Wingate performance, that may reflect a higher glycolysis utilization [12]. Other authors [59,60] observed significantly augmented blood lactate concentrations in taekwondo and Jiu-Jitsu athletes following caffeine supplementation. As before, this effect could be explained by the higher energy expenditures related to increased glycolysis utilization with a greater recruitment of type II motor units [61] (i.e., highly dependent on glycolytic metabolism [62,63]), and by a reduced effect of adenosine on phosphofructokinase inhibition [43].

In comparison to the placebo condition, no differences were noted in the isometric handgrip strength (IHS) with caffeine ingestion (−1.34% versus −0.54%). Our results are similar to previous data with highly resistant training males [64] that reported no differences with caffeine ingestion versus placebo conditions in IHS (1.88%) after a neuromuscular test battery. However, other studies have found improvements in handgrip force after caffeine supplementation [9,60,65,66]. The lack of significant effect of caffeine consumption on isometric strength and the discrepancy observed in the literature may indicate that this ergogenic aid is more effective on dynamic (eccentric and concentric) compared to static (isometric) muscular performance. Moreover, it should take into account that caffeine ingestion stimulates a higher increase in lower body compared to upper body strength performance [67]. Handgrip is not a specific action for boxing athletes and may not be the most appropriate test for them. In fact, we can speculate that another explanation of this result may reside on the differences in muscle recruitment and contraction between the handgrip strength test and how boxers train their hands. While the handgrip strength test required maximal strength of the flexor muscle of the hand, in boxing, other muscles of the forearm are implicated and maximal contraction may not be required. Another explanation may be that the great endurance-strength of these Olympic-level boxers could overcome the fatigue effect of one Wingate test (i.e., focused overall on lower limbs performance). In future studies it should be recommended to determine the ergogenic effects of caffeine on both upper and lower limbs, by subjecting the boxers to several bouts of a specific test that includes the four extremities. In this sense, Negaresh et al. [68], observed during a simulated wrestling tournament that an individualized caffeine supplementation protocol should be implemented when physical performance is expected to be reduced (i.e., usually during the latter combat rounds).

Limitations

Due to the high quality of the sample, its number is limited and could have masked some of the known ergogenic effects of caffeine. Moreover, all the enrolled subjects were male. Lastly, blood samples extraction would help to monitor caffeine presence in plasma in both trials (caffeine and placebo), a procedure that cannot be performed in the present cohort of elite boxers. Future studies using a bigger sample with mixed-gender or female population and blood samples are warranted.

5. Conclusions

The present study has demonstrated that caffeine supplementation (6 mg·kg^{-1}) improves anaerobic performance (i.e., Wingate and CMJ) with a similar electromyographic activity and fatigue levels of lower limbs (i.e., Wingate and CMJ) and enhanced neuromuscular efficiency in some muscles (i.e., vastus lateralis, gluteus maximus and tibialis anterior) in Olympic-level boxers. Further, caffeine consumption enhances reaction speed (i.e., a higher peak power with a lower time to achieve peak power).

Future research should focus on the ergogenic effects of caffeine after repeated bouts of a specific simulated boxing combat test on both the upper and lower extremities and should also address cognitive fatigue.

Author Contributions: P.J. and R.D. conceived and designed the experiments; P.J. and R.D. recruited the subjects and realized the informative session before the starting of the study; P.V.-H. elaborated the supplements, ensured the randomization and he checked that subjects have followed the diet guidelines; A.F.S.J., A.L.-S., P.J., P.L.V., J.R., A.P.-L. and R.D. performed the experiment; A.F.S.J., A.L.-S., P.L.V., J.R. and A.P.-L. extracted the data; A.L.-S., P.V.-H., A.P.-L. and R.D. conducted the statistical analysis; A.S.J.F. and R.D. elaborated tables; A.L.-S. and R.D. elaborated figures; A.F.S.J., A.L.-S. and A.P.-L. wrote the original draft of the manuscript; A.F.S.J., A.L.-S., P.J., P.L.V., J.R., P.V.-H., A.P.-L. and R.D. revised the manuscripts; A.F.S.J., A.L.-S., P.J., P.L.V., J.R., P.V.-H., A.P.-L. and R.D. approved the final version of the manuscript.

Funding: This research was funded by Fundación Universidad Alfonso X el Sabio and Banco Santander.

Acknowledgments: The authors would like to thank the Spanish Boxing Federation and, especially, the Spanish National Coach Rafael Lozano, and Teresa, who allowed the group of elite athletes to attend the sessions, ensuring compliance with all dietary and rest considerations required for participation in the study. We also, want to thank Fernando Mata (NutriScience) for his help during the design and conceptualization of the study.

Conflicts of Interest: The authors declare no conflict of interest.

References

1. Maughan, R.J.; Burke, L.M.; Dvorák, J.; Larson-Meyer, D.E.; Peeling, P.; Phillips, S.M.; Rawson, E.S.; Walsh, N.P.; Garthe, I.; Geyer, H.; et al. IOC Consensus Statement: Dietary Supplements and the High-Performance Athlete. *Int. J. Sport Nutr. Exerc. Metab.* **2018**, *28*, 104–125. [CrossRef]
2. Peeling, P.; Binnie, M.J.; Goods, P.S.; Sim, M.; Burke, L.M. Evidence-Based Supplements for the Enhancement of Athletic Performance. *Int. J. Sport Nutr. Exerc. Metab.* **2018**, *28*, 178–187. [CrossRef]
3. Australian Institute of Sport. ABCD Classification System. Available online: http://www.ausport.gov.au/ais/nutrition/supplements/classification (accessed on 9 March 2018).
4. Graham, T. Caffeine and exercise: Metabolism, endurance and performance. *Sports Med.* **2001**, *31*, 785–807. [CrossRef]
5. Einother, S.J.L.; Giesbrecht, T. Caffeine as an attention enhancer: Reviewing existing assumptions. *Psychopharmacology* **2013**, *225*, 251–274. [CrossRef]
6. McLellan, T.M.; Caldwell, J.A.; Lieberman, H.R. A review of caffeine's effects on cognitive, physical and occupational performance. *Neurosci. Biobehav. Rev.* **2016**, *71*, 294–312. [CrossRef]
7. Williams, J.H. Caffeine, neuromuscular function and high-intensity exercise performance. *J. Sports Med. Phys. Fit.* **1991**, *31*, 481–489.
8. Magkos, F.; Kavouras, S.A. Caffeine Use in Sports, Pharmacokinetics in Man, and Cellular Mechanisms of Action. *Crit. Rev. Food Sci. Nutr.* **2005**, *45*, 535–562. [CrossRef]
9. Cornish, R.S.; Bolam, K.A.; Skiner, T.L. Effect of Caffeine on Exercise Capacity and Function in Prostate Cancer Survivors. *Med. Sci. Sports Exerc.* **2015**, *47*, 468–475. [CrossRef]

10. Dean, S.; Braakhuis, A.; Paton, C. The effects of ECG on fat oxidation and endurance performance in male cyclists. *Int. J. Sport Nutr. Exerc. Metab.* **2009**, *19*, 624–644. [CrossRef]
11. Spriet, L.L. Exercise and Sport Performance with Low Doses of Caffeine. *Sports Med.* **2014**, *44*, 175–184. [CrossRef]
12. Grgic, J. Caffeine ingestion enhances Wingate performance: A meta-analysis. *Eur. J. Sport Sci.* **2018**, *18*, 219–225. [CrossRef]
13. Grgic, J.; Trexler, E.T.; Lazinica, B.; Pedisic, Z. Effects of caffeine intake on muscle strength and power: A systematic review and meta-analysis. *J. Int. Soc. Sports Nutr.* **2018**, *15*, 11. [CrossRef]
14. Mata-Ordoñez, F.; Sanchez-Oliver, A.; Domínguez, R. Importancia de la nutrición en las estrategias de pérdida de pérdida de peso en deportes de combate. *J. Sport Health Res.* **2018**, *10*, 1–12.
15. Campos, F.A.; Bertuzzi, R.; Dourado, A.C.; Santos, V.G.F.; Franchini, E. Energy demands in taekwondo athletes during combat simulation. *Eur. J. Appl. Physiol.* **2012**, *112*, 1221–1228. [CrossRef]
16. Bridge, C.A.; Santos, J.F.D.S.; Chaabene, H.; Pieter, W.; Franchini, E. Physical and Physiological Profiles of Taekwondo Athletes. *Sports Med.* **2014**, *44*, 713–733. [CrossRef]
17. Franchini, E.; Artioli, G.G.; Brito, C.J. Judo combat: Time-motion analysis and physiology. *Int. J. Perform. Anal. Sport* **2013**, *13*, 624–641. [CrossRef]
18. García-Pallarés, J.; López-Gullón, J.M.; Muriel, X.; Diaz, A.; Izquierdo, M. Physical fitness factors to predict male Olympic wrestling performance. *Eur. J. Appl. Physiol.* **2011**, *111*, 1747–1758. [CrossRef]
19. Ratamess, N. Strength and Conditioning for Grappling Sports. *Strength Cond. J.* **2011**, *33*, 18–24. [CrossRef]
20. Aedma, M.; Timpmann, S.; Ööpik, V. Effect of Caffeine on Upper-Body Anaerobic Performance in Wrestlers in Simulated Competition-Day Conditions. *Int. J. Sport Nutr. Exerc. Metab.* **2013**, *23*, 601–609. [CrossRef]
21. Drust, B.; Waterhouse, J.; Atkinson, G.; Edwards, B.; Reilly, T. Circadian Rhythms in Sports Performance—An Update. *Chrono-Int.* **2005**, *22*, 21–44. [CrossRef]
22. Lozano Estevan, M.C.; Martínez, R.C. *Manual de Tecnología Farmacéutica*; Lozano, M.C., Córdoba, D., Córdoba, M., Eds.; Elsevier: Barcelona, Spain, 2012; Chapter 5; pp. 343–353.
23. Harland, B.F. Caffeine and nutrition. *Nutrition* **2000**, *16*, 522–526. [CrossRef]
24. Bar-Or, O. The Wingate anaerobic test. An update on methodology, reliability and validity. *Sports Med.* **1987**, *4*, 381–394. [CrossRef]
25. SENIAM project (Surface ElectroMyoGraphy for the Non-Invasive Assessment of Muscles). Available online: http://www.seniam.org/ (accessed on 1 March 2018).
26. Moritani, T.; Muro, M. Motor unit activity and surface electromyogram power spectrum during increasing force of contraction. *Eur. J. Appl. Physiol. Occup. Physiol.* **1987**, *56*, 260–265. [CrossRef]
27. Lucia, A.; San Juan, A.F.; Montilla, M.; CaNete, S.; Santalla, A.; Earnest, C.; Pérez, M. In professional road cyclists, low pedaling cadences are less efficient. *Med. Sci. Sports Exerc.* **2004**, *36*, 1048–1054. [CrossRef]
28. Hug, F.; Dorel, S. Electromyographic analysis of pedaling: A review. *J. Electromyogr. Kinesiol.* **2009**, *19*, 182–198. [CrossRef]
29. Gorostiaga, E.M.; Asiain, X.; Izquierdo, M.; Postigo, A.; Aguado, R.; Alonso, J.M.; Ibáñez, J. Vertical Jump Performance and Blood Ammonia and Lactate Levels During Typical Training Sessions in Elite 400-m Runners. *J. Strength Cond. Res.* **2010**, *24*, 1138–1149. [CrossRef]
30. Sánchez-Medina, L.; González-Badillo, J.J. Velocity Loss as an indicator of neuromuscular fatigue during resistance training. *Med. Sci. Sports Exerc.* **2011**, *43*, 1725–1734. [CrossRef]
31. López-Samanes, Á.; Moreno-Pérez, D.; Maté-Muñoz, J.L.; Domínguez, R.; Pallarés, J.G.; Mora-Rodriguez, R.; Ortega, J.F. Circadian rhythm effect on physical tennis performance in trained male players. *J. Sports Sci.* **2017**, *35*, 2121–2128. [CrossRef]
32. Lakens, D. Calculating and reporting effect sizes to facilitate cumulative science: A practical primer for t-tests and ANOVAs. *Front. Psychol.* **2013**, *4*, 863. [CrossRef]
33. Cohen, J. *Statistical Power Analysis for the Behavioral Sciences*, 2nd ed.; Routledge, Lawrence Erlbaum Associates Publisher: New York, NY, USA, 1988.
34. Ferguson, C.J. An effect size primer: A guide for clinicians and researchers. *Prof. Psychol. Res. Pract.* **2009**, *40*, 532–538. [CrossRef]
35. Grgic, J.; Grgic, I.; Pickering, C.; Schoenfeld, B.J.; Bishop, D.J.; Pedisic, Z. Wake up and smell the coffee: Caffeine supplementation and exercise performance—An umbrella review of 21 published meta-analyses. *Br. J. Sports Med.* **2019**. bjsports-2018. [CrossRef]

36. López-González, L.M.; Sánchez-Oliver, A.J.; Mata, F.; Jodra, P.; Antonio, J.; Domínguez, R. Acute caffeine supplementation in combat sports: A systematic review. *J. Int. Soc. Sports Nutr.* **2018**, *15*, 60. [CrossRef]
37. Paton, C.D.; Hopkins, W.G. Variation in performance of elite cyclists from race to race. *Eur. J. Sport Sci.* **2006**, *6*, 25–31. [CrossRef]
38. Domínguez, R.; Maté-Muñoz, J.L.; Cuenca, E.; García-Fernández, P.; Mata-Ordoñez, F.; Lozano-Estevan, M.C.; Veiga-Herreros, P.; Da Silva, S.F.; Garnacho-Castaño, M.V. Effects of beetroot juice supplementation on intermittent high-intensity exercise efforts. *J. Int. Soc. Sports Nutr.* **2018**, *15*, 2. [CrossRef]
39. Gaitanos, G.C.; Williams, C.; Boobis, L.H.; Brooks, S. Human muscle metabolism during intermittent maximal exercise. *J. Appl. Physiol.* **1993**, *75*, 712–719. [CrossRef]
40. Parolin, M.L.; Chesley, A.; Matsos, M.P.; Spriet, L.L.; Jones, N.L.; Heigenhauser, G.J.F. Regulation of skeletal muscle glycogen phosphorylase and PDH during maximal intermittent exercise. *Am. J. Physiol. Metab.* **1999**, *277*, E890–E990. [CrossRef]
41. Del Coso, J.; Salinero, J.J.; González-Millán, C.; Abian-Vicen, J.; Pérez-González, B. Dose response effects of a caffeine-containing energy drink on muscle performance: A repeated measures design. *J. Int. Soc. Sports Nutr.* **2012**, *9*, 21. [CrossRef]
42. Faina, I.E. Energy expenditure, aerodynamics and medical problems in cycling: An update. *Sports Med.* **1992**, *14*, 43–63.
43. Simmonds, M.J.; Minahan, C.L.; Sabapathy, S. Caffeine improves supramaximal cycling but not the rate of anaerobic energy release. *Eur. J. Appl. Physiol.* **2010**, *109*, 287–295. [CrossRef]
44. Coswig, V.S.; Gentil, P.; Irigon, F.; Del Vecchio, F.B. Caffeine ingestion changes time-motion and technical-tactical aspects in simulated boxing matches: A randomized double-blind PLA-controlled crossover study. *Eur. J. Sport Sci.* **2018**, *18*, 975–983. [CrossRef]
45. Greer, F.; Morales, J.; Coles, M. Wingate performance and surface EMG frequency variables are not affected by caffeine ingestion. *Appl. Physiol. Nutr. Metab.* **2006**, *31*, 597–603. [CrossRef]
46. Crowe, M.J.; Leicht, A.S.; Spinks, W.L. Physiological and cognitive responses to caffeine during repeated, high-intensity exercise. *Int. J. Sport Nutr. Exerc. Metab.* **2006**, *16*, 528–544. [CrossRef]
47. Keisler, B.D.; Armsey, T.D. Caffeine as an ergogenic aid. *Curr. Sports Med. Rep.* **2006**, *5*, 215–219. [CrossRef]
48. Woolf, K.; Bidwell, W.K.; Carlson, A.G. The effect of caffeine as an ergogenic aid in anaerobic exercise. *Int. J. Sport Nutr. Exerc. Metab.* **2008**, *18*, 412–429. [CrossRef]
49. Lamina, S.; Musa, D.I. Efecto ergogénico de diversas dosis de cafeína en café sobre la potencia aeróbica máxima de jóvenes africanos. *Afr. Health Sci.* **2009**, *10*, 270–274.
50. MacIntosh, B.R.; Neptune, R.R.; Horton, J.F. Cadence, power, and muscle activation in cycle ergometry. *Med. Sci. Sports Exerc.* **2000**, *32*, 1281–1287. [CrossRef]
51. Cortez, L.; Mackay, K.; Contreras, E.; Peñailillo, L. Efecto agudo de la investigación de cafeína sobre el tiempo de reacción y la actividad electromiográfica de la patada circular Dollyo Chagi en taekwondistas. *Rev. Int. Cienc. Del Deport.* **2017**, *13*, 52–62. [CrossRef]
52. Santos, V.G.F.; Santos, V.R.F.; Felippe, L.J.C.; Almeida, J.W.; Bertuzzi, R.; Kiss, M.A.P.D.M.; Lima-Silva, A.E. Caffeine Reduces Reaction Time and Improves Performance in Simulated-Contest of Taekwondo. *Nutrients* **2014**, *6*, 637–649. [CrossRef]
53. Souissi, M.; Abedelmalek, S.; Chtourou, H.; Boussita, A.; Hakim, A.; Sahnoun, Z. Effects of time-of-day and caffeine ingestion on mood states, simple reaction time, and short-term maximal performance in elite judoists. *Boil. Rhythm. Res.* **2013**, *44*, 897–907. [CrossRef]
54. Kalmar, J.M. The Influence of Caffeine on Voluntary Muscle Activation. *Med. Sci. Sports Exerc.* **2005**, *37*, 2113–2119. [CrossRef]
55. Bishop, D. Dietary supplements and team-sport performance. *Sports Med.* **2010**, *40*, 995–1017. [CrossRef]
56. Mohr, M.; Bangsbo, J.; Nielsen, J.J. Caffeine intake improves intense intermittent exercise performance and reduces muscle interstitial potassium accumulation. *J. Appl. Physiol.* **2011**, *111*, 1372–1379. [CrossRef]
57. Glaister, M.; Muniz-Pumares, D.; Patterson, S.D.; Foley, P.; McInnes, G. Caffeine supplementation and peak anaerobic power output. *Eur. J. Sport Sci.* **2015**, *15*, 400–406. [CrossRef]
58. Lopes-Silva, J.P.; Felippe, L.J.C.; Silva-Cavalcante, M.D.; Bertuzzi, R.; Lima-Silva, A.E. Caffeine Ingestion after Rapid Weight Loss in Judo Athletes Reduces Perceived Effort and Increases Plasma Lactate Concentration without Improving Performance. *Nutrients* **2014**, *6*, 2931–2945. [CrossRef]

59. Lopes-Silva, J.P.; Santos, J.F.D.S.; Branco, B.H.M.; Abad, C.C.C.; De Oliveira, L.F.; LoTurco, I.; Franchini, E. Caffeine Ingestion Increases Estimated Glycolytic Metabolism during Taekwondo Combat Simulation but Does Not Improve Performance or Parasympathetic Reactivation. *PLoS ONE* **2015**, *10*, e0142078. [CrossRef]
60. Diaz-Lara, F.J.; Del Coso, J.; García, J.M.; Portillo, L.J.; Areces, F.; Abian-Vicen, J. Caffeine improves muscular performance in elite Brazilian Jiu-jitsu athletes. *Eur. J. Sport Sci.* **2016**, *16*, 1–8. [CrossRef]
61. Esbjörnsson-Liljedahl, M.; Sundberg, C.J.; Norman, B.; Jansson, E. Metabolic response in type I and type II muscle fibers during a 30-s cycle sprint in men and women. *J. Appl. Physiol.* **1999**, *87*, 1326–1332. [CrossRef]
62. Domínguez, R.; Garnacho-Castaño, M.V.; Cuenca, E.; García-Fernández, P.; Muñoz-González, A.; de Jesús, F.; Lozano-Estevan, M.D.C.; Fernandes da Silva, S.; Veiga-Herreros, P.; Maté-Muñoz, J.L. Effects of beetroot juice supplementation on a 30-s high-intensity inertial cycle ergometer test. *Nutrients* **2017**, *9*, 1360. [CrossRef]
63. Cuenca, E.; Jodra, P.; Pérez-López, A.; González-Rodríguez, L.G.; Fernandes da Silva, S.; Veiga-Herreros, P.; Domínguez, R. Effects of Beetroot Juice Supplementation on Performance and Fatigue in a 30-s All-Out Sprint Exercise: A Randomized, Double-Blind Cross-Over Study. *Nutrients* **2018**, *10*, 1222. [CrossRef]
64. Mora-Rodriguez, R.; Pallares, J.G.; López-Samanes, Á.; Ortega, J.F.; Fernandez-Elias, V.E. Caffeine Ingestion Reverses the Circadian Rhythm Effects on Neuromuscular Performance in Highly Resistance-Trained Men. *PLoS ONE* **2012**, *7*, e33807. [CrossRef]
65. Del Coso, J.; Pérez-López, A.; Abian-Vicen, L.; Salinero, J.J.; Lara, B.; Valadés, D. Enhancing physical performance in male volleyball players with a caffeine-containing energy drink. *Int. J. Sports Physiol. Perform.* **2014**, *9*, 1013–1018. [CrossRef]
66. Astley, C.; Souza, D.B.; Polito, M.D. Acute Specific Effects of Caffeine-containing Energy Drink on Different Physical Performances in Resistance-trained Men. *Int. J. Exerc. Sci.* **2018**, *11*, 260–268.
67. Warren, G.L.; Park, N.D.; Marexca, R.D.; McKibans, K.I.; Millard-Stafford, M.L. Effect of caffeine ingestion on muscular strength and endurance: A meta-analysis. *Med. Sci. Sports Exerc.* **2010**, *42*, 1375–1387. [CrossRef]
68. Negaresh, R.; Del Coso, J.; Mokhtarzade, M.; Lima-Silva, A.E.; Baker, J.S.; Willems, M.E.T.; Talebvand, S.; Khodadoost, M.; Farhani, F. Effects of different dosages of caffeine administration on wrestling performance during a simulated tournament. *Eur. J. Sport Sci.* **2019**, *19*, 499–507. [CrossRef]

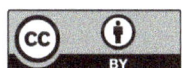

© 2019 by the authors. Licensee MDPI, Basel, Switzerland. This article is an open access article distributed under the terms and conditions of the Creative Commons Attribution (CC BY) license (http://creativecommons.org/licenses/by/4.0/).

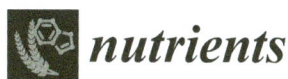

Article

Impact of Caffeine Intake on 800-m Running Performance and Sleep Quality in Trained Runners

Domingo Jesús Ramos-Campo [1], Andrés Pérez [2], Vicente Ávila-Gandía [3,*], Silvia Pérez-Piñero [3] and Jacobo Ángel Rubio-Arias [1]

[1] Faculty of Sports, UCAM, Catholic University San Antonio, 30107 Murcia, Spain
[2] High Performance Research Center (CIARD), UCAM, Catholic University San Antonio, 30107 Murcia, Spain
[3] Department of Exercise Physiology, Catholic University San Antonio, 30107 Murcia, Spain
* Correspondence: vicenteavila@gmail.com or vavila@ucam.edu; Tel./Fax: +34-968-27-87-57

Received: 9 August 2019; Accepted: 22 August 2019; Published: 1 September 2019

Abstract: Background: Caffeine ingestion improves athletic performance, but impairs sleep quality. We aimed to analyze the effect of caffeine intake on 800-m running performance, sleep quality (SQ), and nocturnal cardiac autonomic activity (CAA) in trained runners. Methods: Fifteen male middle-distance runners participated in the study (aged 23.7 ± 8.2 years). In a randomized and comparative crossover study design, the athletes ingested a placebo (PL) or caffeine supplement (CAF; 6 mg·kg^{-1}) one hour before an 800-m running time-trial test in the evening. During the night, CAA and SQ were assessed using actigraphy and a sleep questionnaire. A second 800-m running test was performed 24 h after the first. Time, heart rate, rating of perceived exertion, and blood lactate concentration were analyzed for each running test. Results: No significant differences in CAA and performance variables were found between the two conditions. However, CAF impaired sleep efficiency ($p = 0.003$), actual wake time ($p = 0.001$), and the number of awakenings ($p = 0.005$), as measured by actigraphy. Also, CAF impaired the questionnaire variables of SQ ($p = 0.005$), calm sleep ($p = 0.005$), ease of falling asleep ($p = 0.003$), and feeling refreshed after waking ($p = 0.006$). Conclusion: The supplementation with caffeine (6 mg·kg^{-1}) did not improve the 800-m running performance, but did impair the SQ of trained runners.

Keywords: actigraphy; athletic; coffee; ergogenic aid; supplement

---

1. Introduction

Scientists and coaches are continually looking for techniques to develop more effective and efficient methods to improve exercise performance [1]. One of the popular methods commonly used by athletes to maximize their physical performance is the intake of legal ergogenic aids [2]. In this way, caffeine is frequently used in sport as an ergogenic aid to improve athletic performance and endurance [3]. In fact, it has been reported that 74% of elite athletes may use caffeine as an ergogenic aid prior to or during a competition [4]. Caffeine is a xanthine alkaloid that increases central nervous activity by the blockade of central and peripheral adenosine receptors [5]. This stimulant action produces a greater recruitment of motor units [6], improves the Na$^+$–K$^+$ pump response [7], and increases the rate of calcium release from the sarcoplasmic reticulum [8] and the mobilization of free fatty acids [9]. Also, caffeine enhances adrenaline secretion [10] and reduces ratings of perceived exertion [11]. Therefore, caffeine is administered in order to improve sport performance.

Previous studies that analyzed the effect of caffeine ingestion on runners have shown improvements in running performance compared to placebo [12,13]. It had previously been reported that compared to placebo, the intake of 4.5 mg·kg^{-1} of caffeine increased exercise distance by 2–3 km when running at 85% maximum oxygen uptake until exhaustion [10]. Regarding middle-distance races, compared to placebo, 1500-m [13] or one-mile [14] running performances are improved by 1.3–1.9% after 150–200 mg and 3 mg·kg^{-1} of caffeine intake, respectively. However, another study found similar 800-m running performance in amateur runners after placebo or 5.5 mg·kg^{-1} of caffeine administration [15]. Thus, there is conflicting evidence in relation to the effectiveness of caffeine as an ergogenic aid to improve middle-distance race performance in athletes.

On the other hand, caffeine intake can impair sleep [16], which is considered the most important method for recovery from daily load [17]. Sleep assists in the recovery of the nervous and metabolic cost imposed by the waking state [18]. However, caffeine typically prolongs sleep latency, reduces total sleep time and sleep efficiency, and worsens perceived sleep quality (SQ) [16], particularly if it is administered close to bedtime. Moreover, vigorous-intensity exercise completed close to bedtime increases the latency time and impairs SQ [19]. Therefore, the use of caffeine as an ergogenic aid in a competition performed close to bedtime may decrease SQ and the recovery process, which may decrease athlete performance on the following day. There are some sports modalities, such as athletics, where the athlete needs to perform in qualification races over consecutive days. Some of these races are performed at the end of the evening, and the rest time between the first race (e.g., a semi-final) and the following one (e.g., the final) may be very short. For example, during the Athletics World Championships of 2019, the qualification and the semi-final race of the 800-m event were separated by 24 h. Thus, the administration of caffeine before a qualification race performed in the evening may affect the recovery process and performance in the races on the following day due to sleeping problems. However, there are no studies that have analyzed the effect of caffeine administration to aid performance in a race close to bedtime on SQ and on the running performance the following day.

Therefore, the aim of the present study was to analyze the effect of caffeine intake one hour (19:00 h) before an 800-m race (20:00 h) on actigraphic SQ, subjective SQ, and nocturnal cardiac autonomic activity (CAA), and on the 800-m performance performed 24 h later in trained middle-distance athletes. We hypothesized that the pre-exercise ingestion of 6 mg of caffeine per kg of an athletes's body mass would impair SQ through subjective and actigraphic impairment, but it would not affect the race performance on the following day.

2. Methods

2.1. Design

A randomized and comparative crossover study was conducted to test the effects of caffeine intake or placebo before an 800-m running time trial on actigraphic SQ, the subjective quality of sleep, nocturnal autonomous cardiac activity, countermovement jump (CMJ), and the 800-m performance of athletes at international and national levels. Athletes reported to their usual official athletics track four times over two consecutive weeks. The testing sessions were developed during two consecutive Friday and Saturday evenings in March. Two weeks before the study, the athletes had finished their winter season, performing in the National Indoor Championships. Therefore, the study was developed in a general period training phase.

Upon arrival at the athletics track, runners were given a caffeine or a placebo supplement—placebo (PL) or caffeine (CAF) in randomized order—in experimental Sessions 1 and 3, while no supplements were taken in the experimental Sessions 2 and 4. Forty-five minutes (min) after the intake of the supplements in Sessions 1 and 3, or 45 min after the runners arrived at the athletics track, the participants started the testing session.

An 800-m running time-trial test was performed in each testing session. Performance (time, CMJ height), physiological (peak and mean heart rate and blood lactate concentration), and subjective (rating of perceived exertion) variables were collected during the testing session. The sessions were carried out at 20:00 h and under similar environmental conditions (20–22 °C). In addition, we used actigraphy to monitor the night after PL or CAF ingestion to assess SQ and a sleep questionnaire and to analyze the autonomic modulation.

2.2. Participants

Fifteen male runners in mid-level events participated in the study (age: 23.7 ± 8.2 years; height: 177.4 ± 9.0 cm; weight: 64.6 ± 9.8 kg). Runners performed 9.0 ± 1.8 h per week of training and had at least six years of middle-distance training experience. They were of national and international standard at the 800-m level and their best time at that distance ranged between 1:46.72–2:04.10. Eleven of the runners were of Caucasian race, two were from North Africa (Maghreb race), one was from South America (Latino race), and another was from Central Africa (Black race). All the subjects gave their signed and informed consent, and the study was approved (CE031909) by the Ethics Committee in Institutional Sciences of the University and was in accordance with the Declaration of Helsinki. The subjects were asked to maintain their usual diet and hydration status and not to ingest caffeine or alcohol at least 24 h before each test session or to carry out exhaustive training in the 48 h prior the first and third testing sessions.

2.3. Procedures

Athletes ingested a placebo (sucrose) or caffeine supplement (6 mg·kg^{-1}) in capsules of the same size, color, and smell in a typical double-blind trial, with a 50% chance of ingesting the actual active or placebo substance, avoiding any effects of session or time on the results. The blinding efficacy was checked after the participants had finished their participation. In addition, participants were issued with nutritional guidelines to ensure that they followed a similar diet in the 48 h before each condition session. This diet was the same that runners usually used during competition. The last meal was eaten by runners 3 h before the test. Furthermore, 24 h before each experimental session, caffeine ingestion was restricted. In addition, a caffeine consumption questionnaire [20] was administered to the runners, which showed that all the runners were daily consumers of caffeine (between 250–572 mg of caffeine·day^{-1}) according to classification proposed elsewhere [21]. Also, all the runners were used to ingesting caffeine (6 mg·kg^{-1}) as an ergogenic aid prior to competition.

2.4. Testing Session

During the first visit, body composition was evaluated using a bioimpedance segmental analyzer (Tanita BC-601, Tanita Corp, Tokyo, Japan) following previous recommendations [22]. In addition, 45 min after supplement ingestion, participants performed their traditional competitive warm-up of 15 min duration, including running at low intensity, joint mobility, dynamic stretching, and progressive running sets. After warm-up, a CMJ test was carried out. Two minutes later (~60 min after supplement ingestion), an 800-m time-trial test was performed. Finally, 2 min after the end of the running test, a blood lactate concentration analysis and another CMJ test were carried out. The mean and peak heart rates (Polar RS800, Polar Electro Oy, Kempele, Finland) were recorded during the 800-m running time trial. In addition, ratings of perceived exertion (RPE) were determined using the 10-point Borg scale [23] following the 800 m time trial. The 800-m times were recorded using a Geonaute chronometer Onstart 710 (Decathlon, Villeneuve-d'Ascq, France) by two of the researchers, and the mean of these values was used for analysis. Capillary blood samples (5 µL) were collected by finger prick 2 min after the end of the running test and analyzed for blood lactate concentration ([La–]) using a Lactate Pro analyzer (Lactate Pro, Arkay, Inc., Kyoto, Japan). Countermovement jump heights were performed using a contact platform (Ergotester, Globus, Codogne, Italy). The participants executed two submaximal trials to ensure proper execution of the jumps with 1-min rest between trials. The CMJ height was measured before warm-up and prior to the 800-m time trial, and performed at the center of the platform with the feet placed shoulder-width apart in the standing position. Participants were asked to jump as high as possible with a rapid self-selected countermovement. The depth of the countermovement was self-selected, and participants were asked to try to land close to the take-off point. Each individual's best performed was used for data analysis. The same testing procedure was applied in each testing session.

2.5. Actigraphic Quality of Sleep, Subjective Quality of Sleep, and Autonomous Nocturnal Cardiac Activity

Between the end of testing session and the time to go to bed, the athletes had to do their normal life and record any activity in a diary. Participants were instructed to measure actigraphic sleep quality and nocturnal cardiac autonomic activity (Heart Rate Variability-HRV) during sleep after each day with a training session day. Actigraphic sleep quality was recorded using an actiwatch activity monitoring system (Cambridge Neurotechnology, Cambridge, UK), which measures activity by means of a piezoelectric accelerometer. The movement of the non-dominant wrist of each participant was monitored. A low actigraphic sensitivity threshold (80 counts per epoch) was selected, and the data recorded by the actigraph were analyzed with Actiwatch Sleep Analysis Software. Each subject received a sleep diary to record bedtime, wake-up time, hours napping, hours without wearing the actigraph, and the number of nocturnal awakenings. Data analysis started with the onset of nocturnal rest (bedtime) and ended with the onset of daytime activity (wake time). The following sleep parameters were measured: (I) sleep efficiency (%): percentage of time spent asleep; (II) time in bed (min); (III) actual sleep time (min); (IV) actual wake time (min); (V) number of awakenings; (VI) average time of each awakening(min); and (VII) latency.

Together with the actigraph, during the night, each subject wore an H7 strap Heart monitor (Polar Electro, Kempele, Finland) to evaluate HRV. Variables of cardiac autonomic activity were analyzed for the 4-h period of sleep starting 30 min after the reported bedtime [20]. The R–R series were analyzed using Kubios HRV software (version 2.0, Biosignal Analysis and Medical Imaging Group, University of Kuopio, Finland). The following HRV variables were assessed: (I) low-frequency (LF) band / high-frequency (HF) band ratio; (II) total power (TP); (III) percentage of differences between adjacent normal R–R intervals more than 50 ms (pNN50); (IV) square root of the mean of the sum of the squared differences between adjacent normal R–R intervals (RMSSD); (V) standard deviation of all normal N–N intervals (SDNN); (VI) mean heart rate; and (VII) mean R–R intervals.

Participants were also instructed to evaluate their subjective sleep quality in the morning after awakening using the Karolinska Sleep Diary [24], which analyzes the following questions: (I) sleep quality (very well [5] to very poorly [1]); (II) calm sleep (very calm [5] to very restless [1]); (III) ease of falling asleep (very easy [5] to very difficult [1]); (IV) amount of dreaming (much [3] to none [1]); (V) ease of waking up (very easy [5] to very difficult [1]); (VI) feeling refreshed after awakening (completely [3] to not at all [1]); (VII) slept throughout the time allotted (yes [5] to woke up much too early [1]).

2.6. Statistical Analysis

Statistical analysis of data was performed with SPSS 21.0 software (SPSS 21.0, Chicago, IL, USA) in a Windows environment. Descriptive data are presented as mean ± SD and range. For inferential analysis, a Shapiro–Wilk W-test was performed to establish the normality of the sampling distribution, and Mauchly's W-test analyzed the sphericity between measurements. In addition, analysis of variance for repeated measures (ANOVA) was calculated (general linear model) to analyze the effects of caffeine intake on performance over 800 m, and a paired sample T-test or the nonparametric equivalent (Wilcoxon test) was used to compare the effect of caffeine on heart rate variability and SQ. Effect size (ES) was calculated using partial eta-squared (η^2p) for variance analysis and Cohen's d to indicate the standardized difference between two means. Threshold values for ES were ≥0.1 (small), ≥0.3 (moderate), ≥1.2 (large), and ≥2.0 (very large) [25]. The level of significance was set at $p \leq 0.05$.

3. Results

Table 1 presents the summary statistics for the changes in performance under each of the measured conditions (placebo and caffeine). No significant effects were found in performance (Figure 1).

Significant effects were observed in the variable CMJ (F = 4.564; $p = 0.008$) with a large effect size ($\eta^2p = 0.28$); the pair comparison showed a significant difference between the CMJ results (Δ) on days

1 and 2 when participants took caffeine (mean differences = −6.51, t = −3.14, $p = 0.020$). However, no significant effects were found in in any other variable.

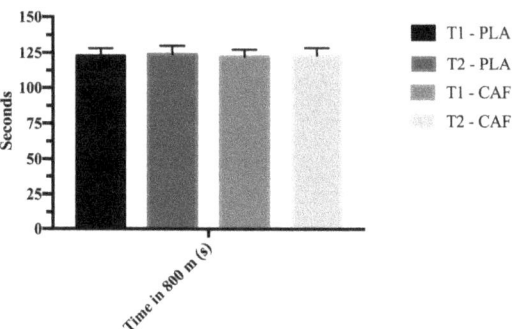

Figure 1. Time in 800 m (s). T1: First test 1; T2: second test; PLA: Placebo; CAF: Caffeine.

Table 1. Results of 800-m running time trial test variables.

	Placebo				Caffeine				ANOVA		
	Test 1		Test 2		Test 1		Test 2				
	mean	SD	mean	SD	mean	SD	mean	SD	F	p	$\eta^2 p$
Time in 800 m (s)	122.6	5.6	123.8	6.2	122.3	5.1	123.3	5.4	2.317	0.12	0.15
RPE (A.U)	8.4	1.1	8.2	1.0	8.3	0.9	8.1	0.9	0.142	0.934	0.01
mean HR in 800 m (bpm)	170.4	9.8	171.4	10.1	172.7	10.6	173.2	9.2	0.625	0.525	0.06
peak HR in 800 m (bpm)	185.8	9.1	184.5	10.1	188.3	8.2	185.5	10.5	0.889	0.395	0.08
CMJ (Δ cm)	−10.2	8.8	−6.8	4.8	−13.3	8.7	−6.8	5.9	4.564	0.008	0.28
Lactate (mmoL/L)	19.1	4.7	19.0	4.2	20.1	4.6	17.8	4.4	0.979	0.413	0.07

RPE: Rate of perceived exertion; CMJ: countermovement jump.

Concerning the SQ results, actigraphic analysis showed significant differences between conditions (placebo versus caffeine) in sleep efficiency ($p = 0.003$; ES = 0.71), actual wake time ($p = 0.001$; ES = −1.18), and number of awakenings ($p = 0.005$; ES = −0.96) (Figure 2 and Table 2).

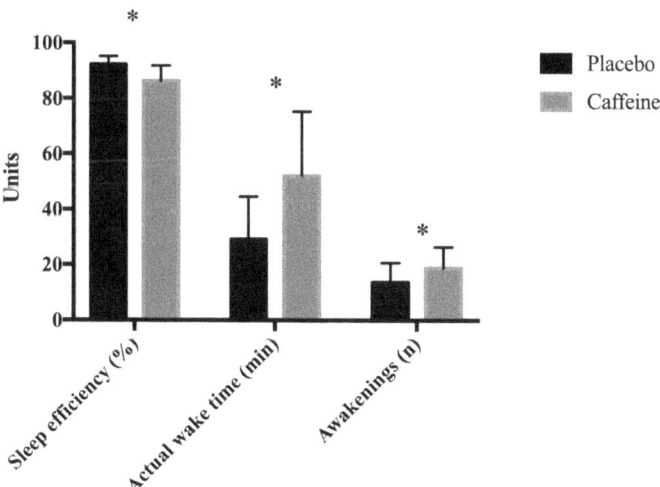

Figure 2. Sleep quality results measured by actigraphy * Significant differences between placebo and caffeine ($p < 0.05$).

Table 2. Sleep quality results.

	Placebo		Caffeine			Effect Size (ES)	95% CI for ES	
	Mean	SD	Mean	SD	p		Lower	Upper
Actigraphic sleep quality								
Latency (min)	6.15	2.79	6.77	2.32	0.290	−0.31	−0.86	0.25
Sleep efficiency (%)	92.2	3.0	86.4	5.5	0.003	0.71	0.27	0.91
Time in bed (min)	470.2	118.3	461.2	128.2	0.641	0.13	−0.42	0.68
Actual sleep time (min)	434.8	119.7	402.3	136.3	0.091	0.51	−0.08	1.08
Actual wake time (min)	29.2	15.4	52.1	23.2	0.001	−1.18	−1.89	−0.45
Awakenings (n)	13.62	7.05	18.85	7.50	0.005	−0.96	−1.61	−0.28
Average time of each awakening (min)	2.79	1.90	3.18	1.72	0.402	−0.24	−0.79	0.32
Karolinska Sleep Questionnaire								
Sleep quality	3.36	0.75	2.21	0.98	0.005	1.11	0.43	1.77
Calm sleep	3.50	1.09	2.36	1.15	0.005	1.11	0.43	1.77
Ease of falling asleep	3.43	1.22	1.57	0.85	0.003	1.38	0.62	2.10
Amount of dreaming	1.43	0.76	1.07	0.48	0.120	0.48	−0.08	1.03
Ease of waking up	3.43	0.76	3.14	0.86	0.395	0.24	−0.30	0.76
Feeling refreshed after awakening	2.07	0.73	1.50	0.65	0.006	1.11	0.43	1.77
Slept throughout the time allotted	3.14	0.86	2.79	1.89	0.389	0.24	−0.30	0.77

In addition, the Karolinska sleep questionnaire showed significant differences between conditions, favoring placebo in SQ ($p = 0.005$; ES = 1.11), calm sleep ($p = 0.005$; ES = 1.11), ease of falling asleep ($p = 0.003$; ES = 1.38), and feeling refreshed after waking ($p = 0.006$; ES = 1.11) (Table 2).

Table 3 shows the summary statistics for heart rate variability during the night. No significant differences were observed between caffeine and placebo.

Table 3. Heart rate variability results during the night after placebo or caffeine ingestion.

	Placebo		Caffeine			Effect Size (ES)	95% CI for ES	
	Mean	SD	Mean	SD	p		Lower	Upper
Mean R-R (ms)	1151.5	114.4	1184.7	131.1	1.000	−0.21	−0.80	0.39
SDNN (ms)	40.4	7.2	36.5	6.7	0.102	0.56	−0.58	0.58
HR (bpm)	52.4	5.7	51.2	6.1	1.000	0.58	−0.01	0.87
RMSSD (ms)	27.1	4.1	26.9	4.0	0.715	0.11	−0.48	0.70
pNN50 (%)	7.1	3.3	7.2	3.1	0.956	−0.02	−0.61	0.58
LF (ms^2)	986.3	617.3	814.0	377.4	0.205	0.41	−0.22	1.02
HF (ms^2)	192.4	111.1	190.7	77.8	0.953	0.02	−0.57	0.61
TP (ms)	1689.1	1094.3	1371.7	639.8	0.214	0.40	−0.23	1.08
LF/HF	5.6	2.5	4.6	2.0	0.182	0.43	−0.20	1.04

SD: standard deviation; SDNN: standard deviation of all normal N–N intervals; HR: mean heart rate; RMSSD: square root of the mean of the sum of the squared differences between adjacent normal R–R intervals; pNN50: percentage of differences between adjacent normal R–R intervals > 50 ms; TP: Total power; LF: low frequency; HF: high frequency (HF).

4. Discussion

To our knowledge, this is the first study to investigate the effects of caffeine intake 1 h (19:00) before an 800-m running time trial (20:00) on actigraphic SQ, subjective SQ, and nocturnal CAA, and on the 800-m performance 24 h later, in trained middle-distance athletes. We found that the ingestion of 6 mg·kg^{-1} of caffeine did not improve the 800-m running performance. In addition, caffeine intake did not modify the 800-m running performance one day after the first 800-m running test. However, regarding SQ, athletes reported significantly worse subjective SQ, calm sleep, ease of falling asleep, and feeling refreshed after waking after CAF ingestion in comparison to PL. In addition, caffeine ingestion impaired the sleep quantity and quality as measured by actigraphy (reducing sleep efficiency, increasing the number of awakenings, and increasing the actual wake time) in 800-m athletes, but did not affect the autonomic nervous system during the night.

Caffeine is a supplement with good-to-strong evidence of achieving benefits in athletic performance when used in specific scenarios across endurance-based situations and in short-term, supramaximal, and/or repeated sprint tasks [26]. However, our findings revealed no significant differences in 800-m times when caffeine ingestion and placebo were compared. These results are in accordance with a study by Marques et al. [15], who found no performance differences between placebo and caffeine conditions in 800-m time-trial running performance in overnight-fasting runners. Furthermore, recent research has shown no positive effect of 5 mg·kg^{-1} intake on anaerobic capacity in recreationally active men. Anaerobic capacity is a key factor in performance in middle-distance sports (e.g., 800 m) [27]. In contrast, there are several studies that have found improvements with the use of caffeine as an ergogenic aid in tests of similar metabolic demands [14,28]. These controversial findings could be due to the characteristics of the subjects, their daily caffeine intake, and their experience in the use of caffeine as an ergogenic aid: previous studies have reported that the ergogenic effect of caffeine in habitual caffeine consumers is diminished [29,30]. In addition, several studies have found significant differences when intake and testing is carried out in the morning versus the evening, showing benefits when the protocol was carried out in the morning, and not when it was carried out in the evening [31,32]. Therefore, this must be considered in our study, because the experimental protocol was performed in the evening, which could diminish the potential effects of caffeine. Finally, the genetic predisposition of athletes has been shown to have a great influence on the responses to the intake of this ergogenic aid [33]. Some genetic polymorphisms affect the speed of metabolism of caffeine (CYP1A2) and the excitability of the nervous system (ADORA2A) [33], and this could affect the results obtained in the present study. Therefore, future studies would assess a genetic test to analyze how these polymorphisms affect 800-m running performance. Finally, regarding RPE, our results showed no significant differences between PL and CAF conditions. These findings are in accordance with the above-mentioned 800-m running study [15]. Moreover, our results agree with a previous meta-analysis that concluded that the intake of caffeine produces a significant reduction in RPE during exercise, but does not produce any change at the end of exhausting exercise [34].

Good sleep is vital in the regulation of hormone secretion and in the restoration of metabolic processes in athletes [35]. However, some factors can impair SQ in athletes before a competition: about 66% of athletes report that they often experience worse sleep than usual on the night(s) before a competition [36] for various reasons, including noise, light, anxiety, and nervousness [37]. Moreover, previous studies report that performing intense exercise close to bedtime impairs SQ [19]. In addition, caffeine ingestion may have adverse effects on SQ [3,16]. Interestingly, the current study, using trained male athletes, found that a 6 mg·kg^{-1} dose of caffeine taken 1 h (19:00) before an 800-m race (20:00) impairs SQ, with lower sleep efficiency and greater actual wake time and number of awakenings. These findings can be due to caffeine promoting wakefulness by antagonizing adenosine A1 and A2A receptors in the brain [38]. These adenosine agonist receptors play a role in arousal and promoting sleep. In addition, 6-sulphatoxymelatonin excretion plays an essential role in in the biological regulation of circadian rhythms, including sleep, and previous studies have reported that caffeine interferes with sleep quantity and quality by the reduction of this substance [39]. Therefore, these physiological responses can explain the SQ results obtained in the present study. Notably, although poor sleep was reported after CAF ingestion, no influence on performance was found. This finding is in accordance with previous studies that reported that disturbed sleep had no influence on sporting performance in competitions [36,40]. Some possible reasons to explain this unchanged exercise performance following a night of poor-quality sleep are that metabolic pathways, rating of perceived exertion, and physiological responses remain largely unaltered [37]. The performance, physiological, and perceptual results of the present study agree with this finding.

Several studies have analyzed the relationship between HRV and caffeine ingestion [41,42], reporting that caffeine seems to produce predominantly a parasympathetic rather than a sympathetic cardiac influence [43]: some studies report that the acute ingestion of caffeine enhances parasympathetic activity [44], and tends to decrease the LF/HF ratio under resting conditions [43], or increase this variable during sleep after caffeine administration [45]. However, other studies found no changes in HRV at rest [46] comparison to placebo. These findings are in accordance with the results of the present study, where no significant differences were observed in HRV variables during sleep after placebo or caffeine ingestion. One possible reason for these findings can be related to the daily caffeine consumption of the participants. Previous studies have reported that the response of the autonomic nervous system to caffeine intake is diminished in habitual caffeine consumers [47]. Therefore, the lack of effect on HRV in the athletes in the present study could be related to the rapid tachyphylaxis of caffeine, as reported [47]. In addition, the effect of caffeine on HRV seems to be time-dependent, resulting in an enhancement of the activity of autonomic nervous system 2.5 h after caffeine ingestion [46]. Thus, in our study the participants ingested the caffeine ~3.5–4.5 h before going to sleep, which could be related to the lack of difference in HRV variables during sleep between the conditions (placebo versus caffeine).

From an application perspective, athletic coaches of middle-distance runners should keep in mind that if the championship has races on consecutive days, the administration of 6 mg·kg^{-1} of caffeine does not improve the 800-m running performance, but can impair sleep quantity and the quality of trained runners who are habitual caffeine consumers.

The main limitation of the present study was that the number of athletes that took part in the study was limited. In addition, our results cannot be generalized to other subjects who ingest lower amounts of caffeine per day (i.e., light caffeine consumers); neither can our findings can be generalized to other athletes' modalities (e.g., long distance) or gender (female athletes). Finally, the results of plasma caffeine concentration were not determined. On the other hand, the main strength of the present study is the level of the athletes who participated and the practical application of the results to the real athletic field. Further research into the influence of caffeine supplementation on running performance and recovery processes (e.g., sleep, using electroencephalography) would be necessary. Moreover, it would be interesting to increase the number of subjects in a future study also comparing subjects with regular and non-regular intake of caffeine.

5. Conclusions

In comparison to placebo, the ingestion of 6 mg·kg^{-1} of caffeine did not improve the 800-m running performance in daily consumers of caffeine trained athletes, and did not modify the performance of a subsequent 800-m running test performed one day after the first. However, caffeine impaired the subjective and actigraphic sleep quantity and quality, but did not affect the autonomic nervous system during the night after the participants had performed the first 800-m running test.

Author Contributions: Conceptualization, D.J.R.-C. and J.A.R.-A.; methodology, D.J.R.-C. and J.A.R.-A.; software, D.J.R.-C., A.P., V.A.-G. and S.P.-P.; validation, D.J.R.-C., A.P., V.A.-G., S.P.-P. and J.A.R.-A.; formal analysis, D.J.R.-C. and J.A.R.-A.; investigation, D.J.R.-C. and J.A.R.-A.; resources, V.A.-G.; data curation, A.P. and D.J.R.-C.; writing—original draft preparation, D.J.R.-C., A.P., V.A.-G. and J.A.R.-A.; writing—review and editing, D.J.R.-C.; visualization, D.J.R.-C., A.P., V.A.-G. and J.A.R.-A.; supervision, D.J.R.-C., V.A.-G. and J.A.R.-A.; project administration, D.J.R.-C.; funding acquisition, D.J.R.-C. and V.A.-G.

Funding: This research received no external funding.

Conflicts of Interest: The authors declare no conflict of interest.

References

1. Ramos-Campo, D.J.; Rubio-Arias, J.; Freitas, T.T.; Camacho, A.; Jiménez-Diaz, J.F.; Alcaraz, P.E. Acute Physiological and Performance Responses to High-Intensity Resistance Circuit Training in Hypoxic and Normoxic Conditions. *J. Strength Cond. Res.* **2017**, *31*, 1040–1047. [CrossRef] [PubMed]
2. Martínez-Sánchez, A.; Ramos-Campo, D.J.; Fernández-Lobato, B.; Rubio-Arias, J.A.; Alacid, F.; Aguayo, E. Biochemical, physiological, and performance response of a functional watermelon juice enriched in L-citrulline during a half-marathon race. *Food Nutr. Res.* **2017**, *61*, 1330098. [CrossRef] [PubMed]
3. Ali, A.; O'Donnell, J.M.; Starck, C.; Rutherfurd-Markwick, K.J. The effect of caffeine ingestion during evening exercise on subsequent sleep quality in females. *Int. J. Sports Med.* **2015**, *36*, 433–439. [CrossRef] [PubMed]
4. Del Coso, J.; Muñoz, G.; Muñoz-Guerra, J. Prevalence of caffeine use in elite athletes following its removal from the World Anti-Doping Agency list of banned substances. *Appl. Physiol. Nutr. Metab.* **2011**, *36*, 555–561. [CrossRef] [PubMed]

5. Mark Davis, J.; Zhao, Z.; Stock, H.S.; Mehl, K.A.; Buggy, J.; Hand, G.A.; Mark, J.; Mehl, K.A. Central nervous system effects of caffeine and adenosine on fatigue. *Am. J. Physiol. Regul. Integr. Comp. Physiol.* **2003**, *284*, R399–R404. [CrossRef] [PubMed]
6. Bazzucchi, I.; Felici, F.; Montini, M.; Figura, F.; Sacchetti, M. Caffeine improves neuromuscular function during maximal dynamic exercise. *Muscle Nerve* **2011**, *43*, 839–844. [CrossRef] [PubMed]
7. Mohr, M.; Nielsen, J.J.; Bangsbo, J. Caffeine intake improves intense intermittent exercise performance and reduces muscle interstitial potassium accumulation. *J. Appl. Physiol.* **2011**, *111*, 1372–1379. [CrossRef]
8. Weber, A.; Herz, R. The relationship between caffeine contracture of intact muscle and the effect of caffeine on reticulum. *J. Gen. Physiol.* **1968**, *52*, 750–759. [CrossRef]
9. Van Soeren, M.H.; Graham, T.E. Effect of caffeine on metabolism, exercise endurance, and catecholamine responses after withdrawal. *J. Appl. Physiol.* **2017**, *85*, 1493–1501. [CrossRef]
10. Graham, T.E.; Hibbert, E.; Sathasivam, P. Metabolic and exercise endurance effects of coffee and caffeine ingestion. *J. Appl. Physiol.* **2017**, *85*, 883–889. [CrossRef]
11. Gonlach, A.R.; Ade, C.J.; Bemben, M.G.; Larson, R.D.; Black, C.D. Muscle Pain as a Regulator of Cycling Intensity. *Med. Sci. Sport. Exerc.* **2016**, *48*, 287–296. [CrossRef] [PubMed]
12. O'Rourke, M.P.; O'Brien, B.J.; Knez, W.L.; Paton, C.D. Caffeine has a small effect on 5-km running performance of well-trained and recreational runners. *J. Sci. Med. Sport* **2008**, *11*, 231–233. [CrossRef] [PubMed]
13. Wiles, J.D.; Bird, S.R.; Hopkins, J.; Riley, M. Effect of caffeinated coffee on running speed, respiratory factors, blood lactate and perceived exertion during 1500-m treadmill running. *Br. J. Sports Med.* **1992**, *26*, 116–120. [CrossRef] [PubMed]
14. Clarke, N.D.; Richardson, D.L.; Thie, J.; Taylor, R. Coffee Ingestion Enhances One-Mile Running Race performance. *Int. J. Sport. Physiol. Perform.* **2018**, *13*, 789–794. [CrossRef] [PubMed]
15. Marques, A.C.; Jesus, A.A.; Giglio, B.M.; Marini, A.C.; Lobo, P.C.B.; Mota, J.F.; Pimentel, G.D. Acute caffeinated coffee consumption does not improve time trial performance in an 800-m run: A randomized, double-blind, crossover, placebo-controlled study. *Nutrients* **2018**, *10*, 657. [CrossRef] [PubMed]
16. Clark, I.; Landolt, H.P. Coffee, caffeine, and sleep: A systematic review of epidemiological studies and randomized controlled trials. *Sleep Med. Rev.* **2017**, *31*, 70–78. [CrossRef]
17. Myllymäki, T.; Kyröläinen, H.; Savolainen, K.; Hokka, L.; Jakonen, R.; Juuti, T.; Martinmäki, K.; Kaartinen, J.; Kinnunen, M.L.; Rusko, H. Effects of vigorous late-night exercise on sleep quality and cardiac autonomic activity. *J. Sleep Res.* **2011**, *20*, 146–153. [CrossRef] [PubMed]
18. Nédélec, M.; Halson, S.; Abaidia, A.E.; Ahmaidi, S.; Dupont, G. Stress, Sleep and Recovery in Elite Soccer: A Critical Review of the Literature. *Sport. Med.* **2015**, *45*, 1387–1400. [CrossRef]
19. Ramos-Campo, D.J.; Ávila-Gandía, V.; Luque, A.J.; Rubio-Arias, J. Effects of hour of training and exercise intensity on nocturnal autonomic modulation and sleep quality of amateur ultra-endurance runners. *Physiol. Behav.* **2019**, *198*, 134–139. [CrossRef]
20. Shohet, K.L.; Landrum, R.E. Caffeine Consumption Questionnaire: A Standardized Measure for Caffeine Consumption in Undergraduate Students. *Psychol. Rep.* **2011**, *89*, 521–526. [CrossRef]
21. Fitt, E.; Pell, D.; Cole, D. Assessing caffeine intake in the United Kingdom diet. *Food Chem.* **2013**, *140*, 421–426. [CrossRef] [PubMed]
22. Ramos-Campo, D.J.; Sánchez, F.M.; García, P.E.; Arias, J.A.R.; Cerezal, A.B.; Clemente-Suarez, V.J.; Díaz, J.F.J. Body composition features in different playing position of professional team indoor players: Basketball, handball and futsal. *Int. J. Morphol.* **2014**, *32*, 1316–1324. [CrossRef]
23. Borg, G.; Hassmén, P.; Lagerström, M. Perceived exertion related to heart rate and blood lactate during arm and leg exercise. *Eur. J. Appl. Physiol. Occup. Physiol.* **1987**, *56*, 679–685. [CrossRef] [PubMed]
24. Åkerstedt, T.; Hume, K.; Minors, D.; Waterhouse, J. The Subjective Meaning of Good Sleep, An Intraindividual Approach Using the Karolinska Sleep Diary. *Percept. Mot. Skills* **2011**, *79*, 287–296. [CrossRef] [PubMed]
25. Hopkins, W.G.; Marshall, S.W.; Batterham, A.M.; Hanin, J. Progressive statistics for studies in sports medicine and exercise science. *Med. Sci. Sports Exerc.* **2009**, *41*, 3–12. [CrossRef] [PubMed]
26. Maughan, R.J.; Burke, L.M.; Dvorak, J.; Larson-Meyer, D.E.; Peeling, P.; Phillips, S.M.; Rawson, E.S.; Walsh, N.P.; Garthe, I.; Geyer, H.; et al. IOC consensus statement: Dietary supplements and the high-performance athlete. *Br. J. Sports Med.* **2018**, *52*, 439–455. [CrossRef]

27. Silveira, R.; Andrade-Souza, V.A.; Arcoverde, L.; Tomazini, F.; Sansonio, A.; Bishop, D.J.; Bertuzzi, R.; Lima-Silva, A.E. Caffeine Increases Work Done above Critical Power, but Not Anaerobic Work. *Med. Sci. Sports Exerc.* **2018**, *50*, 131–140. [CrossRef]
28. Wiles, J.D.; Coleman, D.; Tegerdine, M.; Swaine, I.L. The effects of caffeine ingestion on performance time, speed and power during a laboratory-based 1 km cycling time-trial. *J. Sports Sci.* **2006**, *24*, 1165–1171. [CrossRef]
29. Beaumont, R.; Cordery, P.; Funnell, M.; Mears, S.; James, L.; Watson, P. Chronic ingestion of a low dose of caffeine induces tolerance to the performance benefits of caffeine. *J. Sports Sci.* **2017**, *35*, 1920–1927. [CrossRef]
30. Bell, D.G.; McLellan, T.M. Exercise endurance 1, 3, and 6 h after caffeine ingestion in caffeine users and nonusers. *J. Appl. Physiol.* **2002**, *93*, 1227–1234. [CrossRef]
31. Mora-Rodríguez, R.; Pallarés, J.G.; López-Gullón, J.M.; López-Samanes, Á.; Fernández-Elías, V.E.; Ortega, J.F. Improvements on neuromuscular performance with caffeine ingestion depend on the time-of-day. *J. Sci. Med. Sport* **2015**, *18*, 338–342. [CrossRef] [PubMed]
32. Souissi, M.; Abedelmalek, S.; Chtourou, H.; Boussita, A.; Hakim, A.; Sahnoun, Z. Effects of time-of-day and caffeine ingestion on mood states, simple reaction time, and short-term maximal performance in elite judoists. *Biol. Rhythm Res.* **2013**, *44*, 897–907. [CrossRef]
33. Pickering, C.; Kiely, J. Are the Current Guidelines on Caffeine Use in Sport Optimal for Everyone? Inter-individual Variation in Caffeine Ergogenicity, and a Move Towards Personalised Sports Nutrition. *Sports Med.* **2018**, *48*, 7–16. [CrossRef] [PubMed]
34. Doherty, M.; Smith, P.M. Effects of caffeine ingestion on rating of perceived exertion during and after exercise: A meta-analysis. *Scand. J. Med. Sci. Sport.* **2005**, *15*, 69–78. [CrossRef] [PubMed]
35. Driver, H.S.; Taylor, S.R. Exercise and sleep. *Sleep Med. Rev.* **2000**, *4*, 387–402. [CrossRef]
36. Erlacher, D.; Ehrlenspiel, F.; Adegbesan, O.A.; El-Din, H.G. Sleep habits in German athletes before important competitions or games. *J. Sports Sci.* **2011**, *29*, 859–866. [CrossRef] [PubMed]
37. Fullagar, H.H.K.; Skorski, S.; Duffield, R.; Hammes, D.; Coutts, A.J.; Meyer, T. Sleep and Athletic Performance: The Effects of Sleep Loss on Exercise Performance, and Physiological and Cognitive Responses to Exercise. *Sports Med.* **2015**, *45*, 161–186. [CrossRef]
38. Nehlig, A.; Daval, J.L.; Debry, G. Caffeine and the central nervous system: Mechanisms of action, biochemical, metabolic and psychostimulant effects. *Brain Res. Rev.* **1992**, *17*, 139–170. [CrossRef]
39. Shilo, L.; Sabbah, H.; Hadari, R.; Kovatz, S.; Weinberg, U.; Dolev, S.; Dagan, Y.; Shenkman, L. The effects of coffee consumption on sleep and melatonin secretion. *Sleep Med.* **2002**, *3*, 271–273. [CrossRef]
40. Lastella, M.; Lovell, G.P.; Sargent, C. Athletes' precompetitive sleep behaviour and its relationship with subsequent precompetitive mood and performance. *Eur. J. Sport Sci.* **2014**, *14*, 123–130. [CrossRef]
41. Sondermeijer, H.P.; Van Marle, A.G.J.; Kamen, P.; Krum, H. Acute effects of caffeine on heart rate variability. *Am. J. Cardiol.* **2002**, *90*, 906–907. [CrossRef]
42. Koenig, J.; Jarczok, M.N.; Kuhn, W.; Morsch, K.; Schäfer, A.; Hillecke, T.K.; Thayer, J.F. Impact of Caffeine on Heart Rate Variability: A Systematic Review. *J. Caffeine Res.* **2013**, *3*, 22–37. [CrossRef]
43. Waring, W.S.; Goudsmit, J.; Marwick, J.; Webb, D.J.; Maxwell, S.R.J. Acute Caffeine Intake Influences Central More Than Peripheral Blood Pressure in Young Adults. *Am. J. Hypertens.* **2003**, *16*, 919–924. [CrossRef]
44. Notarius, C.F.; Floras, J.S. Caffeine Enhances Heart Rate Variability in Middle-Aged Healthy, But Not Heart Failure Subjects. *J. Caffeine Res.* **2012**, *2*, 77–82. [CrossRef] [PubMed]
45. Bonnet, M.; Tancer, M.; Uhde, T.; Yeragani, V.K. Effects of caffeine on heart rate and QT variability during sleep. *Depress. Anxiety* **2005**, *22*, 150–155. [CrossRef]
46. Nishijima, Y.; Ikeda, T.; Takamatsu, M.; Kiso, Y.; Shibata, H.; Fushiki, T.; Moritani, T. Influence of caffeine ingestion on autonomic nervous activity during endurance exercise in humans. *Eur. J. Appl. Physiol.* **2002**, *87*, 475–480. [CrossRef]
47. Rauh, R.; Burkert, M.; Siepmann, M.; Mueck-Weymann, M. Acute effects of caffeine on heart rate variability in habitual caffeine consumers. *Clin. Physiol. Funct. Imaging* **2006**, *26*, 163–166. [CrossRef]

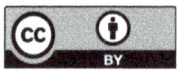 © 2019 by the authors. Licensee MDPI, Basel, Switzerland. This article is an open access article distributed under the terms and conditions of the Creative Commons Attribution (CC BY) license (http://creativecommons.org/licenses/by/4.0/).

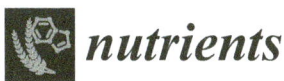

Article

Caffeinated Gel Ingestion Enhances Jump Performance, Muscle Strength, and Power in Trained Men

Sandro Venier [1], Jozo Grgic [2] and Pavle Mikulic [1,*]

[1] Faculty of Kinesiology, University of Zagreb, Zagreb 10000, Croatia; veniersandro@gmail.com
[2] Institute for Health and Sport (IHES), Victoria University, Melbourne 3011, Australia; jozo.grgic@vu.live.edu.au
* Correspondence: pavle.mikulic@kif.hr; Tel.: +385-1-3658-607

Received: 9 April 2019; Accepted: 18 April 2019; Published: 25 April 2019

Abstract: We aimed to explore the effects of caffeinated gel ingestion on neuromuscular performance in resistance-trained men. The participants ($n = 17$; mean ± standard deviation (SD): age 23 ± 2 years, height 183 ± 5 cm, body mass 83 ± 11 kg) completed two testing conditions that involved ingesting a caffeinated gel (300 mg of caffeine) or placebo. The testing outcomes included: (1) vertical jump height in the squat jump (SJ) and countermovement jump (CMJ); (2) knee extension and flexion peak torque and average power at angular velocities of $60°·s^{-1}$ and $180°·s^{-1}$; (3) barbell velocity in the bench press with loads corresponding to 50%, 75%, and 90% of one-repetition maximum (1RM); and (4) peak power output in a test on a rowing ergometer. Compared to the placebo, caffeine improved: (1) SJ ($p = 0.039$; Cohen's d effect size (d) = 0.18; +2.9%) and CMJ height ($p = 0.011$; $d = 0.18$; +3.3%); (2) peak torque and average power in the knee extensors at both angular velocities (d ranged from 0.21 to 0.37; percent change from +3.5% to +6.9%), peak torque ($p = 0.034$; $d = 0.24$; +4.6%), and average power ($p = 0.015$; $d = 0.32$; +6.7%) at $60°·s^{-1}$ in the knee flexors; (3) barbell velocity at 50% 1RM ($p = 0.021$; $d = 0.33$; +3.5%), 75% 1RM ($p < 0.001$; $d = 0.42$; +5.4%), and 90% 1RM ($p < 0.001$; $d = 0.59$, +12.0%). We conclude that the ingestion of caffeinated gels may acutely improve vertical jump performance, strength, and power in resistance-trained men.

Keywords: caffeine; ergogenic aid; resistance training; isokinetic testing

1. Introduction

In the general population, caffeine is a widely consumed food constituent [1]. Caffeine consumption is also widespread among athletes, likely due to its performance-enhancing effects on exercise [2]. In most of the studies that examine the effects of caffeine ingestion on exercise performance, the participants ingest caffeine administered in the form of a capsule and wait 60 min before starting the exercise session [3,4]. This waiting period is used with the idea that plasma levels of caffeine reach their peak values ~60 min following the ingestion of a caffeine-containing capsule [5].

In recent years, however, several studies have explored the effects of alternate sources of caffeine on exercise performance [3]. Some of the alternate sources of caffeine include chewing gums, bars, gels, mouth rinses, energy drinks, aerosols, and coffee [3,6,7]. These sources attracted the attention of researchers, given that they may provide rapid absorption of caffeine in the body. For example, following the consumption of a caffeine-containing gum, increases in caffeine levels in plasma occur within 5 min [8]. This rapid absorption may lead to a faster ergogenic effect, which subsequently may be useful in many situations in sport and in exercise settings.

Wickham and Spriet [3] highlighted that only two studies thus far have examined the effects of caffeinated gels on exercise performance; one reported an ergogenic effect of caffeine on 2000-m rowing-ergometer performance [9], while another stated that caffeine ingestion did not enhance intermittent sprint performance [10]. Due to the scarce and conflicting studies examining the effects of caffeinated gels on exercise performance, it is evident that further research with this source of caffeine is warranted.

Two recent meta-analyses reported that caffeine ingestion acutely enhances muscle strength, as assessed by isokinetic peak torque and jumping performance [11,12]. In both meta-analyses, all included studies explored the effects of caffeine administered in the form of a capsule or liquid.

In resistance exercise, caffeine ingestion may acutely increase muscle strength, muscle endurance, and muscle power [13]. However, the effects of caffeine on muscle power in resistance exercise have been explored the least. Grgic et al. [13] highlighted only four studies [14–17] that have explored the effect of caffeine on power (as assessed by barbell velocity). Grgic et al. [13] suggest that caffeine may have a considerable performance-enhancing effect on barbell velocity in resistance exercise; however, the authors also noted the need for future research on the topic. Given that all four studies that examined the effects of caffeine on muscle power in resistance exercise used caffeine in the form of a capsule, it remains unclear if comparable effects may be observed with caffeinated gel as a source of caffeine. While studies are exploring the effects of caffeine on resistance exercise administered in alternate forms such as coffee and chewing gums [6,7,18], there is a lack of studies utilizing caffeinated gels.

An additional limitation of the current body of evidence that explored the effects of caffeine on power is that almost all studies used performance tests that involved a specific body region in isolation (e.g., upper-body in the bench press exercise). Currently, there is a need for studies that measure power output during exercise tests that require simultaneous coordinated activity of the upper- and lower-body musculature.

This study aimed to explore the effects of caffeinated gel ingestion on: (1) jump performance; (2) isokinetic strength and power of the knee extensor and knee flexor muscles; (3) upper-body power; and (4) whole-body power, in a sample of resistance-trained men. We hypothesized that ingesting a caffeinated gel would acutely enhance exercise performance in all of the employed performance tests compared to the placebo.

2. Materials and Methods

2.1. Study Design

This study employed a randomized, crossover, double-blind, counterbalanced study design. In the first exercise session, participants were familiarized with the performance tests. Following this familiarization session, the participants were randomized to two experimental conditions: caffeinated gel and placebo gel. The dose of caffeinated gel (Smart 1 Energizer Gel, Science in Sport) contained 88 g of carbohydrates and 300 mg of caffeine. The placebo gel (Go Isotonic Energy Gel, Science in Sport) contained the same amount of carbohydrates without any caffeine. Therefore, the only difference in the provided gels was the amount of caffeine.

After ingesting either the placebo or caffeinated gel, the participants were given 10 min to warm-up before the testing session started. All testing sessions were conducted in the morning hours (between 7:00 and 9:00 a.m.) for all participants. The day before each testing session, the participants were requested to maintain their general nutritional and sleep habits, and not to perform any vigorous physical activity. Additionally, the participants were asked to refrain from any caffeine ingestion after 6:00 p.m. on the days before the two experimental conditions. To facilitate this process of caffeine restriction, the participants were provided with a comprehensive list of the most common food and drink products containing caffeine. The participants were also instructed not to ingest any food or drinks (other than plain water) upon waking up; that is, they came to the laboratory in a fasted state. Adherence to these guidelines was established before the start of each testing session. The testing sessions were separated by no less than three and no more than six days. The reliability of the outcomes analyzed in the exercise protocol was established on a pilot sample of five participants that repeated the exercise protocol on two occasions, three days apart (Table 1).

Table 1. Test–retest reliability of the exercise protocol; determined on a pilot sample of five participants.

Exercise Test	Outcome	Average CV
Squat jump (SJ)	Jump height (cm)	1.3%
Countermovement jump (CMJ)	Jump height (cm)	1.3%
Isokinetic knee extension at 60° s^{-1}	Peak torque (Nm)	2.5%
	Average power (W)	1.7%
Isokinetic knee flexion at 60° s^{-1}	Peak torque (Nm)	5.3%
	Average power (W)	4.4%
Isokinetic knee extension at 180° s^{-1}	Peak torque (Nm)	2.1%
	Average power (W)	2.7%
Isokinetic knee flexion at 180° s^{-1}	Peak torque (Nm)	5.9%
	Average power (W)	5.0%
Bench press at 50% 1RM	Barbell velocity (m·s^{-1})	1.7%
Bench press at 75% 1RM	Barbell velocity (m·s^{-1})	3.6%
Bench press at 90% 1RM	Barbell velocity (m·s^{-1})	5.1%
Rowing ergometer test	Peak power (W)	2.5%

1RM: one-repetition maximum; CV: coefficient of variation.

2.2. Participants

The following inclusion criteria was set for this study: (1) apparently healthy men, aged 18–45 years, without any current muscular injuries or other physical limitations; and (2) resistance-trained, defined as having at least one year of resistance exercise experience with a minimal weekly training frequency of two times per week, and by having the ability to successfully lift at least 100% of their current body mass in the bench press exercise.

A power analysis performed prior to the study initiation using the G*Power software indicated that the required sample size for this study is 12 participants. The parameters employed in this analysis were as follows: expected effect f of 0.20 (for barbell velocity in the bench press exercise), alpha of 0.05, statistical power of 0.80, and r of 0.90 [19]. To factor in possible dropouts, we initially recruited a sample of 18 participants. One participant dropped out due to private reasons; 17 participants (mean ± standard deviation (SD): age 23 ± 2 years, height 183 ± 5 cm, body mass 83 ± 11 kg) successfully completed all visits and were included in the analysis. Habitual caffeine intake of the participants was estimated using a validated food frequency questionnaire [20] and amounted to 67 ± 90 mg·day^{-1} (range: 0 to 357 mg·day^{-1}). Of note here, only one participant had a high habitual caffeine intake of 357 mg·day^{-1}; all remaining participants ingested <180 mg·day^{-1} with 12 ingesting <100 mg·day^{-1}. Ethical approval was obtained from the Committee for Scientific Research and Ethics of the Faculty of Kinesiology at the University of Zagreb. Upon informing the participants about the study requirements, benefits, and risks, they provided written informed consent.

2.3. Exercise Tests

2.3.1. Vertical Jump

After the warm-up, the testing protocol started with the assessment of jump performance. The participants performed three squat jumps (SJs) and three countermovement jumps (CMJs) on the force platform (BP600600, AMTI, Inc., Watertown, MA, USA). The force platform was accompanied with a custom-developed software for data acquisition and analysis. Vertical jump height for both the

SJ and the CMJ was automatically calculated by the software from the vertical velocity of the center of mass at take-off data using the following formula [21]:

$$vertical\ jump\ height = TOV^2 / 2g$$

where TOV is the vertical velocity of the center of mass at take-off, and g is the gravitational acceleration (9.81 m·sec^{-2}).

The SJ was performed while starting from an initial semi-squat position (knees ~90° and trunk/hips in a flexed position), with participants holding the position for approximately 2 s before jumping vertically as quickly and as explosively as possible, in order to jump as high as possible in the shortest possible time using a concentric-only muscle action. Hands remained akimbo for the entire movement to eliminate any arm-swing influence. The participants were instructed to maintain fully extended lower limbs throughout the flight period. The CMJ was performed starting from the upright standing position. On the command of the tester, the participants performed a downward countermovement by a fast knee flexion. Immediately after, the vertical jump began by an explosive extension of the legs. The CMJ is characterized by an eccentric–concentric muscle action often referred to as the stretch-shortening cycle muscle action. The participants were instructed that their lowest position should be a semi-squat position (knees ~90° and trunk/hips in a flexed position), and that the jump should be performed as quickly and explosively as possible in order to jump as high as possible in the shortest possible time. One warm-up attempt for both the SJ and CMJ was allowed, during which the correct execution of the jumps was confirmed. Three official attempts followed, with 1 min of rest between the attempts; the highest jumps were used for the analysis.

2.3.2. Isokinetic Strength and Power

The isokinetic dynamometer (System 4 Pro, Biodex Medical Systems, Inc., Shirley, NY, USA) was used for the isokinetic strength and power assessment of the knee extensor and knee flexor muscles. The assessment was performed unilaterally, involving only the dominant leg. The participants were placed in a seated position and stabilization straps were applied to the trunk, waist, thigh, and shin. The lateral femoral epicondyle of the dominant leg was aligned with the dynamometer's axis of rotation. The isokinetic dynamometer was calibrated before each testing session, and the range of motion of the knee joint was set at 80°. Testing was performed at angular velocities of 60°·s^{-1} and 180°·s^{-1}, in that order. At each angular velocity, participants first performed three familiarization repetitions to get accustomed to the speed of the lever arm. Then, following a 30-s rest interval, they performed five maximal knee extensions and flexions. For this exercise, the participants were instructed to extend and flex the knee (to "kick" and "pull") five times as hard and as fast as they could. Peak torque in N·m^{-1} obtained during knee extension and knee flexion movement patterns was used as the measure of the knee extensor and knee flexor muscle strength, respectively. Average power over five repetitions at both angular velocities (i.e., 60°·s^{-1} and 180°·s^{-1}) was also used for the analysis.

2.3.3. Bench Press

The PowerLift mobile phone application was used to measure barbell velocity in the bench press exercise. The PowerLift application has previously been reported as valid, reliable, and accurate for measuring barbell velocity during this exercise [22]. The application allowed video recording of the lift in slow motion. After the recording was complete, the application allowed frame-by-frame inspection of the recorded video material and manual selection of the beginning and the end of the concentric part of the movement. The beginning of the movement was considered as the moment when the barbell left the chest of the participant. The end of the movement was considered as the moment when the participants fully extended the elbows. This distance (d) between the beginning and end of the movement was measured with a measuring tape and entered into the application. The application calculated the time (in ms) between two frames (i.e., the beginning and the end of the movement). The outcome of this test was the mean barbell velocity produced during the press. During each testing session, the participants exercised with loads corresponding to 50%, 75%, and 90% of their one-repetition maximum (1RM; established during the familiarization session), while completing two, one, and one repetition, respectively. During each repetition, the participants were instructed to perform the concentric part of the movement as fast as possible. Three minutes of rest were allowed between repetitions and/or loads.

2.3.4. Rowing Ergometer Test

A test on a rowing ergometer (Model D, Concept II, Inc., Morrisville, VT, USA) was used to assess whole-body power. For this test, the resistance control dial of the ergometer was set at 10 (highest adjustable resistance). First, the participants were given 5 min during which they rowed comfortably at their own pace. No attempts were made to make any corrections in their rowing technique. Then, following a 2-min rest, the participants performed six "introductory" strokes, which were followed by six "all-out" strokes. For the six "all-out" strokes, the participants were instructed to row as hard and as fast as they could. The outcome of the test was peak power output, defined as the highest power output produced during the six "all-out" strokes (expressed in Watts), as shown on the performance monitor of the Concept II ergometer. This test has high test–retest reliability, and was previously validated by a group of physically active individuals by Metikos et al. [23], where it is explained in greater detail.

2.4. Side Effects

Immediately following the completion of the exercise testing session and the morning after the testing, participants completed an eight-item survey regarding their subjective perceptions of side effects that may have occurred ("yes/no" response scale). This scale has been used in previous research that examined the effects of caffeine ingestion on exercise performance [14].

2.5. Assessment of Blinding

We tested the effectiveness of the blinding pre- and post-exercise by asking participants to identify the supplement they had ingested. The question for identification went as follows: "Which supplement do you think you have ingested?" This question had three possible answers: (a) caffeine; (b) placebo; (c) do not know [24].

2.6. Statistical Analysis

A Shapiro–Wilk test was used to assess the normality of distribution. Upon confirming the normality of distribution, a series of one-way repeated measures ANOVAs was used to analyze the differences between conditions (i.e., placebo and caffeine) for all the performance outcomes. The statistical significance threshold was set at $p < 0.05$. Effect sizes (d) were calculated using a Cohen's formula, in which the mean difference between the two measurements is divided by the pooled SD. Trivial, small, moderate, and large effect sizes were considered as <0.20, 0.20–0.49, 0.50–0.79, and ≥0.80, respectively [25]. Percent changes were also calculated. The effectiveness of the blinding was examined using Bang's blinding index (BBI) where -1.0 indicates opposite guessing and 1 complete lack of blinding. A McNemar test was used to explore the differences in the incidence of side effects between the placebo and caffeine conditions. All analyses were performed using Statistica software (StatSoft; Tulsa, OK, USA).

3. Results

3.1. Exercise Tests

3.1.1. Vertical Jump

Compared to placebo, caffeine ingestion improved performance both in the SJ ($p = 0.039$; $d = 0.18$; +2.9%) and in the CMJ ($p = 0.011$; $d = 0.18$; +3.3%).

3.1.2. Lower-Body Isokinetic Strength and Power

Caffeine ingestion had a significant effect on peak torque at the angular velocity of $60°·s^{-1}$, both in the knee extensor ($p = 0.002$; $d = 0.37$; +6.9%) and in the knee flexor muscles ($p = 0.034$; $d = 0.24$; +4.6%). At the angular velocity of $180°·s^{-1}$, caffeine ingestion elicited a significant effect on peak torque in the knee extensor ($p = 0.031$; $d = 0.21$; +3.5%), but not in the knee flexor muscles ($p = 0.168$; $d = 0.17$; +3.0). For average power, at the angular velocity of $60°·s^{-1}$, caffeine had a significant effect in increasing power both in the knee extensor ($p = 0.001$; $d = 0.31$; +6.3%) and the knee flexor muscles ($p = 0.015$; $d = 0.32$; +6.7%). At the angular velocity of $180°·s^{-1}$, a significant effect of caffeine on power produced by the knee extensor muscles was evident ($p = 0.025$; $d = 0.25$; +4.5%); however, the same was not the case for the knee flexor muscles ($p = 0.115$; $d = 0.17$; +3.5) (Table 2).

Table 2. Differences in placebo vs caffeine conditions for the performance outcomes.

Exercise Test	Outcome	Caffeine Condition (mean ± SD)	Placebo Condition (mean ± SD)	d (95% CI)	Relative Effects (%)	p
Squat jump	Jump height (cm)	31.9 ± 4.9	31.0 ± 5.5	0.18 (0.03, 0.32)	+2.9	0.039 *
Countermovement jump	Jump height (cm)	36.4 ± 6.5	35.2 ± 6.5	0.18 (0.05, 0.32)	+3.3	0.011 *
Isokinetic knee extension at 60° s^{-1}	Peak torque (Nm)	256.9 ± 44.5	240.3 ± 45.6	0.37 (0.15, 0.61)	+6.9	0.002 *
	Average power (W)	193.8 ± 36.9	182.3 ± 36.8	0.31 (0.13, 0.50)	+6.3	0.001 *
Isokinetic knee flexion at 60° s^{-1}	Peak torque (Nm)	147.1 ± 24.6	140.7 ± 28.7	0.24 (0.02, 0.46)	+4.6	0.034 *
	Average power (W)	118.7 ± 21.0	111.3 ± 25.9	0.32 (0.01, 0.59)	+6.7	0.015 *
Isokinetic knee extension at 180° s^{-1}	Peak torque (Nm)	180.2 ± 27.8	174.0 ± 31.9	0.21 (0.02, 0.40)	+3.5	0.031 *
	Average power (W)	353.4 ± 57.0	338.1 ± 66.6	0.25 (0.04, 0.46)	+4.5	0.025 *
Isokinetic knee flexion at 180° s^{-1}	Peak torque (Nm)	110.0 ± 18.1	106.8 ± 20.3	0.17 (−0.07, 0.40)	+3.0	0.168
	Average power (W)	212.9 ± 38.0	205.8 ± 46.7	0.17 (−0.04, 0.38)	+3.5	0.115
Bench press at 50% 1RM	Barbell velocity (m·s^{-1})	0.83 ± 0.08	0.80 ± 0.09	0.33 (0.06, 0.61)	+3.5	0.021 *
Bench press at 75% 1RM	Barbell velocity (m·s^{-1})	0.57 ± 0.06	0.54 ± 0.07	0.42 (0.21, 0.64)	+5.4	< 0.001 *
Bench press at 90% 1RM	Barbell velocity (m·s^{-1})	0.39 ± 0.07	0.35 ± 0.07	0.59 (0.27, 0.89)	+12.0	< 0.001 *
Rowing ergometer test	Peak power (W)	725.4 ± 133.5	715.4 ± 106.4	0.08 (−0.27, 0.43)	+1.4	0.647

SD: standard deviation; d: effect size; CI: confidence interval; * denotes statistically significant differences.

3.1.3. Bench Press

For barbell velocity in the bench press exercise, a significant effect of caffeine was observed at 50% of 1RM ($p = 0.021$; $d = 0.33$; +3.5%), at 75% of 1RM ($p < 0.001$; $d = 0.42$; +5.4%), as well as at 90% of 1RM ($p < 0.001$; $d = 0.59$; +12.0%).

3.1.4. Rowing Ergometer Test

No significant effect of caffeine was observed for peak power output on the rowing ergometer test ($p = 0.647$; $d = 0.08$; +1.4).

3.2. Side Effects

The incidence of side effects is presented in Table 3. Based on the results of the McNemar test, none of the comparisons between the caffeine and placebo conditions were significant ($p > 0.05$ for all comparisons).

Table 3. Incidence of side effects reported immediately after and the morning after ingestion of a caffeinated gel or a placebo.

	Placebo	Caffeine	Placebo	Caffeine
	Immediately After Testing Session	Immediately After Testing Session	Morning After Testing Session	Morning After Testing Session
Muscle soreness	0	0	0	0
Increased urine production	0	6	0	6
Tachycardia and heart palpitations	6	12	0	0
Increased anxiety	0	18	0	0
Headache	0	0	0	0
Abdominal/gut discomfort	0	6	0	0
Insomnia	n/a	n/a	0	6
Increased vigor/activeness	12	41	0	0
Perception of improved performance	6	35	n/a	n/a

Data are frequencies for 17 participants, expressed as the percentage of positive cases; none of the comparisons were significant based on the McNemar test.

3.3. Assessment of Blinding

The results from the assessment of blinding pre- and post-exercise are presented in Table 4. When assessed pre-exercise, the BBI for the placebo and caffeine treatments amounted to 0.29 (95% confidence interval (CI): −0.06, 0.65), and 0.24 (95% CI: −0.07, 0.54), respectively. When assessed post-exercise, the BBI for the placebo and caffeine conditions amounted to 0.70 (95% CI: 0.49, 0.93) and 0.35 (95% CI: 0.00, 0.72), respectively. Those that correctly identified caffeine generally reported a "better overall feeling" and "more energy", as well as increased perspiration.

Table 4. Results of the assessment of blinding pre- and post-exercise.

Condition	Responded as Placebo	Responded as Caffeine	Responded as Do not Know	Bang's Blinding Index (Mean and 95% CI)
Pre-Exercise				
Placebo	6	2	9	0.29 (−0.06, 0.65)
Caffeine	3	8	6	0.24 (−0.07, 0.54)
Post-Exercise				
Placebo	12	0	5	0.70 (0.49, 0.93)
Caffeine	3	9	5	0.35 (−0.00, 0.72)

CI: confidence interval.

4. Discussion

The present study aimed to explore the effects of caffeinated gel ingestion on exercise performance of resistance-trained men in tests characterized by a very short duration and maximal exertion. The results indicate that caffeine ingestion in the form of a caffeinated gel had performance-enhancing effects on: (1) vertical jump performance in the SJ and CMJ tests; (2) lower-body isokinetic strength and power; and (3) power of the upper-body musculature. Whole-body power, as assessed on a rowing ergometer test, did not improve following caffeine ingestion. The blinding of the participants was generally effective, and the side effects were minimal.

For the vertical jump performance, our results confirm the recent meta-analytical results by Grgic et al. [11] that caffeine ingestion before exercise may acutely enhance jump height. Indeed, even the effect size in the SJ and CMJ tests that we observed (d of 0.18 for both tests) were very similar to the pooled effect size of 0.17 reported in the meta-analysis. Previous studies that reported ergogenic effects of caffeine on jump performance generally used larger doses of caffeine (e.g., 6 mg·kg^{-1}), as well as a protocol that included a waiting time of 60 min from ingestion to the initiation of the exercise testing [11]. Our results highlight that ingesting even a smaller dose of caffeine (300 mg; ~3.6 mg·kg^{-1}) in the form of a caffeinated gel administered 10 minutes before exercise, may also be ergogenic. These findings mirror those of Bloms et al. [26] who also used both jump techniques and reported that ingesting 5 mg·kg^{-1} of caffeine improved performance both in the SJ and CMJ tests.

A recent meta-analysis [12] reported that caffeine ingestion acutely increases strength, as assessed by an isokinetic dynamometer. Our results provide further support for these findings, given that we observed increases in peak torque following the ingestion of caffeine with d across angular velocities and muscle groups (i.e., knee extensors and knee flexors) ranging from 0.21 to 0.37, and corresponding percent changes ranging from +3.5% to +6.9%. While the ergogenic effects of caffeine were noted at both angular velocities for the knee extensor muscles, a significant effect of caffeine on the knee flexor muscles was observed only at the velocity of 60°·s^{-1}. This divergent effect between muscle groups might be due to the lower level of muscle activation during maximal contractions at baseline in the knee extensor muscles [27]. This naturally occurring lower level of activation may provide a greater "room for improvement" in contraction force following the ingestion of caffeine in this muscle group. Smaller muscle groups may have a higher muscle activation level at baseline and, therefore, are less affected by caffeine ingestion [27]. Caffeine ingestion also improved average power, with a magnitude of improvement similar to that observed for muscle strength.

The ergogenic effect of caffeine on barbell velocity in the bench press exercise was evident across all three employed loads with the effects ranging from small ($d = 0.33$; +3.5%) to moderate ($d = 0.59$; +12.0%). These results provide further support to findings of the previous studies that explored the effects of caffeine on barbell velocity. For example, Mora-Rodriguez et al. [15] reported that caffeine ingestion in a dosage of 3 mg·kg^{-1}, ingested 60 min before exercise, enhanced barbell velocity in the bench press when using external loads amounting to 75% 1RM.

Pallarés et al. [17] suggested that the effects of caffeine on power might be external load- and caffeine dose-dependent. In that study, caffeine ingested in low and moderate doses (3 and 6 mg·kg^{-1}) enhanced barbell velocity in the bench press at loads corresponding to 25% and 50% of 1RM. However, when using loads of 75% of 1RM, only the doses of 6 and 9 mg·kg^{-1} were effective. At the highest load of 90% of 1RM, only 9 mg·kg^{-1} was effective. The findings presented herein are not in full agreement with the work by Pallarés et al. [17] given that, in the present study, an absolute dose of 300 mg (~3.6 mg·kg^{-1}) was ergogenic for barbell velocity across all three loading schemes (including 90% of 1RM).

In contrast to the work by Pallarés et al. [17], the magnitude of effect in the present study increased with an increase in the load that the participants lifted (Table 2). The most pronounced effect across loading schemes, amounting to a +12.0% increase in barbell velocity, was evident for the load corresponding to 90% of 1RM. Based on these results, it seems that the effects of caffeine are more noticeable, at least for this exercise, when requirements for the contraction force are the highest. Given the direct importance of high barbell velocity in the development of power [28], our results suggest that individuals might consider supplementing with caffeine before exercise to achieve acute increases in barbell velocity and, subsequently, stronger stimuli for the development of muscle power.

We did not observe any significant differences between placebo and caffeine conditions in the whole-body power, as assessed by the peak power output produced during the "all-out" rowing ergometer test. Based on these results, it does not seem that caffeine ingestion is ergogenic for whole-body peak power output; however, this could be due to large inter-individual variation in response to caffeine ingestion [29], and therefore needs to be explored in future studies with larger sample sizes.

4.1. Mechanisms of Caffeine

Caffeine produces its ergogenic effects by binding to adenosine receptors [30]. After binding to these receptors, caffeine blunts the fatiguing effects of adenosine and subsequently reduces perceived exertion. Indeed, there is substantial evidence that caffeine's effect of reducing perceived exertion is one of the primary mechanisms for its ergogenic effect on aerobic endurance [31]. However, the ergogenic effect of caffeine on high-intensity, short-duration tests (such as those performed in the current study) may be related to the release of calcium from the sarcoplasmic reticulum, and the subsequent inhibition of its reuptake [30]. These actions may be associated with neuromuscular function changes, as well as increased contractile force in skeletal muscles [32]. For the readers interested, these mechanisms of caffeine are discussed in greater detail elsewhere [30].

4.2. Limitations

The limitations of this study include the following: (1) the sample consisted of trained young men, which limited the generalizability of these results to those who are untrained, of older age, or to women; (2) we did not measure plasma levels of caffeine and, therefore, the amount of caffeine absorbed is not entirely clear; (3) an absolute dose of caffeine was used, whereas a relative dose might have been more appropriate (of note here, an absolute dose was given due to the fixed amount of caffeine per 75-mg gel sachet).

One additional limitation [33] might be that 12 out of 17 participants correctly identified the placebo condition post-exercise; as determined by the 95% CI of the BBI, this identification was not solely due to chance. It is likely that correct identification of the placebo condition in the post-exercise assessment was due to the lack of perceived improvements in performance (only one participant answered "yes" to the perception of improved performance item following the ingestion of placebo). This may especially be evident given the small number of individuals that correctly identified placebos in the pre-exercise evaluation. From that aspect, it is possible that pre-exercise responses are of greater importance than the answers obtained post-exercise. Additionally, based on the findings by Tallis et al. [34], an argument can be made that the correct identification of the placebo did not confound the results. In that study, the participants experienced similar improvements in isokinetic peak torque both when they were told that they were given caffeine and received a dose of caffeine, and when they were told that they ingested the placebo even though the capsule contained caffeine. While the placebo was identified beyond random chance in the post-exercise assessment, correct identification of caffeine in the post-exercise assessment can be attributed solely to chance, as there was a 95% CI overlap with the null value. These results further support an actual ergogenic effect of caffeine.

4.3. Practical Applications

Ingesting a caffeine dose of 300 mg in the form of caffeine gel 10 min before exercise may elicit an acute ergogenic effect on vertical jump height, muscle strength, and power in an isokinetic strength assessment, as well as barbell velocity in the bench press exercise. Due to these ergogenic effects, trained individuals may consider supplementing with caffeinated gels before exercise for acute increases in performance.

5. Conclusions

The ingestion of caffeinated gels with an absolute dose of caffeine of 300 mg may improve aspects of short-term, maximal-exertion exercise performance in resistance-trained men. These improvements are evident in vertical jump performance, strength, and power. These results highlight that individuals seeking acute performance enhancement in jumping, strength, and power may consider ingesting caffeinated gels before exercise.

Author Contributions: Conceptualization, P.M. and J.G.; Data curation, S.V.; Formal analysis, P.M. and J.G.; Investigation, S.V.; Methodology, P.M., J.G., and S.V.; Project administration, P.M.; Resources, P.M.; Supervision, P.M.; Writing—original draft, P.M. and J.G.; Writing—review and editing, P.M., J.G., and S.V.

Funding: This research received no external funding.

Acknowledgments: The authors wish to thank Filip Sabol for his help with the data collection. This paper is a part of the PhD project from the first author (S.V.), supervised by P.M.

Conflicts of Interest: The authors declare no conflict of interest.

References

1. Mitchell, D.C.; Knight, C.A.; Hockenberry, J.; Teplansky, R.; Hartman, T.J. Beverage caffeine intakes in the U.S. *Food Chem. Toxicol.* **2014**, *63*, 136–142. [CrossRef] [PubMed]
2. Del Coso, J.; Muñoz, G.; Muñoz-Guerra, J. Prevalence of caffeine use in elite athletes following its removal from the World Anti-Doping Agency list of banned substances. *Appl. Physiol. Nutr. Metab.* **2011**, *36*, 555–561. [CrossRef] [PubMed]
3. Wickham, K.A.; Spriet, L.L. Administration of caffeine in alternate forms. *Sports Med.* **2018**, *48*, 79–91. [CrossRef]
4. Grgic, J.; Grgic, I.; Pickering, C.; Schoenfeld, B.J.; Bishop, D.J.; Pedisic, Z. Wake up and smell the coffee: Caffeine supplementation and exercise performance-an umbrella review of 21 published meta-analyses. *Br. J. Sports Med.* **2019**. [CrossRef] [PubMed]
5. Graham, T.E. Caffeine and exercise: Metabolism, endurance and performance. *Sports Med.* **2001**, *31*, 785–807. [CrossRef] [PubMed]
6. Hodgson, A.B.; Randell, R.K.; Jeukendrup, A.E. The metabolic and performance effects of caffeine compared to coffee during endurance exercise. *PLoS ONE* **2013**, *8*, e59561. [CrossRef] [PubMed]
7. Richardson, D.L.; Clarke, N.D. Effect of Coffee and Caffeine Ingestion on Resistance Exercise Performance. *J. Strength Cond. Res.* **2016**, *30*, 2892–2900. [CrossRef] [PubMed]
8. Kamimori, G.H.; Karyekar, C.S.; Otterstetter, R.; Cox, D.S.; Balkin, T.J.; Belenky, G.L.; Eddington, N.D. The rate of absorption and relative bioavailability of caffeine administered in chewing gum versus capsules to normal healthy volunteers. *Int. J. Pharm.* **2002**, *234*, 159–167. [CrossRef]
9. Scott, A.T.; O'Leary, T.; Walker, S.; Owen, R. Improvement of 2000-m rowing performance with caffeinated carbohydrate-gel ingestion. *Int. J. Sports Physiol. Perform.* **2015**, *10*, 464–468. [CrossRef] [PubMed]

10. Cooper, R.; Naclerio, F.; Allgrove, J.; Larumbe-Zabala, E. Effects of a carbohydrate and caffeine gel on intermittent sprint performance in recreationally trained males. *Eur. J. Sport Sci.* **2014**, *14*, 353–361. [CrossRef]
11. Grgic, J.; Trexler, E.T.; Lazinica, B.; Pedisic, Z. Effects of caffeine intake on muscle strength and power: A systematic review and meta-analysis. *J. Int. Soc. Sports Nutr.* **2018**, *15*, 11. [CrossRef] [PubMed]
12. Grgic, J.; Pickering, C. The effects of caffeine ingestion on isokinetic muscular strength: A meta-analysis. *J. Sci. Med. Sport* **2019**, *22*, 353–360. [CrossRef] [PubMed]
13. Grgic, J.; Mikulic, P.; Schoenfeld, B.J.; Bishop, D.J.; Pedisic, Z. The influence of caffeine supplementation on resistance exercise: A review. *Sports Med.* **2019**, *49*, 17–30. [CrossRef] [PubMed]
14. Diaz-Lara, F.J.; Del Coso, J.; García, J.M.; Portillo, L.J.; Areces, F.; Abián-Vicén, J. Caffeine improves muscular performance in elite Brazilian Jiu-jitsu athletes. *Eur. J. Sport Sci.* **2016**, *16*, 1079–1086. [CrossRef]
15. Mora-Rodríguez, R.; García Pallarés, J.; López-Samanes, Á.; Ortega, J.F.; Fernández-Elías, V.E. Caffeine ingestion reverses the circadian rhythm effects on neuromuscular performance in highly resistance-trained men. *PLoS ONE* **2012**, *7*, e33807.
16. Mora-Rodríguez, R.; Pallarés, J.G.; López-Gullón, J.M.; López-Samanes, Á.; Fernández-Elías, V.E.; Ortega, J.F. Improvements on neuromuscular performance with caffeine ingestion depend on the time-of-day. *J. Sci. Med. Sport* **2015**, *18*, 338–342. [CrossRef] [PubMed]
17. Pallarés, J.G.; Fernández-Elías, V.E.; Ortega, J.F.; Muñoz, G.; Muñoz-Guerra, J.; Mora-Rodríguez, R. Neuromuscular responses to incremental caffeine doses: Performance and side effects. *Med. Sci. Sports Exerc.* **2013**, *45*, 2184–2192. [CrossRef]
18. Venier, S.; Grgic, J.; Mikulic, P. Acute Enhancement of Jump Performance, Muscle Strength, and Power in Resistance-Trained Men After Consumption of Caffeinated Chewing Gum. *Int. J. Sports Physiol. Perform.* **2019**. [CrossRef]
19. Grgic, J.; Mikulic, P. Caffeine ingestion acutely enhances muscular strength and power but not muscular endurance in resistance-trained men. *Eur. J. Sport Sci.* **2017**, *17*, 1029–1036. [CrossRef] [PubMed]
20. Bühler, E.; Lachenmeier, D.W.; Schlegel, K.; Winkler, G. Development of a tool to assess the caffeine intake among teenagers and young adults. *Ernährungs Umschau* **2014**, *61*, 58–63.
21. Moir, G.L. Three different methods of calculating vertical jump height from force platform data in men and women. *Meas. Phys. Educ. Exerc. Sci.* **2008**, *12*, 207–218. [CrossRef]
22. Balsalobre-Fernández, C.; Marchante, D.; Baz-Valle, E.; Alonso-Molero, I.; Jiménez, S.L.; Muñóz-López, M. Analysis of wearable and smartphone-based technologies for the measurement of barbell velocity in different resistance training exercises. *Front. Physiol.* **2017**, *8*, 649. [CrossRef] [PubMed]
23. Metikos, B.; Mikulic, P.; Sarabon, N.; Markovic, G. Peak power output test on a rowing ergometer: A methodological study. *J. Strength Cond. Res.* **2015**, *29*, 2919–2925. [CrossRef] [PubMed]
24. Saunders, B.; de Oliveira, L.F.; da Silva, R.P.; de Salles Painelli, V.; Gonçalves, L.S.; Yamaguchi, G.; Mutti, T.; Maciel, E.; Roschel, H.; Artioli, G.G.; et al. Placebo in sports nutrition: A proof-of-principle study involving caffeine supplementation. *Scand. J. Med. Sci. Sports* **2017**, *27*, 1240–1247. [CrossRef] [PubMed]
25. Cohen, J. *Statistical power analysis for the behavioural sciences*, 2nd ed.; L. Erlbaum Associates: Hillsdale, NJ, USA, 1988; p. 481.
26. Bloms, L.P.; Fitzgerald, J.S.; Short, M.W.; Whitehead, J.R. The effects of caffeine on vertical jump height and execution in collegiate athletes. *J. Strength Cond. Res.* **2015**, *30*, 1855–1861. [CrossRef] [PubMed]
27. Warren, G.L.; Park, N.D.; Maresca, R.D.; McKibans, K.I.; Millard-Stafford, M.L. Effect of caffeine ingestion on muscular strength and endurance: A meta-analysis. *Med. Sci. Sports Exerc.* **2010**, *42*, 1375–1387. [CrossRef] [PubMed]
28. Tufano, J.J.; Brown, L.E.; Haff, G.G. Theoretical and practical aspects of different cluster set structures: A systematic review. *J. Strength Cond. Res.* **2017**, *31*, 848–867. [CrossRef]
29. Grgic, J. Are There Non-Responders to the Ergogenic Effects of Caffeine Ingestion on Exercise Performance? *Nutrients* **2018**, *10*, 1736. [CrossRef]
30. McLellan, T.M.; Caldwell, J.A.; Lieberman, H.R. A review of caffeine's effects on cognitive, physical and occupational performance. *Neurosci. Biobehav. Rev.* **2016**, *71*, 294–312. [CrossRef]
31. Doherty, M.; Smith, P.M. Effects of caffeine ingestion on rating of perceived exertion during and after exercise: A meta-analysis. *Scand. J. Med. Sci. Sports* **2005**, *15*, 69–78. [CrossRef]
32. Tarnopolsky, M.A. Effect of caffeine on the neuromuscular system–potential as an ergogenic aid. *Appl. Physiol. Nutr. Metab.* **2008**, *33*, 1284–1289. [CrossRef] [PubMed]

33. Grgic, J. Caffeine ingestion enhances Wingate performance: A meta-analysis. *Eur. J. Sport Sci.* **2018**, *18*, 219–225. [CrossRef] [PubMed]
34. Tallis, J.; Muhammad, B.; Islam, M.; Duncan, M.J. Placebo effects of caffeine on maximal voluntary concentric force of the knee flexors and extensors. *Muscle Nerve* **2016**, *54*, 479–486. [CrossRef] [PubMed]

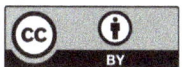

© 2019 by the authors. Licensee MDPI, Basel, Switzerland. This article is an open access article distributed under the terms and conditions of the Creative Commons Attribution (CC BY) license (http://creativecommons.org/licenses/by/4.0/).

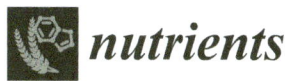

Article

The Acute Effect of Various Doses of Caffeine on Power Output and Velocity during the Bench Press Exercise among Athletes Habitually Using Caffeine

Michal Wilk *, Aleksandra Filip, Michal Krzysztofik, Adam Maszczyk and Adam Zajac

Institute of Sport Sciences, Jerzy Kukuczka Academy of Physical Education in Mikolowska 72a, 40-065 Katowice, Poland
* Correspondence: m.wilk@awf.katowice.pl; Tel.: +48-32-207-52-80

Received: 7 June 2019; Accepted: 25 June 2019; Published: 27 June 2019

Abstract: Background: Previously studies confirm ergogenic effects of caffeine (CAF); however there is no available scientific data regarding the influence of acute CAF intake on power output in athletes habitually consuming CAF. The main goal of this study was to assess the acute effect of 3, 6, 9 mg/kg/b.m. doses of CAF intake on power output and bench press bar velocity in athletes habitually consuming CAF. Methods: The study included 15 healthy strength-trained male athletes (age = 26.8 ± 6.2 years, body mass = 82.6 ± 9.7 kg; BMI = 24.8 ± 2.7; bench press 1RM = 122.3 ± 24.5 kg). All participants were habitual caffeine consumers (5.2 ± 1.2 mg/kg/b.m.; 426 ± 102 mg of caffeine per day). This study had a randomized, crossover, double-blind study design where each participant performed four different experimental sessions, with one week interval between each trial. In every experimental session participants performed bench press, three sets of five repetitions at 50% 1RM. The power output and bar velocity assessments under four different conditions: a placebo (PLAC), and three doses of caffeine ingestion: 3 mg/kg/b.m. (CAF-3), 6 mg/kg/b.m. (CAF-6) and 9 mg/kg/b.m. (CAF-9). Results: The statistical significance was set at $p < 0.05$. The repeated measures ANOVA between PLAC and CAF-3; CAF-6; CAF-9 revealed no statistically significant differences in power output and velocity of the bar during the bench press exercise. A large effect size (ES) in mean power-output was found between PLAC and CAF-9 in Sets 1 and 2. A large ES in peak power-output was found between PLAC and CAF-6 in Set 2, and between PLAC and CAF-9 in Sets 1 and 2. A large ES in peak velocity was found between PLAC and CAF-9 in Sets 1–3. Conclusion: The results of the present study indicate that acute doses of CAF before exercise does not have a significant effect on power output and bar velocity in a group of habitual caffeine users.

Keywords: supplement; resistance exercise; speed; repetition

1. Introduction

Resistance training is a significant component of conditioning programs in competitive sports. The ability to generate high values of power output is one of the most significant factors determining success in numerous sport disciplines [1]. Power output can be described by the relationship between the force generated by the muscles and movement velocity [2]. Particular attention in studies concerning the development of power and high speed of movement has been directed at exercise volume with specific intensity of effort [3,4]. In addition to training, nutrition and supplementation also have a significant effect on adaptation and post-exercise responses [5–9].

Caffeine (CAF) is among the most often used and widely studied supplements in competitive sports. Mechanisms responsible for ergogenic effects of CAF are linked to the impact on various tissues, organs and systems of the human body. In the central nervous system (CNS), CAF acts through interactions with adenosine receptors that influence the release of noradrenaline, dopamine, acetylcholine and serotonin [10–13] and consequently, increase muscle tension [14]. Increased muscle activation can lead to a greater energy demand during exercise, thus leading to a faster depletion of energy substrates in muscle cells [15].

Numerous studies have examined the acute performance-enhancing effects of CAF intake on human physical fitness and exercise performance [16–24]. The most frequently consumed dose of caffeine ranges from 3 to 9 mg/kg body mass (b.m.), ingested in the form of capsules 30 to 90 minutes before exercise. However, the optimal dose may differ based on exercise choice, volume, intensity, and the type of muscle contraction [23,25–28]. Additionally, participants characteristics, such as gender, age and training experience can affect both, power output and the ergogenic effects of CAF intake. Although ergogenic effect of CAF is well-established in many aspects, much controversy remains about the effectiveness of different doses of caffeine on power output of the upper limbs.

Previous studies showed positive acute effects of 3 mg/kg b.m. of CAF on resistance exercise performance and power output, suggesting that this dose has significant ergogenic properties [25,29,30]. However a dose of 3 mg/kg b.m. is sufficient to increase movement velocity at loads of 25–50%1RM, whereas a higher caffeine dose (9 mg/kg b.m.) is necessary when submaximal loads (90%1RM), are used despite the appearance of adverse side effects [25]. Grgic and Mikulic [24] showed an increase in power output during a medicine ball throw following CAF intake (6 mg/kg b.m.). Pallarés et al. [25] also showed significantly increased movement velocity and power output at loads of 25–50%1RM after different doses of CAF ingestion (3, 6, 9 mg/kg b.m.), however, at the load of 75% 1RM, a CAF dose of 3 mg/kg b.m. did not improve power output in the bench press exercise. On the contrary, the study of Wilk et al. [20] did not show changes in concentric power output and bar velocity during the bench press to concentric muscle failure, following the intake of 5 mg/kg/b.m. of CAF compared to a placebo.

Furthermore, one should emphasize that most of the previous studies on CAF intake and the level of power output concerned participants with low daily CAF intake. In competitive athletes the use of CAF before resistance exercise is particularly common. As a result, research suggesting 75–90% of athletes consume CAF before or during training sessions and competitive events [31,32]. According to Svenningsson et al. [33], Fredholm et al. [34] habitual CAF intake modifies physiological responses to acute ingestion by the up-regulation of adenosine receptors. Furthermore, constant exposure to CAF could impact metabolic pathways by inducing cytochrome P450 1A2 and increased induction speed of that enzyme which may alter the rate of CAF metabolism. However based on the available evidence, it does not seem that habitual caffeine ingestion reduces the ergogenic benefits of acute CAF supplementation [35–37]. Evans et al. [38] suggested that non-habitual CAF (<40 mg/day) users experience a greater magnitude of the ergogenic effect compared with CAF habitual users (>130 mg/day). However, Gonçalves et al. [36] indicate that habitual CAF intake (low = 58; moderate = 143; high = 351 mg/day) did not influence exercise performance, suggesting that CAF habituation has no detrimental impact on CAF ergogenesis. Likewise Dodd et al. [35] also did not show any differences in time to exhaustion after acute doses of CAF (placebo; 3 mg/kg/b.m.; 5 mg/kg/b.m.), between a non-habitual user group (<25 mg/day) and habitual CAF consumers (>300 mg/day). The basic source of variability of results among scientists investigating habitual caffeine use, is the division of subjects into low, moderate, and high habitual caffeine consumption groups. Some studies have defined high caffeine use as >100 mg/day [39], while others have defined it as >300 mg/day [35] or even >750 mg/day [40]. Inconsistency in these caffeine intake reference values makes the interpretation and cross-comparison of results difficult. Furthermore, daily doses of CAF intake are reported in values of mg/day [36,38,41], which lacks precision and may be very misleading when athletes with different body mass are considered. This lack of consistency in caffeine use levels has been noted before, and yet, to our knowledge, no one has proposed reference values for caffeine use.

Since there is no available scientific data regarding the influence of acute CAF intake on power output in athletes habitually consuming CAF, with a precisely determined intake of CAF in relation to body mass (mg/day/kg/b.m.) the main goal of this study was to assess the acute effect of various doses of CAF on power output and bar velocity in athletes habitually consuming CAF (4–6 mg/day/kg/b.m.).

2. Materials and Methods

2.1. Study Participants

Fifteen ($n = 15$) healthy strength-trained male basketball and handball athletes participated in the study after completing an ethical consent form (age = 26.8 ± 6.2 years, body mass = 82.6 ± 9.7 kg, BMI = 24.8 ± 2.7, bench press 1RM = 122.3 ± 24.5 kg; data presented as mean ± standard deviation [SD]) with a minimum 3 years of strength training experience (4.2 ± 1.23 years). All participants were habitual caffeine consumers (5.2 ± 1.2 mg/kg/b.m., 426 ± 102 mg of caffeine per day). The inclusion criteria were as follows: (a) free from neuromuscular and musculoskeletal disorders, (b) the participants were able to perform the bench press exercise with a load of at least 120% of their body mass [42], (c) habitual caffeine intake in the range of 4–6 mg/kg/b.m., ~300–500 mg of caffeine per day. The study protocol was approved by the Bioethics Committee for Scientific Research, at the Academy of Physical Education in Katowice, Poland (10/2018) according to the ethical standards of the Declaration of Helsinki, 1983.

2.2. Habitual Caffeine Intake Measurement

Habitual caffeine intake was assessed by a specific Food Frequency Questionnaire (FFQ) adapted from a previously questionnaires [43] under the supervision of a qualified nutritionist. The questionnaire was employed to assess the habitual consumption of dietary products rich in caffeine. Portions, in household measures, were used to assess the amount of food consumed according to the following frequency of consumption: a) more than three times a day, b) two to three times a day, c) once a day, d) five to six times a week, e) two to four times per week, f) once a week, g) three times per month, h) rarely or never. The list was composed of dietary products with high caffeine content including different types of coffees, teas, energy drinks, cocoa's products, popular beverages, medications and caffeine supplements. Previously published information and nutritional tables were used for database construction [17,44,45]. Based on the answers in FFQ, a qualified nutritionist estimated the habitual caffeine intake.

2.3. Experimental Designed

This study used a randomized, crossover, double-blind design where each participant performed a familiarization session with a 1RM test on one day, and four different experimental sessions with one week interval between each trial. The randomization was conducted by a member of the research team that was not directly involved in the data collection. Participants underwent the power output and bar velocity assessments under four different conditions: a placebo (PLAC), and three doses of caffeine ingestion: 3 mg/kg/b.m. (CAF-3), 6 mg/kg/b.m. (CAF-6) and 9 mg/kg/b.m. (CAF-9). CAF or a PLAC were administered orally 60 minutes before each exercise protocol to allow peak blood caffeine concentration and at least 2 hours after the last meal to maintain the same time of absorption. CAF was provided in the form of standard capsules containing 300 mg of CAF, as well as those specifically prepared for the research, containing 100, 50 and 5 mg doses of CAF. The PLAC was provided in identical capsules as CAF (all-purpose flour). All CAF and PLAC capsules were manufactured by Olimp Laboratories. Subjects refrained from physical activity other than that required by the experimental trials and withdrew from alcohol, tobacco and other drugs and supplements during the study. The participants were instructed to maintain their usual hydration, dietary habits including habitual caffeine intake during the entire experiment and keep track of their calorie intake using the "Myfitness pal" software [46] every 24 hours before the testing procedure. There were no differences between individually calorie intake between particular sessions. The subjects were also asked to refrain from heavy exercise for 48 hours and to refrain from caffeine intake 12 hours before each trial. All testing was performed in the Strength and Power Laboratory at the Jerzy Kukuczka Academy of Physical Education in Katowice.

2.4. Familiarization Session and One Repetition Maximum Test

A familiarization session preceded the one repetition maximum testing. The participants arrived at the laboratory at the same time of day as the upcoming experimental sessions (in the morning between 9:00 and 10:00 am) and cycled on an ergometer for 5 minutes at an intensity that resulted in a heart rate of around 130 bpm, followed by a general upper body warm-up. Next, the participants performed 15, 10, and 5 repetitions of the bench press exercise using 20%, 40%, and 60% of their estimated 1RM with a 2/0/X/0 tempo of movement [42]. The sequence of digits describing the tempo of movement (2/0/X/0) represents a 2 second eccentric phase, in which 0 represents a pause during the transition phase, X represents maximum possible tempo of movement during the concentric phase, and the last digit represents no pause at the end of movement. The participants then executed single repetitions with a 5 minutes rest interval between successful trials. The load for each subsequent attempt was increased by 2.5 kg, and the process was repeated until failure. Hand placement on the barbell was individually selected with a grip width on the barbell of 150% individual bi-acromial distance (BAD). BAD was determined by palpating and marking the acromion with a marker, and then measuring the distance between these points with a standard anthropometric tape. The positioning of the hands was recorded to ensure consistent hand placement during all testing sessions. No bench press suits, weightlifting belts, or other supportive garments were permitted. Three spotters were present during all attempts to ensure safety and technical proficiency.

2.5. Experimental Protocol

Four testing sessions were used for the experimental trials. All testing took place between 9.00 and 11.00 a.m. to avoid circadian variation. The general warm-up for the experimental sessions was identical to the one used for the familiarization session. After the warm-up, participants started the main examinations and performed three set of the bench press with 5 repetitions in each set at 50%1RM. The concentric phase of movement was performed at maximal possible velocity, while the eccentric phase with a 2 second duration (2/0/X/0). All repetitions were performed without bouncing the barbell off the chest, without intentionally pausing at the transition between the eccentric and concentric phases, and without raising the lower back off the bench. The time between each session of the experiment was 7 days. During the experimental trials the participants were encouraged to perform at maximal engagement according to the recommendations by Brown and Weir [47]. A linear position transducer system "Tendo Power Analyzer" (Tendo Sport Machines, Trencin, Slovakia) was used for the evaluation of bar velocity. The Tendo Power Analyzer is a reliable system for measuring movement velocity and power output [48,49]. The system consists of a velocity sensor connected to the load by a kevlar cable which, through an interface, instantly transmits the vertical velocity of the bar to a specific software installed in the computer (Tendo Power Analyzer Software 5.0). The system measures upward vertical average and peak velocity of the movement. Using a set external load, the system calculates average peak power and peak velocity in the concentric phase of the movement. The measurement was made independently for each repetition and automatically converted into the values of peak power output (PP), mean power output (MP), peak velocity (PV), mean velocity (MV). All participants completed the described testing protocol.

2.6. Side Effects

Immediately and after 24 hours following each testing procedures participants answered a side effects questionnaire, included nine items on a yes/no scale of caffeine ingestion [25,50–52].

Statistical Analysis

The Shapiro–Wilk, Levene and Mauchly´s tests were used in order to verify the normality, homogeneity and sphericity of the sample data variances. Verification of differences between the PLAC and CAF-3, CAF-6, CAF-9 was performed using ANOVA with repeated measures. Effect sizes (Cohen's

d) were reported where appropriate. Parametric effect sizes (ES), were defined as large for d > 0.8, as moderate between 0.8 and 0.5, and as small for <0.5 [52,53], and was calculated at 95% confidence intervals. The statistical significance was set at $p < 0.05$. All statistical analyses were performed using Statistica 9.1 and Microsoft Office, and were presented as means with standard deviations.

3. Results

The repeated measures ANOVA between PLAC and CAF-3; CAF-6; CAF-9 revealed no statistically significant differences in MP (Table 1), PP (Table 2), MV (Table 3) as well PV (Table 4). No significant differences in PP, MP, PV, MV between PLAC and CAF-3; CAF-6; CAF-9 were observed for Sets 1–3. However, a large effect size (ES) in MP was found between PLAC and CAF-9 in Set 1 and 2 (Table 1). Similarly, the large ES in PP was found between PLAC and CAF-6 in Set 2, and between PLAC and CAF-9 in Set 1 and 2 (Table 2). Additionally, the large ES in PV was found between PLAC and CAF-9 in Sets 1–3 (Table 4).

Table 1. Results of mean power output in three successive sets of the bench press exercise in the group that ingested different doses of caffeine, and the placebo group.

	Mean Power [W]										
	Placebo (95% CI)	Caffeine 3 mg (95% CI)	p	ES	Caffeine 6 mg (95% CI)	p	ES	Caffeine 9 mg (95% CI)	p	ES	F
Set 1	445 ± 98 (403; 508)	453 ± 96 (402; 504)	0.99	0.51	462 ± 92 (413; 511)	0.99	0.55	464 ± 98 (411; 516)	0.99	0.93	0.04
Set 2	456 ± 92 (407; 505)	465 ± 97 (413; 516)	0.99	0.48	474 ± 98 (422; 526)	0.94	0.47	457 ± 77 (416; 498)	0.99	0.82	0.13
Set 3	463 ± 93 (413; 513)	456 ± 93 (407; 506)	0.99	0.42	469 ± 99 (416; 522)	0.99	0.36	473 ± 102 (418; 528)	0.99	0.58	0.08

Notes: mean ± standard deviation [SD]; CI: confidence interval.

Table 2. Results of peak power output in three successive sets of the bench press exercise in the group that ingested different doses of caffeine, and the placebo group.

	Peak Power [W]										
	Placebo (95% CI)	Caffeine 3 mg (95% CI)	p	ES	Caffeine 6 mg (95% CI)	p	ES	Caffeine 9 mg (95% CI)	p	ES	F
Set 1	831 ± 171 (740; 922)	874 ± 202 (767; 982)	0.90	0.59	843 ± 167 (754; 932)	0.99	0.61	848 ± 169 (752; 945)	0.99	0.8	0.16
Set 2	819 ± 172 (727; 911)	874 ± 198 (768; 979)	0.81	0.41	879 ± 175 (785; 973)	0.76	0.93	821 ± 136 (752; 899)	0.99	0.81	0.54
Set 3	858 ± 181 (728; 921)	846 ± 176 (752; 941)	0.98	0.46	871 ± 173 (779; 963)	0.88	0.62	869 ± 172 (773; 968)	0.99	0.72	0.22

Notes: mean ± standard deviation [SD]; CI: confidence interval.

Table 3. Results of mean velocity in three successive sets of the bench press exercise in the group that ingested different doses of caffeine, and the placebo group.

	Mean Velocity [m/s]										
	Placebo (95% CI)	Caffeine 3 mg (95% CI)	p	ES	Caffeine 6 mg (95% CI)	p	ES	Caffeine 9 mg (95% CI)	p	ES	F
Set 1	0.94 ± 0.08 (0.90; 0.99)	0.90 ± 0.07 (0.86; 0.94)	0.35	0.53	0.93 ± 0.06 (0.89; 0.96)	0.90	0.51	0.91 ± 0.05 (0.88; 0.94)	0.62	0.73	1.01
Set 2	0.94 ± 0.08 (0.90; 0.99)	0.93 ± 0.09 (0.88; 0.98)	0.98	0.50	0.95 ± 0.07 (0.91; 0.99)	0.99	0.51	0.90 ± 0.06 (0.87; 0.94)	0.53	0.77	0.96
Set 3	0.95 ± 0.08 (0.91; 1.00)	0.92 ± 0.09 (0.87; 0.97)	0.69	0.44	0.94 ± 0.08 (0.90; 0.99)	0.99	0.52	0.93 ± 0.05 (0.90; 0.96)	0.88	0.61	0.47

Notes: mean ± standard deviation [SD]; CI: confidence interval.

Table 4. Results of peak velocity in three successive sets of the bench press exercise in the group that ingested different doses of caffeine, and the placebo group.

	Peak Velocity [m/s]										
	Placebo (95% CI)	Caffeine 3 mg (95% CI)	p	ES	Caffeine 6 mg (95% CI)	p	ES	Caffeine 9 mg (95% CI)	p	ES	F
Set 1	1.42 ± 0.16 (1.33; 1.51)	1.42 ± 0.16 (1.33; 1.50)	0.99	0.41	1.38 ± 0.12 (1.31; 1.44)	0.81	0.79	1.38 ± 0.11 (1.32; 1.45)	0.89	0.81	0.37
Set 2	1.40 ± 0.16 (1.31; 1.49)	1.43 ± 0.16 (1.34; 1.52)	0.96	0.64	1.44 ± 0.16 (1.35; 1.52)	0.93	0.71	1.36 ± 0.14 (1.28; 1.44)	0.88	0.92	0.68
Set 3	1.42 ± 0.16 (1.34; 1.51)	1.43 ± 0.20 (1.32; 1.54)	0.99	0.51	1.43 ± 0.14 (1.35; 1.51)	0.99	0.55	1.41 ± 0.13 (1.34; 1.48)	0.99	0.82	0.05

Notes: mean ± standard deviation [SD]; CI: confidence interval.

Caffeine Side Effects

Table 5 details the nine different side effects assessed immediately and 24 hours later. Immediately after the PLAC trial, subjects reported a very low frequency of side effects (0%–13%; QUEST + 0 hours). The CAF-3 treatments produced very similar side effects (0%–20%; QUEST + 0 hours), compared with the PLAC trial. The CAF-6 treatments produced greater value of side effects (0%–47%; QUEST + 0 hours). The greatest value of side effect was recorded for perception of performance and increased vigor (40%–47%; QUEST + 0 hours). Finally, the CAF-9 trial produced a drastic increase in the reported frequency of side effects (0%–87%; QUEST + 0 hours) (Table 5).

The following morning of each experimental trial (QUEST + 24 hours), very few participants (0%–7%) reported that PLAC treatment produced residual side effects. The CAF-3 trial produced very similar side effects to PLAC (0%–13%; QUEST + 24 hours). The CAF-6 trial showed greater frequency of side effects, with increased urine output and headaches in comparison with the PLAC and CAF-3 conditions, although with a frequency lower than 33% of the subjects. Finally, CAF-9 increased the frequency of all adverse side effects, with a frequency of appearance from 0 to 73%. In the group ingesting the highest dose of CAF, 67%–73% of participants reported tachycardia, anxiety or nervousness, gastrointestinal problems, and 53% had increased urine output (Table 5).

Table 5. Side effects reported by participants immediately after the testing protocol (QUEST + 0 hours) and 24 hours later (QUEST + 24 hours).

Side Effects	Doses of CAF Intake During Testing Protocol							
	PLAC		CAF 3 mg/b.m.		CAF 6 mg/b.m.		CAF 9 mg/b.m.	
	+0 h	+24 h	+0 h	+24 h	+0 h	+24 h	+0 h	+24 h
Muscle soreness	0	0	0	0	0	0	0	0
Increased urine output	1 (7%)	1 (7%)	3 (20%)	2 (13%)	6 (40%)	5 (33%)	10 (67%)	8 (53%)
Tachycardia and heart palpitations	2 (13%)	1 (7%)	3 (20%)	2 (13%)	6 (40%)	3 (20%)	12 (80%)	11 (73%)
Anxiety or nervousness	1 (7%)	1 (7%)	2 (13%)	7 (7%)	3 (20%)	2 (13%)	10 (67%)	3 (20%)
Headache	2 (13%)	1 (7%)	3 (20%)	1 (7%)	2 (13%)	4 (26%)	3 (20%)	6 (40%)
Gastrointestinal problems	0	1 (7%)	2 (13%)	1 (7%)	4 (26%)	2 (13%)	6 (40%)	11 (73%)
Perception of performance improvement	2 (13%)	-	3 (20%)	-	6 (40%)	-	13 (87%)	-
Increased vigor/activeness	2 (13%)	1 (7%)	2 (13%)	1 (7%)	7 (47%)	2 (13%)	13 (87%)	6 (40%)
Insomnia	-	0	-	0	-	2 (13%)	-	4 (26%)

Data are presented as number of person (n) as well the percentage of prevalence (%).

4. Discussion

The main finding of the study was that acute CAF intake has no significant effect on PP, MP, PV, MV in habitual users of caffeine. Significant changes in PP, MP, PV, MV were not registered after CAF intake with doses of 3, 6 or 9 mg/kg/b.m. compared to PLAC. Despite the fact that the results of our study are inconsistent with previous findings [24–26] it should be emphasized that this is the first scientific study which considers the acute effect of different doses of CAF intake on power output and bar velocity changes during the bench press exercise in habitual CAF users.

Previous research showed that acute CAF intake increase power output [24,25]. However, most of the studies concerned participants with low daily CAF intake. Actually, there are only a few studies analyzing acute effects of CAF intake in habitual users; however, the results are not conclusive and mostly refer to aerobic endurance exercises [35,36,41]. To the best of our knowledge, only one study analyzed power output changes of the upper limbs after different doses of acute CAF intake in group of habitual users [26]. The study of Sabol et al. [26] showed an increase in medicine ball throwing distance in subjects ingesting 6 mg/kg/b.m. of CAF compared to a PLAC. However the differences were non-significant between the intake of PLAC and 2 mg/kg/b.m. as well between PLAC and 4 mg/kg/b.m. It is worth noting that the study of Sabol et al. [26] did not show significant differences in responses to acute CAF ingestion between the groups of low and moderate-to-high habitual CAF users. On the contrary, the result of our study did not show any significant changes in power output and bar velocity after the intake of CAF with a dose of 3, 6 or 9 mg compared to the PLAC. However, it must be indicated that in the study of Sabol et al. [26] only six participants were classified as those with moderate-to-high habitual CAF intake. Furthermore, this group had a very wide range of daily CAF intake (CAF = 358 ± 210 mg/day; range = 135 to 642 mg/day), which limits the reliability of results.

Our study is the first of its kind with a homogeneous research group ($n = 15$) with study participants consuming CAF in the range of 4 to 6 mg/kg/b.m. (~300–500 mg/day). Differences related to the daily CAF intakes limit the possibility to compare our results to those of Sabol et al. [26]. Other previous studies with habitual CAF users, also used different criteria for daily CAF intake. Gonçalves et al. [36] applied the following reference values for daily CAF intake: low = 58 ± 29 mg/day;

moderate = 143 ± 25 mg/day; high = 351 ± 139 mg/day. On the other hand Sabol et al. [26] considered high consumers as subjects ingesting >100 mg/day of CAF, however in the study of Dodd et al. [35] habitual CAF users were defined as subjects that consumed > 300 mg/day. Differences in daily CAF consumption as well lack of reference values to body mass limits the possibility of comparing previous research results. Furthermore, our study is the first in which the daily intake of CAF was determined in relation to body mass.

The physiological effects of acute CAF intake in habitual caffeine consumers is relatively unstudied. Previous research has suggested that high habitual caffeine intake may reduce the ergogenic effects of acute CAF supplementation on exercise performance [54], what was confirmed in our study. However Pickering and Kiely [54] suggested that reductions after acute CAF intake in habitual users can be modified by using pre-trial doses, substantially greater than habitual intake. While this idea has been perpetuated in the scientific literature, the results of our study confirmed this statement. The result of our study did not show significant changes in PP, MP, PV, MV after acute CAF intake compared to PLAC, even when greater pre-trial doses (CAF-9) were used compared to habitual daily intake (4–6 mg/kg/b.m./day).

The results of our study showed that the habitual caffeine intake limits physiological responses to acute CAF doses, in agreement with Svenningsson et al. [33] and Fredholm et al. [34]. Caffeine is an adenosine receptor antagonist, and when ingested, it binds to adenosine receptors [55]. In animal models, studies reported that chronic caffeine intake increases adenosine receptor concentration and this increase attenuates caffeine's effects [33]. In humans, given that the ergogenic effects of caffeine are strongly linked to its effects on adenosine receptors, it has been suggested that habitual caffeine users may experience smaller enhancement in performance following acute CAF intake as compared to non-users [41]. However, exercise itself may alter the sensitivity of adenosine receptors and lower the threshold concentration such that a smaller dose provided during or at the beginning of exercise may be equally or more effective than similar or larger doses provided 1 hour prior to exercise [56,57]. Likewise, smaller doses provided during warm-up exercise immediately prior to performance testing [58], or immediately prior to and during exercise [59] can be ergogenic and may be as effective as a single larger dose ingested 1 hour prior to exercise [60]. However there is no data available about changes in sensitivity of adenosine receptors in physically active, habitual CAF users.

Despite the fact that our study did not show significant changes in power output and bar velocity after acute CAF intake compared to PLAC, it should be noted that there was a large ES in MP, PP, PV between CAF-9 and PLAC which, indicates an acute ergogenic effect. While such changes in power output and bar velocity might be considered as small in statistical terms, this difference may be of great significance in training of elite athletes as well as in scientific research. It is known that plasma levels of caffeine needed to induce tissue changes are significantly higher than those required to affect adenosine receptors in the brain and peripheral nervous system [61,62], which may explain the occurrence of side effects using acute intake of CAF-6 and CAF-9 (Table 5), despite the lack of significant changes in power output and bar velocity. Therefore it can be concluded that acute intake of CAF in habitual users is to some extent ergogenic.

The variety of methodological approaches and results obtained make meaningful conclusions and recommendations for athletes difficult. Furthermore, it is hard to isolate the direct effects of CAF from systematic effects due to the number of potential mechanisms evoked from its wide distribution within the body. Although there is some controversy in regard to caffeine dose–response relationship, it is suggested that caffeine intake increases adrenaline release, evokes greater Ca^{2+} release from the sarcoplasmic reticulum, improves the function of the Na^+/K^+ pump, reduces pain perception and increases plasma fatty acid concentration [63,64]. The present study has several limitations which should be addressed. There were no genetic assessments related to CAF intolerance in the tested athletes. However, according to studies of Cornelis et al. [65] genetic variation in the A2A receptor, the main target of caffeine action in the CNS, is associated with caffeine consumption. Probability of having the ADORA2A 1083TT genotype associated with caffeine-induced anxiety [66] decreases as the caffeine intake increases in a population, and subjects with that genotype are more likely to limit their caffeine intake. People who were homozygous for the 1083T allele experienced greater anxiety after consuming 150 mg of caffeine [66]. Furthermore, before the start of our experiment no study participant reported any side effects after consumption of caffeine within the previous six months.

5. Conclusions

The results of the present study indicate that acute doses of CAF before exercise does not have a significant effect on power output and bar velocity of the bar during the bench press exercise in a group of habitual caffeine users. No significant changes in the above mentioned variables were observed at each of the three doses of CAF administered (3, 6, 9 mg/kg/b.m.). However the results of our study refer only to power output and bar velocity of the upper limbs during the bench press exercise with an external load of 50%1RM. These results therefore may not translate to other forms, volumes, or intensities of exercise.

Author Contributions: Conceptualization, A.F. and M.K.; Methodology, A.F. and M.K.; Software, A.F. and M.W.; Validation, M.W.; Formal Analysis, A.M.; Investigation, M.W., A.F., M.K.; Resources, A.F., M.K.; Data Curation, A.M.; Writing—Original Draft Preparation, M.W.; Writing—Review and Editing, A.F., M.K., A.Z.; Supervision, A.Z.; Project Administration, A.F.; Funding Acquisition, A.Z.

Acknowledgments: This study would not have been possible without our participants' commitment, time and effort. The study was supported and funded by the statutory research of the Jerzy Kukuczka Academy of Physical Education in Katowice, Poland, as well as by the grant of the Ministry of Science and Higher Education in Poland NRSA4 040 54.

Conflicts of Interest: The authors declare that they have no conflicts of interest.

References

1. Kawamori, N.; Haff, G.G. The optimal training load for the development of muscular power. *J. Strength Cond. Res.* **2004**, *18*, 675–684. [PubMed]
2. Argus, C.K.; Gill, N.D.; Keogh, J.W.; Hopkins, W.G. Assessing the variation in the load that produces maximal upper-body power. *J. Strength Cond. Res.* **2014**, *28*, 240–244. [CrossRef] [PubMed]
3. Thomas, G.A.; Kraemer, W.J.; Spiering, B.A.; Volek, J.S.; Anderson, J.M.; Maresh, C.M. Maximal power at different percentages of one repetition maximum: Influence of resistance and gender. *J. Strength Cond. Res.* **2007**, *21*, 336–342. [CrossRef] [PubMed]
4. Jandacka, D.; Uchytil, J. Optimal load maximizes the mean mechanical power output during upper extremity exercise in highly trained soccer players. *J. Strength Cond. Res.* **2011**, *25*, 2764–2772. [CrossRef] [PubMed]
5. Wilk, M.; Michalczyk, M.; Gołaś, A.; Krzysztofik, M.; Maszczyk, A.; Zając, A. Endocrine responses following exhaustive strength exercise with and without the use of protein and protein-carbohydrate supplements. *Biol. Sport* **2018**, *35*, 399–405. [CrossRef]
6. Williams, A.G.; Ismail, A.N.; Sharma, A.; Jones, D.A. Effects of resistance exercise volume and nutritional supplementation on anabolic and catabolic hormones. *Eur. J. Appl. Physiol.* **2002**, *86*, 315–321. [CrossRef]
7. Bosse, J.D.; Dixon, B.M. Dietary protein in maximize resistance training: A review and examination of protein spread and change theories. *J. Int. Soc. Sports Nutr.* **2012**, *9*, 42. [CrossRef]
8. Cermak, N.M.; Res, P.T.; de Groot, L.C.; Saris, W.H.; van Loon, L.J. Protein supplementation augments the adaptive response of skeletal muscle to resistance-type exercise training: A meta-analysis. *Am. J. Clin. Nutr.* **2012**, *96*, 1454–1464. [CrossRef]
9. Burke, L.M. Practical issues in evidence-based use of performance supplements: Supplement interactions, repeated use and individual responses. *Sports Med.* **2017**, *47*, 79–100. [CrossRef]
10. Daly, J.W.; Shi, D.; Nikodijevic, O.; Jacobson, K.A. The role of adenosine receptors in the central action of caffeine. *Pharmacopsychoecologia* **1994**, *7*, 201–213.
11. Davis, J.M.; Zhao, Z.; Stock, H.S.; Mehl, K.A.; Buggy, J.; Hand, G.A. Central nervous system effects of caffeine and adenosine on fatigue. *Am. J. Physiol. Regul. Integr. Comp. Physiol.* **2003**, *284*, 399–404. [CrossRef] [PubMed]

12. Goldstein, E.; Jacobs, P.L.; Whitehurst, M.; Penhollow, T.; Antonio, J. Caffeine enhances upper body strength in resistance-trained women. *J. Int. Soc. Sports Nutr.* **2010**, *7*, 18. [CrossRef] [PubMed]
13. Ferré, S. Mechanisms of the psychostimulant effects of caffeine: Implications for substance use disorders. *Psychopharmacology* **2016**, *233*, 1963–1979. [CrossRef] [PubMed]
14. Behrens, M.; Mau-Moeller, A.; Weippert, M.; Fuhrmann, J.; Wegner, K.; Skripitz, R.; Bader, R.; Bruhn, S. Caffeine-induced increase in voluntary activation and strength of the quadriceps muscle during isometric, concentric and eccentric contractions. *Sci. Rep.* **2015**, *13*, 10209. [CrossRef] [PubMed]
15. Bogdanis, G.C. Effects of physical activity and inactivity on muscle fatigue. *Front. Physiol.* **2012**, *3*, 142. [CrossRef] [PubMed]
16. Davis, J.K.; Green, J.M. Caffeine and anaerobic performance: Ergogenic value and mechanisms of action. *Sports Med.* **2009**, *39*, 813–832. [CrossRef] [PubMed]
17. Burke, L.M. Caffeine and sports performance. *Appl. Physiol. Nutr. Metab.* **2008**, *33*, 1319–1334. [CrossRef]
18. Tarnopolsky, M.A. Caffeine and creatine use in sport. *Ann. Nutr. Metab.* **2010**, *57*, 1–8. [CrossRef]
19. Warren, G.L.; Park, N.D.; Maresca, R.D.; McKibans, K.I.; Millard-Stafford, M.L. Effect of caffeine ingestion on muscular strength and endurance: A meta-analysis. *Med. Sci. Sports Exerc.* **2010**, *42*, 1375–1387. [CrossRef]
20. Wilk, M.; Krzysztofik, M.; Maszczyk, A.; Chycki, J.; Zając, A. The acute effects of caffeine intake on time under tension and power generated during the bench press movement. *J. Int. Soc. Sports Nutr.* **2019**, *16*, 8. [CrossRef]
21. Da Silva, V.L.; Messias, F.R.; Zanchi, N.E.; Gerlinger-Romero, F.; Duncan, M.J.; Guimarães-Ferreira, L. Effects of acute caffeine ingestion on resistance training performance and perceptual responses during repeated sets to failure. *J. Sports Med. Phys. Fit.* **2015**, *55*, 383–389.
22. Duncan, M.J.; Thake, C.D.; Downs, P.J. Effect of caffeine ingestion on torque and muscle activity during resistance exercise in men. *Muscle Nerve* **2014**, *50*, 523–527. [CrossRef] [PubMed]
23. Grgic, J.; Trexler, E.T.; Lazinica, B.; Pedisic, Z. Effects of caffeine intake on muscle strength and power: A systematic review and meta-analysis. *J. Int. Soc. Sports Nutr.* **2018**, *15*, 11. [CrossRef] [PubMed]
24. Grgic, J.; Mikulic, P. Caffeine Ingestion acutely enhances muscular strength and power but not muscular endurance in resistance-trained men. *Eur. J. Sport Sci.* **2017**, *17*, 1029–1036. [CrossRef] [PubMed]
25. Pallarés, J.G.; Fernández-Elías, V.E.; Ortega, J.F.; Muñoz, G.; Muñoz-Guerra, J.; Mora-Rodríguez, R. Neuromuscular responses to incremental caffeine doses: Performance and side effects. *Med. Sci. Sports Exerc.* **2013**, *45*, 2184–2192. [CrossRef] [PubMed]
26. Sabol, F.; Grgic, J.; Mikulic, P. The effects of three different doses of caffeine on jumping and throwing performance: A randomized, double-blind, crossover study. *Int. J. Sports Physiol. Perform.* **2019**, *31*, 1–25. [CrossRef] [PubMed]
27. Grgic, J.; Mikulic, P.; Schoenfeld, B.J.; Bishop, D.J.; Pedisic, Z. The influence of caffeine supplementation on resistance exercise: A review. *Sports Med.* **2019**, *49*, 17–30. [CrossRef]
28. Tallis, J.; Yavuz, H.C.M. The effects of low and moderate doses of caffeine supplementation on upper and lower body maximal voluntary concentric and eccentric muscle force. *Appl. Physiol. Nutr. Metab.* **2018**, *43*, 274–281. [CrossRef] [PubMed]
29. Mora-Rodríguez, R.; García Pallarés, J.; López-Samanes, Á.; Ortega, J.F.; Fernández-Elías, V.E. Caffeine ingestion reverses the circadian rhythm effects on neuromuscular performance in highly resistance-trained men. *PLoS ONE* **2012**, *7*, e33807. [CrossRef]
30. Diaz-Lara, F.J.; Del Coso, J.; García, J.M.; Portillo, L.J.; Areces, F.; Abián-Vicén, J. Caffeine improves muscular performance in elite brazilian jiu-jitsu athletes. *Eur. J. Sport Sci.* **2016**, *16*, 1079–1086. [CrossRef]
31. Del Coso, J.; Muñoz, G.; Muñoz-Guerra, J. Prevalence of caffeine use in elite athletes following its removal from the world anti-doping agency list of banned substances. *Appl. Physiol. Nutr. Metab.* **2011**, *36*, 555–561. [CrossRef] [PubMed]
32. Desbrow, B.; Leveritt, M. Awareness and use of caffeine by athletes competing at the 2005 ironman triathlon world championships. *Int. J. Sport Nutr. Exerc. Metab.* **2006**, *16*, 545–558. [CrossRef] [PubMed]
33. Svenningsson, P.; Nomikos, G.G.; Fredholm, B.B. The stimulatory action and the development of tolerance to caffeine is associated with alterations in gene expression in specific brain regions. *J. Neurosci.* **1999**, *19*, 4011–4022. [CrossRef]
34. Fredholm, B.B.; Bättig, K.; Holmén, J.; Nehlig, A.; Zvartau, E.E. Actions of caffeine in the brain with special reference to factors that contribute to its widespread use. *Pharmacol. Rev.* **1999**, *51*, 83–133. [PubMed]

35. Dodd, S.L.; Brooks, E.; Powers, S.K.; Tulley, R. The effects of caffeine on graded exercise performance in caffeine naive versus habituated subjects. *Eur. J. Appl. Physiol. Occup. Physiol.* **1991**, *62*, 424–429. [CrossRef]
36. Gonçalves, L.S.; Painelli, V.S.; Yamaguchi, G.; Oliveira, L.F.; Saunders, B.; da Silva, R.P.; Maciel, E.; Artioli, G.G.; Roschel, H.; Gualano, B. Dispelling the myth that habitual caffeine consumption influences the performance response to acute caffeine supplementation. *J. Appl. Physiol. (1985)* **2017**, *123*, 213–220. [CrossRef] [PubMed]
37. Glaister, M.; Howatson, G.; Abraham, C.S.; Lockey, R.A.; Goodwin, J.E.; Foley, P.; McInnes, G. Caffeine supplementation and multiple sprint running performance. *Med. Sci. Sports Exerc.* **2008**, *40*, 1835–1840. [CrossRef] [PubMed]
38. Evans, M.; Tierney, P.; Gray, N.; Hawe, G.; Macken, M.; Egan, B. Acute ingestion of caffeinated chewing gum improves repeated sprint performance of team sport athletes with low habitual caffeine consumption. *Int. J. Sport Nutr. Exerc. Metab.* **2018**, *28*, 221–227. [CrossRef]
39. Fine, B.J.; Kobrick, J.L.; Lieberman, H.R.; Marlowe, B.; Riley, R.H.; Tharion, W.J. Effects of caffeine or diphenhydramine on visual vigilance. *Psychopharmacology* **1994**, *114*, 233–238. [CrossRef] [PubMed]
40. Winston, A.P.; Hardwick, E.; Jaberi, N. Neuropsychiatric effects of caffeine. *Adv. Psychiatr. Treat.* **2005**, *11*, 432–439. [CrossRef]
41. Bell, D.G.; McLellan, T.M. Exercise endurance 1, 3, and 6 h after caffeine ingestion in caffeine users and nonusers. *J. Appl. Physiol. (1985)* **2002**, *93*, 1227–1234. [CrossRef] [PubMed]
42. Wilk, M.; Golas, A.; Krzysztofik, M.; Nawrocka, M.; Zając, A. The effects of eccentric cadence on power and velocity of the bar during the concentric phase of the bench press movement. *J. Sports Sci. Med.* **2019**, *18*, 191–197. [PubMed]
43. Bühler, E.; Lachenmeier, D.W.; Schlegel, K.; Winkler, G. Development of a tool to assess the caffeine intake among teenagers and young adults. *Ernahrungs Umschau* **2014**, *61*, 58–63.
44. Frankowski, M.; Kowalski, A.; Ociepa, A.; Siepak, J.; Niedzielski, P. Caffeine levels in various caffeine-rich and decaffeinated coffee grades and coffee extracts marketed in Poland. *Bromat. Chem. Toksykol.* **2008**, *1*, 21–27.
45. SELF Nutrition Data. Available online: https://nutritiondata.self.com/ (accessed on 2 April 2019).
46. Teixeira, V.; Voci, S.M.; Mendes-Netto, R.S.; da Silva, D.G. The relative validity of a food record using the smartphone application MyFitnessPal. *Nutr. Diet.* **2018**, *75*, 219–225. [CrossRef]
47. Brown, L.E.; Weir, J.P. ASEP procedures recommendation I: Accurate assessment of muscular strength and Power. *J. Exerc. Physiol. Online* **2001**, *4*, 1–21.
48. García-Ramos, A.; Haff, G.G.; Padial, P.; Feriche, B. Reliability and validity assessment of a linear position transducer. *Sports Biomech.* **2018**, *17*, 117–130. [CrossRef]
49. Goldsmith, J.A.; Trepeck, C.; Halle, J.L.; Mendez, K.M.; Klemp, A.; Cooke, D.M.; Haischer, M.H.; Byrnes, R.K.; Zoeller, R.F.; Whitehurst, M.; et al. Validity of the open barbell and tendo weightlifting analyzer systems versus the optotrak certus 3d motion-capture system for barbell velocity. *Int. J. Sports Physiol. Perform.* **2019**, *14*, 540–543. [CrossRef]
50. Childs, E.; de Wit, H. Subjective, behavioral, and physiological effects of acute caffeine in light, nondependent caffeine users. *Psychopharmacology* **2006**, *185*, 514–523. [CrossRef]
51. Desbrow, B.; Leveritt, M. Well-trained endurance athletes' knowledge, insight, and experience of caffeine use. *Int. J. Sport Nutr. Exerc. Metab.* **2007**, *17*, 28–39. [CrossRef]
52. Cohen, J. *Statistical Power Analysis for the Behavioral Sciences*, 2nd ed.; Hillsdale, N.J., Ed.; L. Erlbaum Associates: Mahwah, NJ, USA, 1988; p. 567.
53. Maszczyk, A.; Gołaś, A.; Pietraszewski, P.; Roczniok, R.; Zając, A.; Stanula, A. Application of neural and regression models in sports results prediction. *Procedia Soc. Behav. Sci.* **2014**, *117*, 482–487. [CrossRef]
54. Pickering, C.; Kiely, J. Are the current guidelines on caffeine use in sport optimal for everyone? Inter-individual variation in caffeine ergogenicity, and a move towards personalised sports nutrition. *Sports Med.* **2018**, *48*, 7–16. [CrossRef] [PubMed]
55. McLellan, T.M.; Caldwell, J.A.; Lieberman, H.R. A review of caffeine's effects on cognitive, physical and occupational performance. *Neurosci. Biobehav. Rev.* **2016**, *71*, 294–312. [CrossRef] [PubMed]
56. Cox, G.R.; Desbrow, B.; Montgomery, P.G.; Anderson, M.E.; Bruce, C.R.; Macrides, T.A.; Martin, D.T.; Moquin, A.; Roberts, A.; Hawley, J.A.; et al. Effect of different protocols of caffeine intake on metabolism and endurance performance. *J. Appl. Physiol. (1985)* **2002**, *93*, 990–999. [CrossRef] [PubMed]

57. Ryan, E.J.; Kim, C.H.; Fickes, E.J.; Williamson, M.; Muller, M.D.; Barkley, J.E.; Gunstad, J.; Glickman, E.L. Caffeine gum and cycling performance: A timing study. *J. Strength Cond. Res.* **2013**, *27*, 259–264. [CrossRef] [PubMed]
58. Lane, S.C.; Hawley, J.A.; Desbrow, B.; Jones, A.M.; Blackwell, J.R.; Ross, M.L.; Zemski, A.J.; Burke, L.M. Single and combined effects of beetroot juice and caffeine supplementation on cycling time trial performance. *Appl. Physiol. Nutr. Metab.* **2014**, *39*, 1050–1057. [CrossRef]
59. Hogervorst, E.; Bandelow, S.; Schmitt, J.; Jentjens, R.; Oliveira, M.; Allgrove, J.; Carter, T.; Gleeson, M. Caffeine Improves physical and cognitive performance during exhaustive exercise. *Med. Sci. Sports Exerc.* **2008**, *40*, 1841–1851. [CrossRef]
60. Conway, K.J.; Orr, R.; Stannard, S.R. Effect of a divided caffeine dose on endurance cycling performance, postexercise urinary caffeine concentration, and plasma paraxanthine. *J. Appl. Physiol. (1985)* **2003**, *94*, 1557–1562. [CrossRef]
61. Fredholm, B.B. Astra Award Lecture. Adenosine, adenosine receptors and the actions of caffeine. *Pharmacol Toxicol.* **1995**, *76*, 93–101. [CrossRef]
62. Nehlig, A. Are we dependent upon coffee and caffeine? A review on human and animal data. *Neurosci. Biobehav. Rev.* **1999**, *23*, 563–576. [CrossRef]
63. Graham, T.E.; Spriet, L.L. Metabolic, catecholamine, and exercise performance responses to various doses of caffeine. *J. Appl. Physiol. (1985)* **1995**, *78*, 867–874. [CrossRef] [PubMed]
64. O'Connor, P.J.; Motl, R.W.; Broglio, S.P.; Ely, M.R. Dose-dependent effect of caffeine on reducing leg muscle pain during cycling exercise is unrelated to systolic blood pressure. *Pain* **2004**, *109*, 291–298. [CrossRef] [PubMed]
65. Cornelis, M.C.; El-Sohemy, A.; Campos, H. Genetic polymorphism of the adenosine a2a receptor is associated with habitual caffeine consumption. *Am. J. Clin. Nutr.* **2007**, *86*, 240–244. [CrossRef] [PubMed]
66. Alsene, K.; Deckert, K.; Sand, P.; de Wit, H. Association between a2a receptor gene polymorphisms and caffeine-induced anxiety. *Neuropsychopharmacology* **2003**, *28*, 1694–1702. [CrossRef]

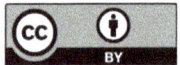

© 2019 by the authors. Licensee MDPI, Basel, Switzerland. This article is an open access article distributed under the terms and conditions of the Creative Commons Attribution (CC BY) license (http://creativecommons.org/licenses/by/4.0/).

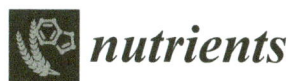

Article

The Effect of Caffeine on the Velocity of Half-Squat Exercise during the Menstrual Cycle: A Randomized Controlled Trial

Blanca Romero-Moraleda [1], Juan Del Coso [2,*], Jorge Gutiérrez-Hellín [1,3] and Beatriz Lara [1]

[1] Exercise Physiology Laboratory, Camilo José Cela University, 28692 Madrid, Spain
[2] Centre for Sport Studies, Rey Juan Carlos University, Fuenlabrada, 28943 Madrid, Spain
[3] Exercise and Sport Sciences, Faculty of Health Sciences, Universidad Francisco de Vitoria, 28224 Pozuelo, Spain
* Correspondence: juan.delcoso@urjc.es; Tel.: +34-918444694

Received: 30 September 2019; Accepted: 31 October 2019; Published: 4 November 2019

Abstract: Recent literature confirms the ergogenic effect of acute caffeine intake to increase muscle strength and power in men. However, the information about the effect of caffeine on muscle performance in women is uncertain and it is unknown whether its ergogenicity is similar during the menstrual cycle. The goal of this investigation was to assess the effect of acute caffeine intake on mean and peak velocity of half-squat exercise during three different phases of the menstrual cycle. Thirteen trained eumenorrheic athletes (age = 31 ± 6 years; body mass = 58.6 ± 7.8 kg) participated in a double-blind, crossover and randomized experimental trial. In the early follicular (EFP), late follicular (LFP) and mid luteal phases (MLP), participants either ingested a placebo (cellulose) or 3 mg/kg/bm of caffeine in an opaque and unidentifiable capsule. In each trial, participants performed a half-squat exercise at maximal velocity with loads equivalent to 20%, 40% 60% and 80% of one repetition maximum (1RM). In each load, mean and peak velocity were measured during the concentric phase of the exercise using a rotatory encoder. In comparison to the placebo, a two-way ANOVA showed that the ingestion of 3 mg/kg/bm of caffeine increased mean velocity at 60% 1RM in EFP (Δ = 1.4 ± 2.7%, p = 0.04; ES: 0.2 ± 0.2) and LFP (Δ = 5.0 ± 10.4%, p = 0.04; ES: 0.3 ± 0.4). No other statistical differences were found for the caffeine-placebo comparison for mean velocity, but caffeine induced an ergogenic effect of small magnitude in all of the menstrual cycle phases. These results suggest that the acute intake of 3 mg/kg/bm of caffeine induces a small effect to increase movement velocity during resistance exercise in eumenorrheic female athletes. The positive effect of caffeine was of similar magnitude in all the three phases of the menstrual cycle.

Keywords: women; resistance exercise; exercise training; velocity; ergogenic aid; muscle function

1. Introduction

Despite the equivocal findings of previous original investigations [1–4], emerging literature using meta-analysis suggests that acute caffeine intake is able to increase muscle strength and power [5,6]. This new information has given support to consider caffeine as an effective strategy to increase performance in resistance exercise with a relatively low prevalence of side effects when taken in the recommended doses (i.e., 3 to 9 mg per kilogram of body mass: mg/kg/bm [7]). However, most of this body of research has been carried out only on male samples. For example, in the meta-analyses by Grgic et al., about caffeine ergogenicity on muscle performance [5,6], only 9.7%–22.2% of the total sample used for these analyses were women. In fact, a detailed analysis of [5] revealed a significant increase in upper body muscle performance with caffeine in men while this effect was not present in women. Thus, caution is needed when assuming that the ergogenicity of caffeine for resistance exercise is also present in women [7].

Although some investigations have found an ergogenic effect of caffeine on muscle performance in women [1,8,9], this has not always been the case [10]. In general terms, it seems that the effectiveness of caffeine in increasing resistance exercise performance is lower in women than in men [11]. Sabblah et al. (2015) examined the effects of 5 mg/kg/bm of caffeine on the bench press and squat one repetition maximum (1RM) in both men and women and found there was a tendency towards an ergogenic effect of caffeine in the weight lifted in males only. Nevertheless, one common limitation of these investigations is that none of the studies controlled for the potential effects of the menstrual cycle on muscle performance [12] nor for the possible interaction of caffeine with the fluctuations of female sex hormones during the menstrual cycle [13,14].

Although the pharmacokinetics of acute caffeine intake are similar in the follicular, ovulatory and luteal phases [15,16], ethinylestradiol might induce an inhibition of the activity of CYP1A2, an enzyme responsible for the metabolism of caffeine [17]. In this sense, the administration of low-doses of estrogen-containing oral contraceptives reduces the rate of plasma clearance of caffeine and increases the time necessary to reach peak plasma caffeine concentration [18]. Then, the ergogenicity of caffeine to increase muscle strength might be higher in the days when the concentration of natural estrogens is higher (i.e., late follicular phase) because the serum caffeine concentration would remain longer than in the menstrual cycle phases were serum estrogen concentrations are low (i.e., menses and luteal phase) [19]. In addition, previous investigations have reported higher caffeine-induced effects on cardiovascular and subjective variables in the follicular phase than in the luteal phase [13,20]. With this background of knowledge, to date it is difficult to ascertain whether acute caffeine intake could improve muscle performance in women during resistance exercise. Furthermore, it is unknown if the potential ergogenic effect of caffeine on muscle performance is present, and of similar magnitude, during all the different phases of the menstrual cycle. Therefore, the main aim of this investigation was to determine the effect of caffeine intake on muscle performance during the early follicular, late follicular and mid-luteal phases of the menstrual cycle in eumenorrheic females.

2. Materials and Methods

2.1. Participants

Thirteen healthy trained women volunteered to participate in this study (age = 31 ± 6 years; body mass = 58.6 ± 7.8 kg; body height = 1.66 ± 0.06 m; body fat percentage = 14.5 ± 6.5%). All of the participants were competitive athletes and fulfilled the following inclusion criteria: a) age between 18 and 40 years; b) active training (including a combination of running, cycling and swimming practice) of ~2 h/day, at least 5 days/week for the previous two months; c) low caffeine consumption (i.e., <100 mg/day); and d) steady duration of their menstrual cycle for the previous 4 months. Participants were excluded if they reported a) any type of injury within the previous six months; b) a positive smoking status; c) medication usage within the previous month; d) previous history of cardiopulmonary diseases; e) oral contraceptive use; f) allergy to caffeine; or g) any type of menstrual disorders such as dysmenorrhea, amenorrhea, or strong symptoms associated with pre-menstrual syndrome. Participants were included if they had at least six months of resistance training experience (16 ± 8 months of experience in this sample), and were familiar with the half-squat exercise. All this information was obtained from a pre-participation screening that included a medical and training history as well as a food frequency questionnaire. One week before the experiment protocol, participants were fully informed of the procedures and the risks associated with the experiment. Participants signed their informed written consent prior to participating in the investigation. The study was approved by the Camilo José Cela University Research Ethics Committee. All research protocols were in accordance with the latest version of the Declaration of Helsinki.

2.2. Experimental Design

A double-blind, placebo-controlled, crossover and randomized experimental design was used in this investigation. In each of the following three phases of the menstrual cycle: early follicular (EFP), late follicular (LFP) and the mid-luteal (MLP), each participant completed 2 experimental trials making a total of 6 identical experimental trials (Figure 1). In each trial, leg muscle performance was measured using a half-squat exercise at maximal velocity with loads equivalent to 20%, 40% 60% and 80% of one repetition maximum (1RM). In each load, mean and peak velocity were measured during the concentric phase of the exercise. During each of these three menstrual cycle phases, and in a randomized order, participants ingested an opaque and unidentifiable capsule containing either caffeine (3 mg/kg/bm; 100% purity, Bulk Powders, UK) or an inert substance as a placebo (e.g., cellulose; 100% purity, Guinama, Spain). These two trials within each phase were separated by 48 h to allow recovery, testing reproducibility, and substance elimination. The first menstrual cycle phase under investigation was randomly assigned, and a similar number of participants started in EFP (5 participants), LFP (4 participants) and MLP (4 participants). An alphanumeric code was assigned to each trial by a person independent of the study. This was done in order to double-blind the participants and researchers to the trial order and substances. Menstrual cycle phase identification was carefully conducted according to the methodological considerations raised by Janse de Jonge [21] and with the help of a period tracker application, tympanic temperature, body mass changes and assessment of the urinary peak of the luteinizing hormone.

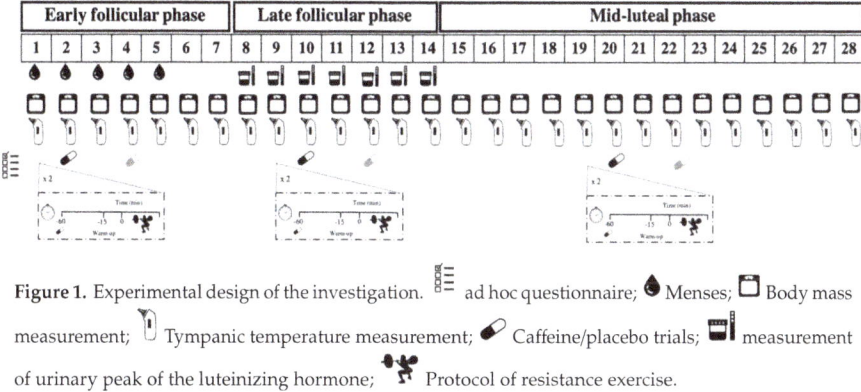

Figure 1. Experimental design of the investigation. ad hoc questionnaire; Menses; Body mass measurement; Tympanic temperature measurement; Caffeine/placebo trials; measurement of urinary peak of the luteinizing hormone; Protocol of resistance exercise.

This image displays the protocol followed by an athlete with a 28 day menstrual cycle. After participants had recorded the regularity and length of their menstrual cycles for 4 months, caffeine (3 mg/kg/bm) or a placebo was administered in three different phases of the menstrual cycle: early follicular, late follicular and mid-luteal. Muscle performance were measured 60 min after the assigned capsule was ingested. They then measured their basal tympanic temperature, body mass, and increases in luteinizing hormone using urine test strips to determine the onset of each menstrual cycle phase.

2.3. Standardizations, Familiarization and Pre-Experimental Trial

Once participants had fulfilled all the inclusion/exclusion criteria and signed the informed consent, they were encouraged to avoid nutritional supplements and sympathetic-adrenergic stimulants for the duration of the study. Participants were explicitly encouraged to avoid any nutritional source of caffeine (coffee, tea, soft and energy drinks, chocolate), and were informed about the necessity of maintaining their habitual training routines and a stable state of physical fitness during the experiment. Two weeks before the onset of the experiment, participants performed two familiarization sessions with the testing protocol in order to minimize any learning effects during the experiment. One week before the experiment, a 1RM test was performed to standardize the loads in the subsequent experimental sessions. For this 1RM measurement, participants commenced with sets of increasing loads estimated to be between 20% and 90% of 1RM, as previously described by Banyard et al. [22]. Then, the first 1RM attempt was performed with a maximum of five 1RM attempts permitted. After any successful 1RM attempt, the barbell load was increased between 0.5 and 2.5 kg until the last successful lift with a correct technique was obtained, which was categorized as 1RM (96.5 ± 17.1 kg). Two minutes of recovery were taken between 1RM attempts. On this day, participants were nude-weighed (±50 g, Radwag, Poland) in order to properly calculate caffeine dosage. The day before each trial, participants performed light, standardized training and a self-selected precompetitive diet/fluid routine was kept and recorded for replication. Participants were also required to refrain from intaking alcohol and to maintain a sleep pattern with at least 8 h of sleep the day before each trial.

2.4. Experimental Protocol

Participants performed six identical experimental trials starting with the menstrual cycle phase that was randomly assigned. Trials were performed in a laboratory, in the morning (between 09:00 and 11:00) and under similar environmental conditions (22–23 °C and 60% humidity; OH1001, OH Haus, Spain). Participants arrived at the laboratory in a fed state (~3 h after their last meal). In each experimental trial, the participants were nude-weighed after voiding (Tanita BF 350, Tanita Corporation, Tokyo, Japan), and then ingested the assigned capsule with caffeine or a placebo—and rested supine for 45 min. They subsequently performed a standardized 15 min warm-up protocol that included pedaling on a cycle ergometer and a submaximal attempt on the half squat machine. Then, participants performed two attempts of the half-squat exercise with loads that represented 20%, 40%, 60% and 80% of their 1RM—measured in the pre-experimental trial. The testing was performed on a Smith Machine (Technogym, Barcelona, Spain) in which 2 vertical guides regulated the barbell movement. Participants were encouraged to produce each repetition at their maximal velocity, and they could repeat any attempt if they considered that this was not maximal. Two minutes of passive rest were allocated between the attempts with the same load and three minutes of resting between different loads. The complete range of motion for the half squat exercise consisted of lowering the body by bending the knees to a 90° angle until touching a bench with the buttocks. In this position, participants executed a maximal velocity knee extension and thus, the concentric phase of the exercise was isolated and measured. Execution technique and motivation were standardized and monitored by 2 experienced researchers for reliability of the experimental conditions. In each attempt, barbell displacement in the concentric phase of the movement was recorded with a rotatory encoder and associated software (Isocontrol, EV-Pro, Spain) and mean and peak velocity (in m/s) were measured. The attempt with the highest barbell displacement velocity in each load was used for statistical analysis. With this information, the estimated 1RM was calculated [23] in all phases to ensure that 1RM remained unchanged throughout the experiment (EFP: 97.0 ± 23.2 kg; LFP: 98.5 ± 18.1 kg; MLP: 98.1 ± 22.2 kg).

2.5. Determination of Menstrual Cycle Phase

The EFP, LFP and MLP phases were selected for investigation because they represent main events occurring during the menstrual cycle (i.e., menses, pre-ovulation and peak progesterone concentration, respectively). The duration of the menstrual cycle and the onset of each phase were accurately determined by using (a) a period tracker application; (b) measurement of basal tympanic temperature and body mass changes; and (c) assessment of the urinary peak of the luteinizing hormone, following established recommendations [21]. The duration of each participant's menstrual cycle was recorded for a minimum of 4 months prior to the onset of the experiment for a valid characterization of length. This information was obtained using a mobile application (Mycalendar®, Period-tracker, Hong Kong, China) together with a menstruation diary, which included the date of menses, length of menses, and discomfort in the days preceding and during the menses. All participants had a regular menstrual cycle for the four months previous to the experiment (27 ± 2 days, range = 24–31 days) and were considered as eumenorrheic. During the familiarization period, participants were trained on how to measure their own basal tympanic temperature and to obtain valid body mass measurements. A digital thermometer (model HDT8208C, Nursal Ear Thermometer, Dongguan, China) and a digital scale (BT200, Daga, Barcelona, Spain) were provided for each participant to obtain data every morning immediately after waking up. Participants obtained these data for one complete menstrual cycle, starting with the phase randomly allocated (tympanic temperature; EFP: 36.34 ± 0.42; LFP: 36.43 ± 0.62; MLP: 36.42 ± 0.47 °C, body mass; EFP: 58.86 ± 9.28; LFP: 58.89 ± 9.14; MLP: 59.03 ± 9.11 kg). In addition, participants were supplied with 7 reactive test strips (One Step Ovulation LH Test Strip; CVS Health, Woonsocket, RI, US) to assess any increase in the luteinizing hormone in the first-morning urine sample. With all this information, the following events were used to determine the onset of each phase, as follows: EFP was indicated by the onset of menses; LFP was indicated by a positive test for urinary luteinizing hormone; MLP was determined to be between 70% and 75% of the individual menstrual cycle length (i.e., from the 20th to 22th day of the menstrual cycle for a regular cycle of 28 days [21]). All these protocols helped to align the participants' cycles and therefore, despite different cycle lengths, participants performed the testing in the same cycle phases.

2.6. Statistical Analysis

Data were collected as previously indicated and the results of each test were blindly introduced into the statistical package SPSS v 20.0 (IBM company, New York City, NY, US) for later analysis. Normality was tested for each variable with the Shapiro–Wilk test. All included variables in this investigation presented a normal distribution ($P > 0.05$) and parametric statistics were used to determine the ergogenicity of caffeine. The caffeine-placebo differences in mean and peak velocity were identified using a two-way ANOVA with repeated measures (treatment × load). After a significant F test, differences among means were identified using the Bonferroni post hoc procedure. The significance level was set at $P \leq 0.05$. The results are presented as means ± SD. To improve the identification of meaningful differences, the effect size was also calculated in all caffeine-placebo pairwise comparisons to allow a magnitude-based inference approach [24]. The effect-size statistic ±90% confidence intervals (CI) was used on log transformed data to reduce bias due to non-uniformity of error. The smallest significant standardized effect threshold was set as 0.2. Ranges of likelihood <1% indicated almost certainly no chances of change; 1% to 5%, very unlikely; 5% to 25%, unlikely; 25% to 75%, possible; 75% to 95%, likely; 95% to 99%, very likely; >99%, most likely. Differences were rated as unclear when likelihood exceeded >5% in both positive/negative directions. Effect sizes were interpreted according to the following ranges: <0.2, trivial; 0.2–0.6, small; 0.6–1.2, moderate; 1.2–2.0, large; 2.0–4.0, very large and; >4.0, extremely large [24].

3. Results

Figure 2 displays mean and peak velocity differences between caffeine and the placebo for all the loads under investigation. In comparison to the placebo, the two-way ANOVA showed that the ingestion of 3 mg/kg/bm of caffeine increased mean velocity at 60% 1RM in EFP ($\Delta = 1.4 \pm 2.7\%$, $P = 0.04$) and LFP ($\Delta = 5.0 \pm 10.4\%$, $P = 0.04$). No other differences were identified with the two-way ANOVA in mean or peak velocity. However, the magnitude-based inference approach showed that, in EFP, mean velocity was likely higher at 20% 1RM ($\Delta = 2.9 \pm 4.0\%$, chance% as positive/trivial/negative = 55/45/0%) with placebo than with caffeine. In EFP, mean velocity was possibly higher at 40% 1RM ($\Delta = 3.1 \pm 5.7\%$; 55/44/1%) with caffeine than with the placebo (Figure 2, panel A). In LFP, mean velocity was possibly higher at 40% 1RM with caffeine than with the placebo ($\Delta = 3.7 \pm 8.7\%$; 63/35/2%). In MLP, mean velocity was likely higher at 20% ($\Delta = 5.4 \pm 8.7\%$; 85/14/1%), and 40% 1RM ($\Delta = 6.1 \pm 9.1\%$, 85/15/0%) and possibly higher at 60% ($\Delta = 5.3 \pm 12.1\%$; 70/28/2%), and 80% 1RM ($\Delta = 4.7 \pm 14.7\%$; 54/43/3%) with caffeine than with the placebo.

For peak velocity, it was very likely that this variable was higher with placebo at 20% 1RM ($\Delta = 3.1 \pm 5.7\%$, 55/44/1%) and possibly higher with caffeine at 40% 1RM ($\Delta = 3.1 \pm 5.7\%$; 55/44/1%)

in the EFP (Figure 2, panel B). Caffeine induced possible ergogenic effects on peak velocity at 20% (Δ = 3.1 ± 4.3%, 53/47/0%), 40% (Δ = 3.9 ± 7.9%, 63/35/1%), and 60% 1RM (Δ = 2.8 ± 7.7%, 60/36/4%) in the LFP with no trivial or unclear effects in the MLP.

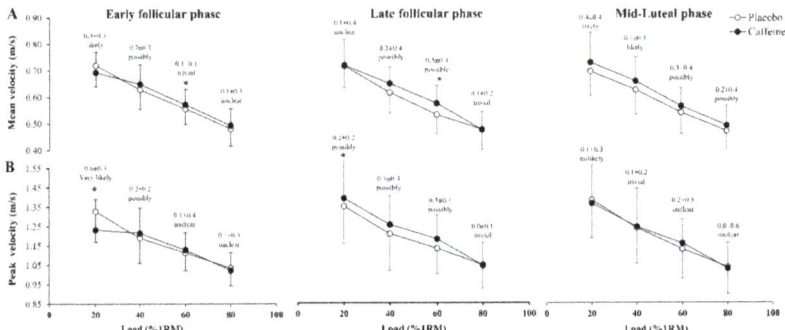

Figure 2. Changes induced with the ingestion of 3 mg/kg/bm of caffeine on mean velocity (**A**) and peak velocity (**B**) during the concentric phase of the Smith machine half-squat exercise of increasing loads (20%, 40%, 60% and 80% of one repetition maximum; 1RM) in each phase of the menstrual cycle. Data are mean ± standard deviation from 13 eumenorrheic athletes. The information over the data corresponds to the caffeine-placebo effect size statistic ±90% confidence intervals and magnitude base inference of this comparison. (*) Caffeine different from placebo within the same menstrual cycle phase at $P < 0.05$.

4. Discussion

The current body of evidence has found that acute caffeine intake (i.e., 5–6 mg/kg/bm) is able to increase muscle strength and power in women [1,8–10], although the ergogenic effect of this substance was small in all these investigations. However, previous research protocols on this topic did not consider the menstrual cycle phase in which the caffeine ergogenicity was found, despite the potential interaction between female sex hormones and caffeine [13,14]. To the authors' knowledge, this is the first study to directly compare the ergogenic response to caffeine on resistance exercise performance during the different phases of the menstrual cycle. Using a repeated-measures design in which the onset of the menstrual cycle phase was carefully delimited, caffeine-placebo comparisons were made in the early follicular, late follicular and mid-luteal phases while muscle performance was measured during a half squat force-velocity relationship. By using a traditional statistical approach, the two-way ANOVA revealed only subtle ergogenic effects of caffeine on mean and peak velocity in the half squat exercise. However, the magnitude-based inference approach indicated that caffeine was able to produce small ergogenic effects on mean and peak velocity at several loads (Figure 2) with a tendency to move the force-velocity relationship upwards in all phases of the menstrual cycle. Overall, the magnitude of these effects was comparable in all the three menstrual cycle phases under investigation. Taken together, these data suggest that caffeine might have a potential to enhance maximal velocity of movement in half-squat exercise. Although this effect was equally present during the menstrual cycle, the effect was catalogued as of small magnitude.

The concentration of the main female sex hormones fluctuates during different phases of the menstrual cycle provoking changes in physiological functions and performance [25–27]. The ovarian hormones estrogen and progesterone provoke opposing physiological functions—while estrogen is a hormone with a purported anabolic function, progesterone has been related to catabolic pathways [21,28]. For this reason, it has been speculated that muscle performance and muscle adaptations might be favored when estrogen concentration is high and progesterone is low (i.e., follicular phase). In fact, although muscle performance seems unaffected during the menstrual cycle [29], concentrating most of the resistance training in the follicular phase induces greater changes in muscle strength and hypertrophy compared to concentrating resistance training in the luteal phase [30]. In addition, the intake of 2 mg/kg/bm of caffeine produces greater caffeine-induced cardiovascular and mood changes in the follicular vs. the luteal phase [13,20]. Together, these effects might indicate that acute caffeine intake will produce a higher caffeine ergogenicity in the follicular phase.

Interestingly, this speculation was not confirmed by our data because caffeine presented a similar ergogenic effect to increase mean velocity in the early follicular, late follicular and mid luteal phases (Figure 2). Caffeine produced a negative effect on peak velocity at 20% 1RM in the early follicular phase of the menstrual cycle. However, this negative effect was not found in the remaining loads of this menstrual cycle phase nor in peak velocity values of the late follicular and mid luteal phases. In the author's opinion, this lack of effect of acute caffeine intake at 20% 1RM in the early follicular phase is anecdotical and does not alter the overall positive effect of caffeine to increase velocity during half-squat exercise (Figure 2). Caffeine produced this positive effect in the mid-luteal phase despite the probable high serum concentration of progesterone at this time of the menstrual cycle [15]. Although we did not assess serum caffeine concentrations, it is presumable that the stable caffeine metabolism during the menstrual cycle in these women who were not taken oral contraceptives [15,16] produced comparable serum caffeine concentrations in the early follicular, late follicular and mid luteal phases that promoted comparable ergogenicity for muscle performance. This finding is novel and reflects the high potential capacity of acute caffeine intake to produce increases in muscle performance in women, as previously found in other exercise and sport disciplines [31–33]. In this case, these data are novel because suggests that the magnitude of the caffeine ergogenic effect is comparable across the menstrual cycle.

Nevertheless, it is very important to take into account the individual responses during the menstrual cycle. In the current investigation, eumenorrheic women with no menstrual disorders were selected as the study sample to avoid the possible effects of these symptoms on the results of the pairwise caffeine-placebo comparisons. However, there is a high percentage of athletes who report premenstrual symptoms that might ultimately decrease performance [34]. Unfortunately, the results of this investigation cannot be used to ascertain whether caffeine might be used to avoid or to reduce the performance detriments produced by any menstrual disorder and further investigation about the effects of caffeine in these populations is warranted. The ergogenic effect of caffeine on muscle performance in women taking oral contraceptives should also be investigated because ethinylestradiol, one of the substances included in contraceptive pills, decreases caffeine metabolism [17].

There are several limitations to this experiment that should be mentioned and discussed to understand its scope. Firstly, to determine the onset of the menstrual cycle phases there was no measure of the concentration and/or quantity of female steroids hormones. However, we used a menstrual period tracker application, and measured changes in tympanic temperature and body mass. In addition, we also used luteinizing hormone urine test strips, as previously recommended [12,35]. Secondly, although the participants who underwent this protocol had at least six months of resistance training experience, they had no experience in velocity-based training. Lastly, we only used a dose of 3 mg/kg/bm of caffeine which is lower than the 5–6 mg/kg/bm used in previous investigations on caffeine effects on muscle performance. In addition, we selected low caffeine users while it is possible that higher doses are necessary to find an ergogenic effect of caffeine in women habituated to caffeine intake, as this has been demonstrated in male athletes [36]. Thus, it is possible that the magnitude of the ergogenic effect on mean and peak velocity found in this investigation was affected by the dose and the lack of tolerance to this drug.

5. Conclusions

In summary, the pre-exercise ingestion of 3 mg/kg/bm of caffeine increased, to a similar extent, mean and peak velocity in the half squat exercise at increasing loads in the early follicular, late follicular, and mid luteal phases of eumenorrheic trained athletes. Thus, in eumenorrheic women, caffeine might have the potential of increasing muscle performance during the menstrual cycle, although

3 mg/kg/bm would produce an effect of small magnitude. The outcomes of this investigation suggest that eumenorrheic female athletes might use acute caffeine intake to increase movement velocity during resistance training routines. The use of caffeine might be used to increase maximal strength values on different strength-based exercises [37]. In addition, it has been recently found that resistance training performed at fast movement velocities offers superior muscular strength gains than resistance training with slow-to-moderate velocities [38]. Thus, the use of caffeine before resistance training might be effective to enhance muscle adaptation derived from long-term strength training, although such hypothesis deserves further confirmation. In this sense, caffeine ergogenicity for resistance exercise can be equally obtained in all phases of the menstrual cycle and then, the supplementation with caffeine can be used to design strength training programs without any interference with athletes' menstrual cycle.

Author Contributions: B.R.-M., J.D.C. and B.L. conceived and designed the investigation, analyzed and interpreted the data, drafted the paper, and approved the final version submitted for publication. J.G.-H. participated in data gathering, critically reviewed the paper and approved the final version submitted for publication.

Funding: The study was part of the CAFTRI project supported by a grant from the Spanish National Sports Council conceded to the Spanish Federation of Triathlon, which supported the expenses necessary to carry out this project.

Acknowledgments: The authors would like to thank the participants for their invaluable contribution to this study.

Conflicts of Interest: The authors declare no conflict of interest with the finding reported in this study.

References

1. Ali, A.; O'Donnell, J.; Foskett, A.; Rutherfurd-Markwick, K. The influence of caffeine ingestion on strength and power performance in female team-sport players. *J. Int. Soc. Sports Nutr.* **2016**, *13*, 46. [CrossRef]
2. Astorino, T.A.; Rohmann, R.L.; Firth, K. Effect of caffeine ingestion on one-repetition maximum muscular strength. *Eur. J. Appl. Physiol.* **2008**, *102*, 127–132. [CrossRef]
3. Diaz-Lara, F.J.; Del Coso, J.; García, J.M.; Portillo, L.J.; Areces, F.; Abián-Vicén, J. Caffeine improves muscular performance in elite Brazilian Jiu-jitsu athletes. *Eur. J. Sport Sci.* **2016**, *16*, 1079–1086. [CrossRef]
4. Grgic, J.; Mikulic, P. Caffeine ingestion acutely enhances muscular strength and power but not muscular endurance in resistance-trained men. *Eur. J. Sport Sci.* **2017**, *17*, 1029–1036. [CrossRef]
5. Grgic, J.; Trexler, E.T.; Lazinica, B.; Pedisic, Z. Effects of caffeine intake on muscle strength and power: A systematic review and meta-analysis. *J. Int. Soc. Sports Nutr.* **2018**, *15*, 11. [CrossRef]
6. Grgic, J.; Pickering, C. The effects of caffeine ingestion on isokinetic muscular strength: A meta-analysis. *J. Sci. Med. Sport* **2019**, *22*, 353–360. [CrossRef]
7. Grgic, J.; Mikulic, P.; Schoenfeld, B.J.; Bishop, D.J.; Pedisic, Z. The Influence of Caffeine Supplementation on Resistance Exercise: A Review. *Sports Med.* **2019**, *49*, 17–30. [CrossRef]
8. Goldstein, E.; Jacobs, P.L.; Whitehurst, M.; Penhollow, T.; Antonio, J. Caffeine enhances upper body strength in resistance-trained women. *J. Int. Soc. Sports Nutr.* **2010**, *7*, 18. [CrossRef]
9. Sabblah, S.; Dixon, D.; Bottoms, L. Sex differences on the acute effects of caffeine on maximal strength and muscular endurance. *Comp. Exerc. Physiol.* **2015**, *11*, 89–94. [CrossRef]
10. Arazi, H.; Hoseinihaji, M.; Eghbali, E. The effects of different doses of caffeine on performance, rating of perceived exertion and pain perception in teenagers female karate athletes. *Braz. J. Pharm. Sci.* **2016**, *52*, 685–692. [CrossRef]
11. Mielgo-Ayuso, J.; Marques-Jiménez, D.; Refoyo, I.; Del Coso, J.; León-Guereño, P.; Calleja-González, J. Effect of Caffeine Supplementation on Sports Performance Based on Differences Between Sexes: A Systematic Review. *Nutrients* **2019**, *11*, 2313. [CrossRef] [PubMed]
12. Bambaeichi, E.; Reilly, T.; Cable, N.T.; Giacomoni, M. The isolated and combined effects of menstrual cycle phase and time-of-day on muscle strength of eumenorrheic females. *Chronobiol. Int.* **2004**, *21*, 645–660. [CrossRef]
13. Temple, J.L.; Ziegler, A.M.; Martin, C.; de Wit, H. Subjective Responses to Caffeine Are Influenced by Caffeine Dose, Sex, and Pubertal Stage. *J. Caffeine Res.* **2015**, *5*, 167–175. [CrossRef] [PubMed]
14. Temple, J.L.; Ziegler, A.M. Gender Differences in Subjective and Physiological Responses to Caffeine and the Role of Steroid Hormones. *J. Caffeine Res.* **2011**, *1*, 41–48. [CrossRef] [PubMed]

15. Kamimori, G.H.; Joubert, A.; Otterstetter, R.; Santaromana, M.; Eddington, N.D. The effect of the menstrual cycle on the pharmacokinetics of caffeine in normal, healthy eumenorrheic females. *Eur. J. Clin. Pharmacol.* **1999**, *55*, 445–449. [CrossRef]
16. McLean, C.; Graham, T.E. Effects of exercise and thermal stress on caffeine pharmacokinetics in men and eumenorrheic women. *J. Appl. Physiol.* **2002**, *93*, 1471–1478. [CrossRef]
17. Granfors, M.T.; Backman, J.T.; Laitila, J.; Neuvonen, P.J. Oral contraceptives containing ethinyl estradiol and gestodene markedly increase plasma concentrations and effects of tizanidine by inhibiting cytochrome P450 1A2. *Clin. Pharmacol. Ther.* **2005**, *78*, 400–411. [CrossRef]
18. Abernethy, D.R.; Todd, E.L. Impairment of caffeine clearance by chronic use of low-dose oestrogen-containing oral contraceptives. *Eur. J. Clin. Pharmacol.* **1985**, *28*, 425–428. [CrossRef]
19. Temple, J.L.; Bernard, C.; Lipshultz, S.E.; Czachor, J.D.; Westphal, J.A.; Mestre, M.A. The Safety of Ingested Caffeine: A Comprehensive Review. *Front. Psychiatry* **2017**, *8*, 80. [CrossRef]
20. Temple, J.L.; Ziegler, A.M.; Graczyk, A.; Bendlin, A.; Sion, T.; Vattana, K. Cardiovascular responses to caffeine by gender and pubertal stage. *Pediatrics* **2014**, *134*, e112–e119. [CrossRef]
21. De Jonge, X.A.J. Effects of the Menstrual Cycle on Exercise Performance. *Sport Med.* **2003**, *33*, 833–851. [CrossRef] [PubMed]
22. Banyard, H.G.; Nosaka, K.; Haff, G.G. Reliability and Validity of the Load-Velocity Relationship to Predict the 1RM Back Squat. *J. Strength Cond. Res.* **2017**, *31*, 1897–1904. [CrossRef] [PubMed]
23. Bazuelo-Ruiz, B.; Padial, P.; García-Ramos, A.; Morales-Artacho, A.J.; Miranda, M.T.; Feriche, B. Predicting Maximal Dynamic Strength from the Load-Velocity Relationship in Squat Exercise. *J. Strength Cond. Res.* **2015**, *29*, 1999–2005. [CrossRef] [PubMed]
24. Hopkins, W.; Marshall, S.; Batterham, A.; Hanin, J. Progressive Statistics for Studies in Sports Medicine and Exercise Science. *Med. Sci. Sports Exerc.* **2009**, *41*, 3–13. [CrossRef]
25. Ansdell, P.; Brownstein, C.G.; Škarabot, J.; Hicks, K.M.; Simoes, D.C.M.; Thomas, K.; Howatson, G.; Hunter, S.K.; Goodall, S. Menstrual cycle associated modulations in neuromuscular function and fatigability of the knee extensors in eumenorrheic females. *J. Appl. Physiol.* **2019**, *126*, 1701–1712. [CrossRef]
26. Wikström-Frisén, L.; Boraxbekk, C.J.; Henriksson-Larsén, K. Effects on power, strength and lean body mass of menstrual/oral contraceptive cycle based resistance training. *J. Sports Med. Phys. Fit.* **2017**, *57*, 43–52.
27. Isacco, L.; Boisseau, N. Sex Hormones and Substrate Metabolism During Endurance Exercise. In *Sex Hormones, Exercise and Women*; Springer International Publishing: Cham, Switzerland, 2017; pp. 35–58.
28. Hackney, A.C. *Sex Hormones, Exercise and Women*; Springer International Publishing: Cham, Switzerland, 2016; ISBN 978-3-319-44557-1.
29. Romero-Moraleda, B.; Del Coso, J.; Gutiérrez-Hellín, J.; Ruiz-Moreno, C.; Grgic, J.; Lara, B. The Influence of the Menstrual Cycle on Muscle Strength and Power Performance. *J. Hum. Kinet.* **2019**, *68*, 123–133. [CrossRef]
30. Sung, E.; Han, A.; Hinrichs, T.; Vorgerd, M.; Manchado, C.; Platen, P. Effects of follicular versus luteal phase-based strength training in young women. *Springerplus* **2014**, *3*, 668. [CrossRef]
31. Lara, B.; Gonzalez-Millán, C.; Salinero, J.J.; Abian-Vicen, J.; Areces, F.; Barbero-Alvarez, J.C.; Muñoz, V.; Portillo, L.J.; Gonzalez-Rave, J.M.; Del Coso, J. Caffeine-containing energy drink improves physical performance in female soccer players. *Amino Acids* **2014**, *46*, 1385–1392. [CrossRef]
32. Pérez-López, A.; Salinero, J.J.; Abian-Vicen, J.; Valadés, D.; Lara, B.; Hernandez, C.; Areces, F.; González, C.; Del Coso, J. Caffeinated energy drinks improve volleyball performance in elite female players. *Med. Sci. Sports Exerc.* **2015**, *47*, 850–856. [CrossRef]
33. Del Coso, J.; Portillo, J.; Muñoz, G.; Abián-Vicén, J.; Gonzalez-Millán, C.; Muñoz-Guerra, J. Caffeine-containing energy drink improves sprint performance during an international rugby sevens competition. *Amino Acids* **2013**, *44*, 1511–1519. [CrossRef] [PubMed]
34. Czajkowska, M.; Drosdzol-Cop, A.; Gałazka, I.; Naworska, B.; Skrzypulec-Plinta, V. Menstrual Cycle and the Prevalence of Premenstrual Syndrome/Premenstrual Dysphoric Disorder in Adolescent Athletes. *J. Pediatr. Adolesc. Gynecol.* **2015**, *28*, 492–498. [CrossRef] [PubMed]
35. Tenan, M.S.; Hackney, A.C.; Griffin, L. Maximal force and tremor changes across the menstrual cycle. *Eur. J. Appl. Physiol.* **2016**, *116*, 153–160. [CrossRef] [PubMed]

36. Wilk, M.; Filip, A.; Krzysztofik, M.; Maszczyk, A.; Zajac, A. The Acute Effect of Various Doses of Caffeine on Power Output and Velocity during the Bench Press Exercise among Athletes Habitually Using Caffeine. *Nutrients* **2019**, *11*, 1465. [CrossRef]
37. Grgic, J.; Sabol, F.; Venier, S.; Tallis, J.; Schoenfeld, B.J.; Del Coso, J.; Mikulic, P. Caffeine Supplementation for Powerlifting Competitions: An Evidence-Based Approach. *J. Hum. Kinet.* **2019**, *68*, 37–48. [CrossRef]
38. Davies, T.B.; Kuang, K.; Orr, R.; Halaki, M.; Hackett, D. Effect of movement velocity during resistance training on dynamic muscular strength: A systematic review and meta-analysis. *Sport Med.* **2017**, *47*, 1603–1617. [CrossRef]

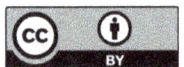

© 2019 by the authors. Licensee MDPI, Basel, Switzerland. This article is an open access article distributed under the terms and conditions of the Creative Commons Attribution (CC BY) license (http://creativecommons.org/licenses/by/4.0/).

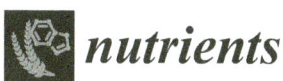

Article

The Effects of High Doses of Caffeine on Maximal Strength and Muscular Endurance in Athletes Habituated to Caffeine

Michal Wilk [1,*], Michal Krzysztofik [1], Aleksandra Filip [1], Adam Zajac [1] and Juan Del Coso [2]

1. Institute of Sport Sciences, Jerzy Kukuczka Academy of Physical Education, 40-065 Katowice, Poland
2. Exercise Physiology Laboratory, Camilo José Cela University, 28692 Madrid, Spain
* Correspondence: m.wilk@awf.katowice.pl; Tel.: +48-32-207-52-80

Received: 23 July 2019; Accepted: 13 August 2019; Published: 15 August 2019

Abstract: Background: The main goal of this study was to assess the acute effects of the intake of 9 and 11 mg/kg/ body mass (b.m.) of caffeine (CAF) on maximal strength and muscle endurance in athletes habituated to caffeine. Methods: The study included 16 healthy strength-trained male athletes (age = 24.2 ± 4.2 years, body mass = 79.5 ± 8.5 kg, body mass index (BMI) = 24.5 ± 1.9, bench press 1RM = 118.3 ± 14.5 kg). All participants were habitual caffeine consumers (4.9 ± 1.1 mg/kg/b.m., 411 ± 136 mg of caffeine per day). This study had a randomized, crossover, double-blind design, where each participant performed three experimental sessions after ingesting either a placebo (PLAC) or 9 mg/kg/b.m. (CAF-9) and 11 mg/kg/b.m. (CAF-11) of caffeine. In each experimental session, participants underwent a 1RM strength test and a muscle endurance test in the bench press exercise at 50% 1RM while power output and bar velocity were measured in each test. Results: A one-way repeated measures ANOVA revealed a significant difference between PLAC, CAF-9, and CAF-11 groups in peak velocity (PV) ($p = 0.04$). Post-hoc tests showed a significant decrease for PV ($p = 0.04$) in the CAF-11 compared to the PLAC group. No other changes were found in the 1RM or muscle endurance tests with the ingestion of caffeine. Conclusion: The results of the present study indicate that high acute doses of CAF (9 and 11 mg/kg/b.m.) did not improve muscle strength nor muscle endurance in athletes habituated to this substance.

Keywords: bench press; upper limb; resistance exercise; ergogenic substances; time under tension; 1RM test

---

1. Introduction

Caffeine (CAF) is one of the most widely consumed drugs in the world and has become a popular ergogenic aid for many athletes due to its properties to improve several aspects of physical performance. The acute intake of CAF has been effective to enhance exercise performance in a wide range of sport specific tasks [1], muscular endurance [2–4], and strength-power exercise modalities [4,5]. The ergogenic effect of caffeine has been found when consumed at doses ranging from 3 to 9 mg/kg body mass (b.m.) and ingested in the form of capsules 30 to 90 minutes before exercise [6]. Mechanisms responsible for ergogenic effect of caffeine are linked to the impact of this substance on various tissues, organs, and systems of the human body [4,7–10]. However, there is a growing consensus to consider that caffeine's ergogenicity lies in its tendency to bind to adenosine A_1 and A_{2A} receptors [11].

Although studies have confirmed the ergogenic effects of caffeine in many aspects, much controversy remains about the effects of acute CAF intake on maximal strength (1-repetition maximum (1RM)) and local muscle endurance. Several investigations have found that the acute intake of 3–6 mg/kg/b.m. of CAF produces an increase in 1RM test performance [3,12–14], and in the total number of repetitions performed (T-REP) [12,13,15]. However, other investigations have found that the same dosage did not produce such effects [2,3,5,15,16], suggesting that other factors such as the type of testing, the muscle mass involved, and the athlete's experience in strength training might affect the ergogenic effect of caffeine on muscle performance. Furthermore, Wilk et al. [2] observed a positive effect of CAF intake on time under tension (TUT) in a muscle endurance test, but no significant effect in the T-REP. According to Wilk et al. [17] and Burd et al. [18], TUT might be the most reliable indicator to assess exercise volume in resistance exercise regardless of the number of repetitions performed. Based on literature review, it can be concluded that previous results of studies on the acute effects of CAF intake on muscle strength and endurance are inconclusive.

Most investigations on the effects of caffeine intake on muscle performance have used participants unhabituated to caffeine or with low-to-moderate daily consumption of caffeine from 58 to 250 mg/day [3,12,16]. However, caffeine is an ergogenic aid frequently used in training and competition and it seems that athletes seeking for caffeine ergogenicity are already habituated to caffeine. There are reports indicating that 75–90% of athletes consume CAF before or during training sessions and competitive events [19–21], which indicates that studies on the effectiveness of acute CAF intake are particularly important in habitual caffeine users.

According to Svenningsson et al. [22] and Fredholm et al. [23], habitual caffeine intake modifies physiological responses to acute ingestion of CAF by the up-regulation of adenosine receptors. Furthermore, constant exposure to caffeine could impact caffeine metabolism by inducing an accelerated conversion of caffeine into dimethylxanthines by the cytochrome P450. Therefore, progressive habituation to the performance benefits of caffeine intake has been recognized in humans when it is consumed chronically [24]. However, the evidence to certify the existence of habituation to the ergogenic benefits is still inconclusive because it was found that low caffeine consumers benefited from the acute intake of 3–6 mg/kg/b.m. of CAF to a similar extent as individuals habituated to caffeine [25,26]. Lara et al. [27] found that caffeine ergogenicity was lessened when the substance was ingested daily (3 mg/day/kg/b.m.) for 20 days but it was still ergogenic after this period. In contrast, Beaumont et al. [28] observed that caffeine's ergogenicity practically disappeared after 28 days of daily ingestion (1.5–3 mg/day/kg/b.m.). Interestingly, all these investigations tested tolerance to caffeine's ergogenicity using endurance exercise protocols, while only one of them used muscle performance tests. Wilk et al. [5] showed that neither 3, 6, nor 9 mg/kg/b.m. of CAF intake enhanced power output and bar velocity during bench press exercise in strength-trained male athletes habituated to caffeine. However, there are no available data regarding the influence of acute CAF intake on maximal strength and muscular endurance in athletes habitually consuming caffeine.

Due to the aforementioned contrasting results, the main goal of this study was to assess the acute effect of high doses of CAF (9 and 11 mg/kg/b.m.) on maximal strength and muscle endurance assessed on the basis of T-REP and TUT in athletes habituated to CAF (4–6 mg/day/kg/b.m.). We hypothesized that high doses of caffeine, exceeding athletes' usual daily consumption of caffeine, would enhance muscle strength and muscular endurance. Since the value of daily habitual intake of caffeine may significantly modify the acute ergogenic effects of CAF ingestion, we used doses of CAF significantly above daily consumption in this investigation.

2. Materials and Methods

2.1. Study Participants

Sixteen healthy strength-trained male athletes (age: 24.2 ± 4.2 years, body mass: 79.5 ± 8.5 kg, body mass index (BMI): 24.5 ± 1.9, bench press 1RM: 118.3 ± 14.5 kg; mean ± standard deviation) volunteered to participate in the study after completing an ethical consent form. Participants had a minimum of 3 years of strength training experience (4.1 ± 1.4 years) and practiced team sports. All participants were classified as high habitual caffeine consumers according to the classification recently proposed by Gonçalves et al. [26]. The participants self-reported their daily ingestion of CAF (4.9 ± 1.1 mg/kg/b.m., 411 ± 136 mg of caffeine per day) based on the Food Frequency Questionnaire

(FFQ) with their average consumption assessed for four weeks before the start of the experiment. The inclusion criteria were as follows: (a) Free from neuromuscular and musculoskeletal disorders, (b) performance of the bench press exercise with a load of at least 120% of body mass, (c) habitual caffeine intake in the range of 4–6 mg/day/kg/b.m., ~300–500 mg of caffeine per day. Participants were excluded when they suffered from any pathology or injury. Additionally, they were required to refrain from alcohol and tobacco consumption and were asked not to take any medications or dietary supplements as well as other ergogenic substances during and two weeks prior to the experiment. The study protocol was approved by the Bioethics Committee for Scientific Research at the Academy of Physical Education in Katowice, Poland, according to the ethical standards of the latest version of the Declaration of Helsinki, 2013.

2.2. Habitual Caffeine Intake Assessment

Habitual caffeine intake was assessed by an adapted version of the Food Frequency Questionnaire (FFQ) proposed by Bühler et al. [29]. The FFQ was completed individually with the supervision of a qualified nutritionist. The FFQ was employed to assess the habitual consumption of dietary products containing caffeine. Portions, in household measures, were used to assess the amount of food consumed according to the following frequency of consumption: a) More than three times a day, b) two to three times a day, c) once a day, d) five to six times a week, e) two to four times per week, f) once a week, g) three times per month, h) rarely or never. The list was composed of dietary products with moderate-to-high caffeine content including different types of coffee, tea, energy drinks, cocoa products, popular beverages, medications, and caffeine supplements. Previously published information and nutritional tables were used for database construction [1,30,31]. Based on the answers in the FFQ, a qualified nutritionist estimated the habitual caffeine intake for each participant.

2.3. Experimental Design

This study used a randomized, double-blind, placebo-controlled crossover design where each participant acted as his own control. Participants performed a familiarization session with a preliminary 1RM test on one day and three different experimental sessions with a one-week interval between sessions to allow complete recovery and substances wash-out. The blinding and randomization of the sessions was conducted by a member of the research team that was not directly involved in data collection.

During the three experimental sessions, participants either ingested a placebo (PLAC), 9 mg/kg/b.m. of CAF (CAF-9) or 11 mg/kg/b.m. of CAF (CAF-11). After 60 minute of absorbing the substances, participants underwent a 1RM strength test and a muscle endurance test with the bench press exercise. During each test, power output and bar velocity were measured. Both CAF and PLAC were administered orally 60 minute before each exercise protocol to allow peak blood caffeine concentration and at least 2 hours after the last meal to maintain the same time of absorption. CAF was provided in the form of capsules containing the individual dose of CAF (Caffeine Kick®, Olimp Laboratories, Dębica, Poland). The producer also prepared identical PLAC capsules filled out with an inert substance (all-purpose flour). Participants refrained from physical activity the day before testing and they kept their habitual training routines during the study period. In addition, participants were instructed to maintain their usual hydration and dietary habits during the study period including habitual caffeine intake and register their calorie intake using "Myfitness pal" software [32] every 24 hours before the testing procedure. The average calorie intake was ~3300 kcal/day and it was similar before the three experimental trials. Participants were also asked to refrain from caffeine intake 12 hours before each trial. All testing was performed at the Strength and Power Laboratory at the Jerzy Kukuczka Academy of Physical Education in Katowice, Poland.

2.4. Familiarization Session and One Repetition Maximum Test

A familiarization session preceded the preliminary one repetition maximum testing. Participants arrived at the laboratory at the same time of day as in the upcoming experimental sessions (in the morning, between 9:00 and 10:00). Upon arrival, participants cycled on an ergometer for 5 minutes at an intensity that resulted in a heart rate of approximately 130 bpm, followed by a general upper body warm-up. Next, participants performed 15, 10, 5, and 3 repetitions of the bench press exercise using 20, 40, 60, and 80% of their estimated 1RM with a 2/0/X/0 tempo of movement. The sequence of digits describing the tempo of movement (2/0/X/0) referred to a 2 seconds eccentric phase, 0 represented a pause during the transition phase, X referred to the maximum possible tempo of movement during the concentric phase, and the last digit indicated no pause at the end of movement [33]. Participants then executed single repetitions of the bench press exercise with a 5 minutes rest interval between successful trials. The load for each subsequent attempt was increased by 2.5 to 5 kg, and the process was repeated until failure. Hand placement on the barbell was individually selected with a grip width on the barbell of 150% individual bi-acromial distance (BAD). BAD was determined by palpating and marking the acromion with a marker, and then measuring the distance between these points with a standard anthropometric tape. The positioning of the hands was recorded to ensure consistent hand placement during all testing sessions. No bench press suits, weightlifting belts, or other supportive garments were permitted. Three spotters were present during all attempts to ensure safety and technical proficiency.

2.5. Experimental Protocol

Three testing sessions were used for the experimental trials and the protocols were identical. All testing took place between 9.00 and 11.00 to avoid circadian variation. The general warm-up for the experimental sessions was identical to the one used for the familiarization session. After warming up, participants performed the 1RM bench press test to assess upper-body maximal muscle strength. For the 1RM test, the first warm-up set included eight to ten repetitions with 50% 1RM determined during the familiarization session. The second set included three to five repetitions with 75% 1RM. Participants then completed one repetition with 95% 1RM. Based on whether the participant successfully lifted the load or not, the weight was increased or decreased (2.5 to 5 kg) in subsequent attempts until the 1RM value for the session was obtained. Three- to five–minute rest intervals were allowed between the 1RM attempts, and all 1RM values were obtained within five attempts. After a five-minute rest interval, muscle endurance was assessed with one 'all-out' set using a load of 50% of participants' 1RM measured in the previous 1RM test. The end of the muscle endurance test was assumed when momentary concentric failure occurred. The concentric phase of the bench press movement was performed at maximal possible velocity in each repetition, while the eccentric phase was performed with 2 seconds duration (2/0/X/0). During the muscle endurance test, the following variables were registered:

- T-REP—total number of repetitions [n];
- TUT_{CON}—time under tension of concentric contractions [s];
- PP—peak concentric power [W];
- MP—mean concentric power [W];
- PV—peak concentric velocity [m/s];
- MV—mean concentric velocity [m/s].

All repetitions were performed without bouncing the barbell off the chest, without intentionally pausing at the transition between the eccentric and concentric phases, and without raising the lower back off the bench. During the experimental trials, participants were encouraged to perform at maximal effort according to the recommendations by Brown and Weir [34]. A linear position transducer system (Tendo Power Analyzer, Tendo Sport Machines, Trencin, Slovakia) was used for the evaluation of bar velocity. The Tendo Power Analyzer is a reliable system for measuring movement velocity and to estimate power output [35,36]. The system consists of a velocity sensor connected to the load by a

Kevlar cable which, through an interface, instantly transmits the vertical velocity of the bar to specific software installed in the computer (Tendo Power Analyzer Software 5.0). The system measures upward vertical mean and peak velocity of the movement. Using a set external load, the system calculates mean and peak power output in the concentric phase of the movement. The measurement was made independently in each repetition and automatically converted into the values of power (max, mean) and concentric velocity (max, mean). All familiarization and experimental sessions were recorded by means of a Sony camera (Sony FDR191 AX53). Time under tension and the number of performed repetitions was obtained manually from the recorded data using slow speed playback (1/5 speed). In order to ensure the reliability of manual data collection, four independent observers performed data analysis from the Sony camera. There were no significant differences in TUT [s] nor in T-REP [n] between the data collected by 4 evaluators. All participants completed the described testing protocol that was carefully replicated in the subsequent experimental sessions.

2.6. Side Effects

Immediately after finishing testing, and after 24 hours, participants answered a side effects questionnaire (QUEST), which is a nine-item measure with a dichotomous (yes/no) response scale of caffeine ingestion [20,37,38].

2.7. Statistical Analysis

The Shapiro-Wilk, Levene, and Mauchly's tests were used in order to verify the normality, homogeneity and sphericity of the sample data variance. Verification of differences between the PLAC vs. CAF-9 and CAF-11 groups was performed using one-way ANOVA. In the event of a significant main effect, post-hoc comparisons were conducted using the Tukey's test. Percent relative effects and the 95% confidence intervals were also calculated. Effect Sizes (Cohen's d) were reported where appropriate. Parametric effect sizes (ES) were defined as large for $d > 0.8$, moderate between 0.8 and 0.5, and small for <0.5 [39]. Statistical significance was set at $p < 0.05$. All statistical analyses were performed using Statistica 9.1 and were presented as means ± standard deviations.

3. Results

The one-way ANOVA revealed a statistically significant difference in PV ($p = 0.04$; Table 1) between PLAC vs. CAF-9 and CAF-11 groups. However, no significant differences in 1RM, T-REP, TUT_{CON}, MP, PP, nor MV between PLAC, CAF-9, and CAF-11 groups were observed among experimental sessions. Next, the Tukey's post-hoc test revealed a significantly lower PV in the CAF-11 when compared to the PLAC group ($p = 0.04$; Table 2).

Table 1. Summary of performance data under the three employed conditions.

Variable	Placebo (95% CI)	CAF-9 (95% CI)	CAF-11 (95% CI)	F	p
1RM [kg]	118.3 ± 14.5 (109.4–125.5)	122.3 ± 15.3 (115.7–132.5)	124.2 ± 11.4 (116.3–135.2)	0.24	0.78
T-REP [n]	25.1 ± 3.2 (23.3–26.8)	25.0 + 4.9 (22.4–27.6)	25.6 ± 3.3 (23.8–27.3)	0.09	0.90
TUT_{CON} [s]	17.1 ± 3.29 (15.3–18.8)	19.1 ± 3.29 (17.3–20.8)	16.9 ± 3.39 (15.1–18.8)	2.01	0.14
MP [W]	348 ± 79 (305–390)	333 ± 72 (294–372)	318 ± 78 (276–360)	0.61	0.54
PP [W]	798 ± 164 (710–886)	766 ± 134 (694–837)	731 ± 186 (632–831)	0.61	0.51

Table 1. *Cont.*

Variable	Placebo (95% CI)	CAF-9 (95% CI)	CAF-11 (95% CI)	F	p
MV [m/s]	0.71 ± 0.10 (0.66–0.76)	0.67 ± 0.08 (0.63–0.72)	0.70 ± 0.07 (0.66–0.74)	0.8	0.45
PV [m/s]	1.39 ± 0.16 (1.31–1.48)	1.37 ± 0.15 (1.29–1.45)	1.25 ± 0.17 (1.16–1.34)	3.43	0.04 *

All data are presented as mean ± standard deviation; CI—confidence interval; * statistically significant difference $p < 0.05$; 1RM: One repetition maximum; T-REP: Total number of repetitions; TUT_{CON}: Time under tension during concentric movement; MP: Mean power output; PP: Peak power output; MV: Mean velocity; PV: Peak velocity.

Table 2. Differences in placebo vs. caffeine conditions between experimental trials.

Variable	Comparison	p	Effect Size (Cohen d)	Relative Effects [%]
1RM [kg]	Placebo vs CAF-9	0.82	0.26—small	3.3 ± 4.1
	Placebo vs CAF-11	0.74	0.45—small	4.7 ± 5.1
T-REP [n]	Placebo vs CAF-9	0.99	−0.02—negative effects	0.4 ± 12.1
	Placebo vs CAF-11	0.93	0.15—small	2.0 ± 11.2
TUT_{CON} [s]	Placebo vs CAF-9	0.22	0.6—moderate	10.5 ± 15.5
	Placebo vs CAF-11	0.99	−0.05—negative effects	−6.2 ± 21.5
MP [W]	Placebo vs CAF-9	0.85	−0.19—negative effects	−1.5 ± 7.6
	Placebo vs CAF-11	0.51	−0.38—negative effects	−9.4 ± 10.5
PP [W]	Placebo vs CAF-9	0.84	−0.21—negative effects	−4.2 ± 8.3
	Placebo vs CAF-11	0.48	−0.38—negative effects	−9.2 ± 11.6
MV [m/s]	Placebo vs CAF-9	0.43	−0.44—negative effects	−6.0 ± 11.8
	Placebo vs CAF-11	0.91	−0.11—negative effects	−1.4 ± 6.6
PV [m/s]	Placebo vs CAF-9	0.90	−0.12—negative effects	−1.5 ± 10.2
	Placebo vs CAF-11	0.04 *	−0.84—negative effects	−11.2 ± 10.7

All data are presented as mean ± standard deviation; * statistically significant difference $p < 0.05$; 1RM: One repetition maximum; T-REP: Total number of repetitions; TUT_{CON}: Time under tension during concentric movement; MP: Mean power output; PP: Peak power output; MV: Mean velocity; PV: Peak velocity.

Side Effects

Table 3 details the occurrence of nine different side effects assessed immediately after and 24 hours after testing. Immediately after the PLAC trial, participants reported a very low frequency of side effects (0–13%; QUEST + 0 hour). After CAF-9 ingestion, there were more severe side effects (0–88%; QUEST + 0 hour) compared to the PLAC trial. The most severe side effects were recorded for increased urine output, tachycardia and heart palpitations, anxiety or nervousness, perception of performance improvement, and increased vigor (63–88%; QUEST + 0 hour). Finally, the CAF-11 trial produced a drastic increase in the intensity and frequency of side effects (0–92%; QUEST + 0 hour; Table 3).

In the morning following testing (QUEST + 24 hours), very few participants (0–13%) reported side effects with the PLAC. The CAF-9 trial showed greater frequency of side effects (0–69%), with increased urine output, tachycardia and heart palpitations, gastrointestinal problems, and increased vigor in comparison with the PLAC trial. Finally, CAF-11 intake increased the frequency and severity of all adverse side effects, with a frequency of appearance from 0 to 88% (Table 3).

Table 3. Number (frequency) of participants that reported side effects immediately after the testing protocol (side effects questionnaire (QUEST) + 0 hour) and 24 hours later (QUEST + 24 hours).

Side Effects	Occurrence of Side Effects in Particular Groups					
	PLAC		CAF-9		CAF-11	
	+0 h	+24 h	+0 h	+24 h	+0 h	+24 h
Muscle soreness	0 (0%)	0 (0%)	0 (0%)	0 (0%)	0 (0%)	0 (0%)
Increased urine output	1 (6%)	1 (6%)	10 (63%)	9 (57%)	10 (63%)	10 (63%)
Tachycardia and heart palpitations	3 (19%)	1 (6%)	12 (76%)	11 (69%)	15 (92%)	13 (81%)
Anxiety or nervousness	1 (6%)	2 (13%)	11 (69%)	4 (25%)	14 (88%)	13 (81%)
Headache	2 (13%)	1 (6%)	3 (19%)	6 (37%)	8 (50%)	8 (50%)
Gastrointestinal problems	0 (0%)	1 (6%)	6 (38%)	10 (63%)	6 (38%)	13 (81%)
Perception of performance improvement	2 (13%)	0 (0%)	14 (88%)	0 (0%)	6 (38%)	0 (0%)
Increased vigor/activeness	2 (13%)	1 (6%)	13 (81%)	8 (50%)	6 (38%)	6 (38%)
Insomnia	0 (0%)	0 (0%)	0 (0%)	4 (25%)	0 (0%)	6 (38%)

Data are presented as the number of participants (frequency) that responded affirmatively to the existence of a side effect.

4. Discussion

The main finding of the study was that, compared to the ingestion of the PLAC, the acute intake of high doses of CAF (9 and 11 mg/kg/b.m.) was not effective to produce any statistically measurable ergogenic effect on the bench press 1RM, T-REP, TUT$_{CON}$, PP, MP, nor MV in individuals habituated to CAF intake. In fact, the intake of 11 mg/kg/b.m. significantly decreased PV during bench press testing performed to concentric muscle failure in these habitual caffeine users. All this information suggests that even high doses of CAF were ineffective to produce ergogenic effects on maximal strength and muscular endurance in high-caffeine consumers. This lack of effect was evident despite the fact that the dosage of caffeine used pre-exercise was well-above their daily intake of this substance. In addition, these data might be indicative of tolerance to caffeine's ergogenicity for muscle performance while the high occurrence of side effects is still maintained with high doses of caffeine.

Previous studies have shown a variety of effects when different doses of CAF were administered to athletes performing testing to assess maximum strength and muscle endurance. Some of them indicated a significant increase in 1RM and T-REP performance [12,13], while others did not confirm such benefits [2,14]. Perhaps differences in the results of previous studies may be attributed to different doses of CAF consumed by study participants, in addition to the use of participants with an uneven habituation to caffeine. Since the value of daily habitual intake of caffeine might significantly modify the acute ergogenic effects of CAF ingestion [40], this investigation was aimed to study the acute effects of high doses (9 and 11 mg/kg/b.m.) of CAF intake on maximal strength and muscle endurance of the upper limbs, using athletes clearly habituated to caffeine.

Previous research using well-controlled caffeine treatments has suggested that the habitual intake of this stimulant might progressively reduce the ergogenic effect of acute CAF supplementation on exercise performance [27,28,40], reductions after acute CAF intake in habitual users can be modified using pre-trial doses which should be greater than the daily habitual intake. However, our results do not support this statement. Despite the fact that the doses of CAF used in our study were much greater (9 and 11 mg/kg/b.m.) than the daily intake of studied athletes (4–6 mg/kg/b.m./day), there were no positive changes in the analyzed strength, endurance, and power variables. In fact, our results indicate a significant decrease in PV after the intake of CAF-11 compared to the PLAC. Previous studies showed that acute CAF intake leads to higher activation of motor units [41] and higher MVIC [10,42]. However in the presented study the supposed effect of increased muscle tension following CAF intake, not only did not increase the power output generated during the CON phase of the movement, but a decrease in PV was observed. A decrease in PV after ingestion of CAF-11 undermines the legitimacy of using high doses of CAF before explosive, high-velocity, low-resistance exercises performed to muscle failure. According to Pallarés et al. [37], explosive, high-velocity, low-resistance actions require a much lower CAF dose (3 mg/kg/b.m.) in individuals with none or low habituation to caffeine. However, in the light of the current results, this statement does not apply to habitual caffeine users. The results of the present study, and especially the decrease in PV after CAF intake (11 mg/kg/b.m.), are particularly important for competitive athletes, since research indicates that 75–90% of athletes consume CAF before or during training sessions and competitive events [19,20]. In this regard, when seeking the benefits of acute caffeine intake to muscle performance, the dishabituation to caffeine should be recommended instead of the use of doses above the daily intake of caffeine. For how long habitual caffeine users should discontinue the intake of caffeine merits further investigation. For now, current evidence suggests that the dishabituation period should be longer than four days [43].

Furthermore, besides statistically significant change in PV, the results of the study showed negative effect sizes (ES) and relative (%) decreases in T-REP, TUT_{CON}, MP, PP, PV, and MV after the intake of CAF-11 compared to the PLAC, as well as relative decreases in MP, PP, PV, MV following the ingestion of CAF-9 compared to the PLAC. Decreased values of T-REP and TUT_{CON} after acute intake of CAF-11 may have resulted from the increased muscle tension generated during the movement [10,42]. A supposed increase of muscle activation can lead to a higher energy demand during exercise, thus leading to a faster depletion of energy substrates in muscle cells [44], which may partially explain a decline in T-REP and TUT_{CON} after the intake of CAF-11. However, the increased muscle tension following CAF intake did not improve the power output generated during the CON phase of the movement. The relative increase in results was observed only in the 1RM test after the intake of CAF-9 and CAF-11 (3.3% and 4.7%, respectively) and in TUT_{CON} after consuming CAF-9 (10.5%). While such an improvement in results of the 1RM test may be considered small in statistical terms, it can be of great significance in training and competition of elite athletes, especially in competitions where success depends on maximal strength production [45]. The relative % increase in results of the 1RM test after the intake of CAF-9 and CAF-11 compared to the PLAC is partly compatible with Pallarés et al. [37] who demonstrated that muscle contractions against heavy loads (75–90% 1RM) required a high CAF dose (9 mg/kg/b.m.) to obtain an ergogenic effect in low caffeine consumers. The results of our research confirm that, also in habitual consumers, high doses of CAF ingestion might be effective in improving maximal strength, although this effect is accompanied by a high occurrence of side effects (Table 3). Additionally, the TUT_{CON} increased by 10.5% after the intake of CAF-9 compared to the PLAC what may be of great significance in training of elite strength athletes. However, the increase in TUT_{CON} in the present study is contrary to the results of Wilk et al. [2], who showed a decrease in TUT during the bench press exercise at 70% 1RM performed to muscle failure after the intake of CAF (5 mg/kg/b.m.) compared to the PLAC. It should be pointed out that differences in the external load used in both exercise protocols (50% 1RM vs. 70% 1RM) could have affected the results following CAF intake [37]. The 10.5% increase in TUT_{CON} in the present study indicates that TUT may be an additional indicator of training volume during resistance training, compared to the T-REP, where a 0.4% decrease in results was registered after the intake of CAF-9 compared to the PLAC.

Furthermore, the results of our study showed that high doses of CAF in habitual caffeine consumers may be ineffective or also have a negative effect on physical performance in athletes. The ingestion of CAF-9 and CAF-11 significantly increased the frequency of self-reported side effects (0–88% for

CAF-9; 0–92% for CAF-11) compared to the PLAC. It has been empirically established that side effects of caffeine intake are severe when doses between 9 and 13 mg/kg/b.m. are used [46]. Increased urine output, tachycardia and heart palpitations, anxiety or nervousness, as well as perception of performance improvement are among the most common adverse effects experienced by athletes when they consume caffeine [47]. The current investigation adds some valuable information as it indicates that these adverse effects are still persistent in individuals habituated to caffeine, at least when they consume a high dose of CAF to exceed their habitual intake of this substance. However, the occurrence of these side effects does not always prevent athletes from improving their performance, as was the case with rowers in Carr et al. [48], who improved their times in a 2000-m ergometer test, or participants in the study of Pallarés et al. [37], who significantly improved their neuromuscular performance after the ingestion of 9 mg/kg/b.m. of CAF. On the contrary, Wilk et al. [5] showed an increased frequency of all adverse side effects after the intake of 9 mg/kg/b.m. of CAF yet with no significant increases in power output and bar velocity during the bench press exercise compared to the PLAC. All this information might be indicative of the necessity of evaluating both performance and side effects when planning to use >9 mg/kg/b.m. of CAF before training or competition.

The duration of adverse effects resulting from CAF intake is another issue to be considered in research and sports training. The present study showed a drastic increase in the reported frequency of side effects 24 hours after ingestion (Table 3). The CAF-9 trial showed a frequency of side effects in the range from 0 to 69%, with increased urine output, tachycardia and heart palpitations, gastrointestinal problems, as well as increased vigor in comparison with the PLAC group. CAF-11 intake increased the frequency of all adverse side effects, with a frequency of appearance from 0 to 88%. It should be stressed that even if caffeine allows for improved physical performance, it can significantly disturb sleep indices at night, such as sleep efficiency and ability to fall asleep, as well as induce an overall decrease in sleep itself [49]. Therefore, athletes who consume CAF to enhance their performance during training and/or competition should take into account its detrimental effects on sleep, especially if subsequent high-intensity exercise is to be performed on the following day.

The present study has several limitations which should be addressed. The procedure of the research assumed all participants were similarly habituated to caffeine despite the fact that their daily intake of caffeine and the duration of this intake presented some inter-individual variation. It has been recently suggested that all individuals respond to caffeine ingestion when caffeine is compared to a placebo using multiple and repeated testing sessions [50]. Although two different tests were used to assess the effect of caffeine intake on muscle performance, the ergogenic effect of CAF was not evident, suggesting that habituation to caffeine precluded the effect of acute CAF intake. However, it is still possible that the use of other muscle strength tests can still show ergogenic effects of high doses of CAF on performance of caffeine-habituated athletes. Furthermore, there were no genetic assessments related to caffeine metabolism in the tested athletes. According to Cornelis et al [51], genetic variation in the A_{2A} receptor (ADORA2A), the main target of caffeine action in the central nervous system, is associated with caffeine consumption. The probability of having the ADORA2A 1083TT genotype associated with caffeine-induced anxiety decreases as the caffeine intake increases in a population, and subjects with that genotype are more likely to limit their caffeine intake. People who were homozygous for the 1083T allele experienced greater anxiety after consuming 150 mg of caffeine [52]. Before the start of our experiment, no study participant reported any side effects after consumption of CAF within the last six months suggesting that the side effects found in this investigation were the result of the high doses used in this study rather than a genetic predisposition.

Practical Applications

The ingesting of high doses of CAF (9 and 11 mg/kg/b.m.) can bring minor benefits during training with near or maximal external loads. However, if explosive, high-velocity, low-resistance exercises are performed to muscle failure, the high doses of CAF (9 and 11 mg/kg/b.m.) are not recommended as they may hinder performance. These suggestions apply only to habitual strength-trained male caffeine users.

5. Conclusions

The results of the present study indicate that acute intake of high doses of CAF (9 and 11 mg/kg/b.m.) before exercise did not produce significant improvements in maximal strength and muscle endurance during the bench press exercise performed to concentric failure in a group of habitual caffeine users. However, it should be noted that slight benefits in 1RM and TUT_{CON} after the intake of high doses of CAF were observed. In addition, the results of this study showed a significant decrease in PV of the bar after the intake of CAF-11 compared to the PLAC. Overall, this investigation indicates that the use of high doses of CAF does not improve significant performance during resistance exercises in high caffeine consumers while it causes a significant increase in the occurrence of side effects. These outcomes undermine the convenience of using high doses of CAF before resistance training performed to momentary muscle failure. However, these results may not translate to other forms, volumes, or intensities of exercise. Future research should compare the inter-subject variation in response to different doses of caffeine. Additionally, as Chtourou and Souissi [53] mention, it would be wise to compare the changes in power-output and strength responses to CAF intake between several time-points following ingestion.

Author Contributions: Conceptualization, A.F. and M.K.; methodology, A.F., M.W., and M.K.; software, A.F. and M.W.; validation, M.W.; formal analysis, M.W.; investigation, M.W., A.F., and M.K.; resources, A.F., M.K.; data curation, M.W.; writing—original draft preparation, M.W., J.D.C.; writing—review and editing, A.F., M.K., A.Z., and J.D.C.; supervision, A.Z.; project administration, A.F.; funding acquisition, A.Z.

Funding: The study was supported and funded by the statutory research of the Jerzy Kukuczka Academy of Physical Education in Katowice, Poland, as well as by the grant of the Ministry of Science and Higher Education in Poland NRSA4 040 54.

Acknowledgments: This study would not have been possible without our participants' commitment, time, and effort.

Conflicts of Interest: The authors declare no conflict of interest.

References

1. Burke, L.M. Caffeine and sports performance. *Appl. Physiol. Nutr. Metab.* **2008**, *33*, 1319–1334. [CrossRef] [PubMed]
2. Wilk, M.; Krzysztofik, M.; Maszczyk, A.; Chycki, J.; Zajac, A. The acute effects of caffeine intake on time under tension and power generated during the bench press movement. *J. Int. Soc. Sports Nutr.* **2019**, *16*, 8. [CrossRef] [PubMed]
3. Grgic, J.; Mikulic, P. Caffeine ingestion acutely enhances muscular strength and power but not muscular endurance in resistance-trained men. *Eur. J. Sport Sci.* **2017**, *17*, 1029–1036. [CrossRef] [PubMed]
4. Goldstein, E.; Jacobs, P.L.; Whitehurst, M.; Penhollow, T.; Antonio, J. Caffeine enhances upper body strength in resistance-trained women. *J. Int. Soc. Sports Nutr.* **2010**. [CrossRef] [PubMed]
5. Wilk, M.; Filip, A.; Krzysztofik, M.; Maszczyk, A.; Zajac, A. The acute effect of various doses of caffeine on power output and velocity during the bench press exercise among athletes habitually using caffeine. *Nutrients* **2019**, *11*, 1465. [CrossRef] [PubMed]
6. Grgic, J.; Grgic, I.; Pickering, C.; Schoenfeld, B.J.; Bishop, D.J.; Pedisic, Z. Wake up and smell the coffee: Caffeine supplementation and exercise performance—An umbrella review of 21 published meta-analyses. *Br. J. Sports Med.* **2019**. [CrossRef] [PubMed]
7. Daly, J.W.; Shi, D.; Nikodijevic, O.; Jacobson, K.A. The role of adenosine receptors in the central action of caffeine. *Pharmacopsychoecologia* **1994**, *7*, 201–213. [PubMed]
8. Davis, J.M.; Zhao, Z.; Stock, H.S.; Mehl, K.A.; Buggy, J.; Hand, G.A. Central nervous system effects of caffeine and adenosine on fatigue. *Am. J. Physiol. Regul. Integr. Comp. Physiol.* **2003**, *284*, R399–R404. [CrossRef] [PubMed]

9. Ferré, S. Mechanisms of the psychostimulant effects of caffeine: Implications for substance use disorders. *Psychopharmacology (Berl.)* **2016**, *233*, 1963–1979. [CrossRef]
10. Behrens, M.; Mau-Moeller, A.; Weippert, M.; Fuhrmann, J.; Wegner, K.; Skripitz, R.; Bader, R.; Bruhn, S. Caffeine-induced increase in voluntary activation and strength of the quadriceps muscle during isometric, concentric and eccentric contractions. *Sci. Rep.* **2015**, *5*, 102–109. [CrossRef]
11. Southward, K.; Rutherfurd-Markwick, K.; Badenhorst, C.; Ali, A. The role of genetics in moderating the inter-individual differences in the ergogenicity of caffeine. *Nutrients* **2018**, *10*, 1352. [CrossRef] [PubMed]
12. Duncan, M.J.; Oxford, S.W. The effect of caffeine ingestion on mood state and bench press performance to failure. *J. Strength Cond. Res.* **2011**, *25*, 178–185. [CrossRef] [PubMed]
13. Diaz-Lara, F.J.; Del Coso, J.; García, J.M.; Portillo, L.J.; Areces, F.; Abián-Vicén, J. Caffeine improves muscular performance in elite Brazilian Jiu-jitsu athletes. *Eur. J. Sport Sci.* **2016**, *16*, 1079–1086. [CrossRef] [PubMed]
14. Beck, T.W.; Housh, T.J.; Schmidt, R.J.; Johnson, G.O.; Housh, D.J.; Coburn, J.W.; Malek, M.H. The acute effects of a caffeine-containing supplement on strength, muscular endurance, and anaerobic capabilities. *J. Strength Cond. Res.* **2006**, *20*, 506–510. [PubMed]
15. Green, J.M.; Wickwire, P.J.; McLester, J.R.; Gendle, S.; Hudson, G.; Pritchett, R.C.; Laurent, C.M. Effects of caffeine on repetitions to failure and ratings of perceived exertion during resistance training. *Int. J. Sports Physiol. Perform.* **2007**, *2*, 250–259. [CrossRef] [PubMed]
16. Astorino, T.A.; Rohmann, R.L.; Firth, K. Effect of caffeine ingestion on one-repetition maximum muscular strength. *Eur. J. Appl. Physiol.* **2008**, *102*, 127–132. [CrossRef] [PubMed]
17. Wilk, M.; Golas, A.; Stastny, P.; Nawrocka, M.; Krzysztofik, M.; Zajac, A. Does tempo of resistance exercise impact training volume? *J. Hum. Kinet.* **2018**, *62*, 241–250. [CrossRef]
18. Burd, N.A.; Andrews, R.J.; West, D.W.D.; Little, J.P.; Cochran, A.J.R.; Hector, A.J.; Cashaback, J.G.A.; Gibala, M.J.; Potvin, J.R.; Baker, S.K.; et al. Muscle time under tension during resistance exercise stimulates differential muscle protein sub-fractional synthetic responses in men. *J. Physiol. (Lond.)* **2012**, *590*, 351–362. [CrossRef] [PubMed]
19. Del Coso, J.; Muñoz, G.; Muñoz-Guerra, J. Prevalence of caffeine use in elite athletes following its removal from the World Anti-Doping Agency list of banned substances. *Appl. Physiol. Nutr. Metab.* **2011**, *36*, 555–561. [CrossRef]
20. Desbrow, B.; Leveritt, M. Awareness and use of caffeine by athletes competing at the 2005 Ironman Triathlon World Championships. *Int. J. Sport Nutr. Exerc. Metab.* **2006**, *16*, 545–558. [CrossRef]
21. Aguilar-Navarro, M.; Muñoz, G.; Salinero, J.; Muñoz-Guerra, J.; Fernández-Álvarez, M.; Plata, M.; Del Coso, J. Urine caffeine concentration in doping control samples from 2004 to 2015. *Nutrients* **2019**, *11*, 286. [CrossRef] [PubMed]
22. Svenningsson, P.; Nomikos, G.G.; Fredholm, B.B. The stimulatory action and the development of tolerance to caffeine is associated with alterations in gene expression in specific brain regions. *J. Neurosci.* **1999**, *19*, 4011–4022. [CrossRef] [PubMed]
23. Fredholm, B.B.; Bättig, K.; Holmén, J.; Nehlig, A.; Zvartau, E.E. Actions of caffeine in the brain with special reference to factors that contribute to its widespread use. *Pharmacol. Rev.* **1999**, *51*, 83–133. [PubMed]
24. Sökmen, B.; Armstrong, L.E.; Kraemer, W.J.; Casa, D.J.; Dias, J.C.; Judelson, D.A.; Maresh, C.M. Caffeine use in sports: Considerations for the athlete. *J. Strength Cond. Res.* **2008**, *22*, 978–986. [CrossRef] [PubMed]
25. Dodd, S.L.; Brooks, E.; Powers, S.K.; Tulley, R. The effects of caffeine on graded exercise performance in caffeine naive versus habituated subjects. *Eur. J. Appl. Physiol. Occup. Physiol.* **1991**, *62*, 424–429. [CrossRef] [PubMed]
26. de Souza Gonçalves, L.; de Salles Painelli, V.; Yamaguchi, G.; de Oliveira, L.F.; Saunders, B.; da Silva, R.P.; Maciel, E.; Artioli, G.G.; Roschel, H.; Gualano, B. Dispelling the myth that habitual caffeine consumption influences the performance response to acute caffeine supplementation. *J. Appl. Physiol.* **2017**, *123*, 213–220.
27. Lara, B.; Ruiz-Moreno, C.; Salinero, J.J.; Del Coso, J. Time course of tolerance to the performance benefits of caffeine. *PLoS ONE* **2019**, *14*, e0210275. [CrossRef] [PubMed]
28. Beaumont, R.; Cordery, P.; Funnell, M.; Mears, S.; James, L.; Watson, P. Chronic ingestion of a low dose of caffeine induces tolerance to the performance benefits of caffeine. *J. Sports Sci.* **2017**, *35*, 1920–1927. [CrossRef]
29. Bühler, E.; Lachenmeier, D.W.; Schlegel, K.; Winkler, G. Development of a tool to assess the caffeine intake among teenagers and young adults. *Ernahrungs Umschau* **2014**, *61*, 58–63.

30. Frankowski, M.; Kowalski, A.; Ociepa, A.; Siepak, J.; Niedzielski, P. Caffeine levels in various caffeine—Rich and decaffeinated coffee grades and coffee extracts marketed in Poland. *Bromat. Chem. Toksykol.* **2008**, *1*, 21–27.
31. Self Nutrition Data. Available online: https://nutritiondata.self.com/ (accessed on 2 April 2019).
32. Teixeira, V.; Voci, S.M.; Mendes-Netto, R.S.; da Silva, D.G. The relative validity of a food record using the smartphone application MyFitnessPal. *Nutr. Diet* **2018**, *75*, 219–225. [CrossRef] [PubMed]
33. Wilk, M.; Golas, A.; Krzysztofik, M.; Nawrocka, M.; Zajac, A. The effects of eccentric cadence on power and velocity of the bar during the concentric phase of the bench press movement. *J. Sports Sci. Med.* **2019**, *18*, 191–197. [PubMed]
34. Brown, L.E.; Weir, J.P. ASEP procedures recommendation I: Accurate assessment of muscular strength and power. *J Exerc. Physiol. Online* **2001**, *4*, 1–21.
35. García-Ramos, A.; Haff, G.G.; Padial, P.; Feriche, B. Reliability and validity assessment of a linear position transducer. *Sports Biomech.* **2018**, *17*, 117–130. [CrossRef] [PubMed]
36. Goldsmith, J.A.; Trepeck, C.; Halle, J.L.; Mendez, K.M.; Klemp, A.; Cooke, D.M.; Haischer, M.H.; Byrnes, R.K.; Zoeller, R.F.; Whitehurst, M.; et al. Validity of the open barbell and tendo weightlifting analyzer systems versus the optotrak certus 3D motion-capture system for barbell velocity. *Int. J. Sports Physiol. Perform.* **2019**, *14*, 540–543. [CrossRef] [PubMed]
37. Pallarés, J.G.; Fernández-Elías, V.E.; Ortega, J.F.; Muñoz, G.; Muñoz-Guerra, J.; Mora-Rodríguez, R. Neuromuscular responses to incremental caffeine doses: Performance and side effects. *Med. Sci. Sports Exerc.* **2013**, *45*, 2184–2192. [CrossRef] [PubMed]
38. Childs, E.; de Wit, H. Subjective, behavioral, and physiological effects of acute caffeine in light, nondependent caffeine users. *Psychopharmacology (Berl.)* **2006**, *185*, 514–523. [CrossRef]
39. Cohen, J. *Statistical Power Analysis for the Behavioral Sciences*, 2nd ed.; Routledge: New York, NY, USA, 2013.
40. Pickering, C.; Kiely, J. Are the current guidelines on caffeine use in sport optimal for everyone? Inter-individual variation in caffeine ergogenicity, and a move towards personalised sports nutrition. *Sports Med.* **2018**, *48*, 7–16. [CrossRef]
41. Duncan, M.J.; Thake, C.D.; Downs, P.J. Effect of caffeine ingestion on torque and muscle activity during resistance exercise in men. *Muscle Nerve.* **2014**, *50*, 523–527. [CrossRef]
42. Park, N.D.; Maresca, R.D.; McKibans, K.I.; Morgan, D.R.; Allen, T.S.; Warren, G.L. Caffeine enhancement of maximal voluntary strength and activation in uninjured but not injured muscle. *Int. J. Sport Nutr. Exerc. Metab.* **2008**, *18*, 639–652. [CrossRef]
43. Irwin, C.; Desbrow, B.; Ellis, A.; O'Keeffe, B.; Grant, G.; Leveritt, M. Caffeine withdrawal and high-intensity endurance cycling performance. *J. Sports Sci.* **2011**, *29*, 509–515. [CrossRef] [PubMed]
44. Bogdanis, G.C. Effects of physical activity and inactivity on muscle fatigue. *Front. Physiol.* **2012**, *3*, 142. [CrossRef] [PubMed]
45. Grgic, J.; Sabol, F.; Venier, S.; Tallis, J.; Schoenfeld, B.J.; Del Coso, J.; Mikulic, P. Caffeine supplementation for powerlifting competitions: An evidence-based approach. *J. Hum. Kinet.* **2019**, *68*, 131–142.
46. Pasman, W.J.; van Baak, M.A.; Jeukendrup, A.E.; de Haan, A. The effect of different dosages of caffeine on endurance performance time. *Int. J. Sports Med.* **1995**, *16*, 225–230. [CrossRef] [PubMed]
47. Salinero, J.J.; Lara, B.; Abian-Vicen, J.; Gonzalez-Millán, C.; Areces, F.; Gallo-Salazar, C.; Ruiz-Vicente, D.; Del Coso, J. The use of energy drinks in sport: Perceived ergogenicity and side effects in male and female athletes. *Br. J. Nutr.* **2014**, *112*, 1494–1502. [CrossRef] [PubMed]
48. Carr, A.J.; Gore, C.J.; Dawson, B. Induced alkalosis and caffeine supplementation: Effects on 2000-m rowing performance. *Int. J. Sport Nutr. Exerc. Metab.* **2011**, *21*, 357–364. [CrossRef] [PubMed]
49. Miller, B.; O'Connor, H.; Orr, R.; Ruell, P.; Cheng, H.L.; Chow, C.M. Combined caffeine and carbohydrate ingestion: Effects on nocturnal sleep and exercise performance in athletes. *Eur. J. Appl. Physiol.* **2014**, *114*, 2529–2537. [CrossRef] [PubMed]
50. Del Coso, J.; Lara, B.; Ruiz-Moreno, C.; Salinero, J. Challenging the myth of non-response to the ergogenic effects of caffeine ingestion on exercise performance. *Nutrients* **2019**, *11*, 732. [CrossRef] [PubMed]
51. Cornelis, M.C.; El-Sohemy, A.; Campos, H. Genetic polymorphism of the adenosine A2A receptor is associated with habitual caffeine consumption. *Am. J. Clin. Nutr.* **2007**, *86*, 240–244. [CrossRef]
52. Alsene, K.; Deckert, J.; Sand, P.; de Wit, H. Association between A2A receptor gene polymorphisms and caffeine-induced anxiety. *Neuropsychopharmacology* **2003**, *28*, 1694–1702. [CrossRef]

53. Chtourou, H.; Souissi, N. The effect of training at a specific time of day: A review. *J. Strength Cond. Res.* **2012**, *26*, 1984–2005. [CrossRef] [PubMed]

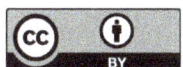 © 2019 by the authors. Licensee MDPI, Basel, Switzerland. This article is an open access article distributed under the terms and conditions of the Creative Commons Attribution (CC BY) license (http://creativecommons.org/licenses/by/4.0/).

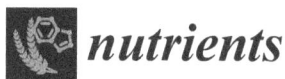

Correction

Correction: Wilk et al. "The Effects of High Doses of Caffeine on Maximal Strength and Muscular Endurance in Athletes Habituated to Caffeine" Nutrients, 2019, 11(8), 1912

Michal Wilk [1,*], Michal Krzysztofik [1], Aleksandra Filip [1], Adam Zajac [1] and Juan Del Coso [2]

[1] Institute of Sport Sciences, Jerzy Kukuczka Academy of Physical Education, 40-065 Katowice, Poland; m.krzysztofik@awf.katowice.pl (M.K.); a.filip@awf.katowice.pl (A.F.); a.zajac@awf.katowice.pl (A.Z.)
[2] Exercise Physiology Laboratory, Camilo José Cela University, 28692 Madrid, Spain; jdelcoso@ucjc.edu
* Correspondence: m.wilk@awf.katowice.pl; Tel.: +48-32-207-52-80

Received: 19 September 2019; Accepted: 27 September 2019; Published: 4 November 2019

The authors wish to make a correction to the published version of their paper [1]. We noticed an error in the statistical analysis that requires correcting, as it may contribute to an incorrect understanding of our study's scientific results and conclusions. In the study Section 2.7 (Statistical Analysis), the identification of differences between the placebo (PLAC) and the two doses of caffeine under experimentation 9 and 11 mg/kg/b.m.; CAF-9 and CAF-11, respectively) was performed using a one-way ANOVA. As the 16 participants of this investigation underwent all the experimental trials and acted as the own controls, the correct statically approach should have included the use of a one-way repeated measures ANOVA. After running this new statistical analysis, some new differences have appeared between PLAC and the use of caffeine, in addition to the new p values for each comparison. The repeated measures ANOVA revealed statistically significant differences in 1RM ($p < 0.01$), MP ($p < 0.01$) and PP ($p = 0.04$) between PLAC vs. CAF-9 and CAF-11, in addition to the difference in PV ($p < 0.01$) that was already presented in the previous version of the manuscript (Table 1). Tukey's post-hoc tests revealed a significantly higher 1RM in CAF-9 and CAF-11 trials when compared to PLAC and significantly lower MP, PP and PV in the CAF-11 trial when compared to PLAC (Table 2).

Table 1. Summary of performance data under the three employed conditions.

Variable	Placebo (95% CI)	CAF-9 (95% CI)	CAF-11 (95% CI)	F	p
1RM [kg]	118.3 ± 14.5 (109.4 – 125.5)	122.3 ± 15.3 (115.7 – 132.5)	124.2 ± 11.4 (116.3 – 135.2)	7.46	0.01 *
T-REP [n]	25.1 ± 3.2 (23.3 – 26.8)	25.0 ± 4.9 (22.4 – 27.6)	25.6 ± 3.3 (23.8 – 27.3)	0.14	0.86
TUT$_{CON}$ [s]	17.1 + 3.29 (15.3 – 18.8)	19.1 ± 3.29 (17.3 – 20.8)	16.9 ± 3.39 (15.1 – 18.8)	2.67	0.08
MP [W]	348 ± 79 (305 – 390)	333 ± 72 (294 – 372)	318 ± 78 (276 – 360)	6.07	0.01 *
PP [W]	798 ± 164 (710 – 886)	766 ± 134 (694 – 837)	731 ± 186 (632 – 831)	3.27	0.04 *

Table 1. Cont.

Variable	Placebo (95% CI)	CAF-9 (95% CI)	CAF-11 (95% CI)	F	p
MV [m/s]	0.71 ± 0.10 (0.66 – 0.76)	0.67 ± 0.08 (0.63 – 0.72)	0.70 ± 0.07 (0.66 – 0.74)	1.39	0.26
PV [m/s]	1.39 ± 0.16 (1.31 – 1.48)	1.37 ± 0.15 (1.29 – 1.45)	1.25 ± 0.17 (1.16 – 1.34)	6.09	0.01 *

All data are presented as mean ± standard deviation; CI—Confidence interval; * statistically significant difference $p < 0.05$; 1RM: One repetition maximum; T-REP: Total number of repetitions; TUT_{CON}: Time under tension during concentric movement; MP: Mean power output; PP: Peak power output; MV: Mean velocity; PV: Peak velocity.

Table 2. Differences in placebo vs. caffeine conditions between experimental trials.

Variable	Comparison	p	Effect Size (Cohen d)	Relative Effects [%]
1RM [kg]	Placebo vs. CAF-9	0.01 *	0.26—small	3.3 ± 4.1
	Placebo vs. CAF-11	0.01 *	0.45—small	4.7 ± 5.1
T-REP [n]	Placebo vs. CAF-9	0.99	−0.02—negative effects	0.4 ± 12.1
	Placebo vs. CAF-11	0.90	0.15—small	2.0 ± 11.2
TUT_{CON} [s]	Placebo vs. CAF-9	0.14	0.6—moderate	10.5 ± 15.5
	Placebo vs. CAF-11	0.99	−0.05—negative effects	−6.2 ± 21.5
MP [W]	Placebo vs. CAF-9	0.21	−0.19—negative effects	−1.5 ± 7.6
	Placebo vs. CAF-11	0.01 *	−0.38—negative effects	−9.4 ± 10.5
PP [W]	Placebo vs. CAF-9	0.44	−0.21—negative effects	−4.2 ± 8.3
	Placebo vs. CAF-11	0.04 *	−0.38—negative effects	−9.2 ± 11.6
MV [m/s]	Placebo vs. CAF-9	0.25	−0.44—negative effects	−6.0 ± 11.8
	Placebo vs. CAF-11	0.86	−0.11—negative effects	−1.4 ± 6.6
PV [m/s]	Placebo vs. CAF-9	0.84	−0.12—negative effects	−1.5 ± 10.2
	Placebo vs. CAF-11	0.01 *	−0.84—negative effects	−11.2 ± 10.7

All data are presented as mean ± standard deviation; * statistically significant difference $p < 0.05$; 1RM: One repetition maximum; T-REP: Total number of repetitions; TUT_{CON}: Time under tension during concentric movement; MP: Mean power output; PP: Peak power output; MV: Mean velocity; PV: Peak velocity.

Although the original experimental results remain unchanged, this new and correct statistical analysis indicates that the acute intake of high doses of CAF (9 and 11 mg/kg/b.m.) was effective to produce statistically measurable ergogenic effect on the bench press 1RM in individuals habituated to CAF intake. In case of muscular endurance, the intake of 11 mg/kg/b.m. significantly decreased MP, PP and PV during bench press testing performed to concentric muscle failure in these habitual caffeine users.

The authors apologize to the readers for any inconvenience caused by this modification. The original manuscript will remain online on the article webpage with a reference to this correction.

Conflicts of Interest: The authors declare no conflict of interest.

Reference

1. Wilk, M.; Krzysztofik, M.; Filip, A.; Zajac, A.; Del Coso, J. The Effects of High Doses of Caffeine on Maximal Strength and Muscular Endurance in Athletes Habituated to Caffeine. *Nutrients* **2019**, *11*, 1912. [CrossRef] [PubMed]

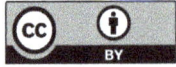

© 2019 by the authors. Licensee MDPI, Basel, Switzerland. This article is an open access article distributed under the terms and conditions of the Creative Commons Attribution (CC BY) license (http://creativecommons.org/licenses/by/4.0/).

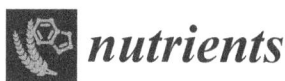

Article

Acute Effects of an "Energy Drink" on Short-Term Maximal Performance, Reaction Times, Psychological and Physiological Parameters: Insights from a Randomized Double-Blind, Placebo-Controlled, Counterbalanced Crossover Trial

Hamdi Chtourou [1,2], Khaled Trabelsi [3], Achraf Ammar [2,4], Roy Jesse Shephard [5] and Nicola Luigi Bragazzi [6,*]

1. Activité Physique, Sport et Santé, UR18JS01, Observatoire National du Sport, Tunis 1003, Tunisia; h_chtourou@yahoo.fr
2. High Institute of Sport and Physical Education, University of Sfax, Sfax 3000, Tunisia; ammar.achraf@ymail.com
3. UR15JS01: Education, Motricité, Sport et Santé (EM2S), High Institute of Sport and Physical Education, University of Sfax, Sfax 3000, Tunisia; trabelsikhaled@gmail.com
4. Institute of Sport Sciences, Otto-von-Guericke University, 39104 Magdeburg, Germany
5. Faculty of Kinesiology and Physical Education, University of Toronto, Toronto, ON M5S 1A1, Canada; royjshep@shaw.ca
6. Department of Health Sciences (DISSAL), Postgraduate School of Public Health, University of Genoa, 16132 Genoa, Italy
* Correspondence: robertobragazzi@gmail.com; Tel.: +39-010-353-8508

Received: 15 April 2019; Accepted: 29 April 2019; Published: 30 April 2019

Abstract: The current study examined the relationships between the effects of consuming a caffeine-containing "energy drink" upon (i) short-term maximal performance, (ii) reaction times, and (iii) psychological factors (i.e., mood state, ratings of perceived exertion (RPE), and affective load) and on physiological parameters (i.e., blood pressure and blood glucose). A randomized, double-blind, placebo-controlled, counterbalanced crossover design was implemented in this study. Nineteen male physical-education students (age: 21.2 ± 1.2 years; height: 1.76 ± 0.08 m; body-mass: 76.6 ± 12.6 kg) performed two test sessions: after drinking the "Red Bull" beverage (RB) and after drinking a placebo (PL). One hour after ingestion of each drink, resting blood glucose and blood pressure were measured and the participants completed the Profile of Mood States questionnaire. Then, after a 5-min warm-up, simple visual reaction time and handgrip force were measured, and the 30-s Wingate test was performed. Immediately after these tests, the RPE, blood glucose, and blood pressure were measured, and the affective load was calculated. Differences between treatments were assessed using two-way repeated measures analyses of variance and paired t-tests, as appropriate. Relationships between the test variables were assessed using Bland–Altman correlations. Significant (i) improvements in peak and mean power output, handgrip force, pre- and post-exercise blood glucose, blood pressure, and vigor and (ii) reductions in reaction times, depression, confusion, fatigue, anger, anxiety, RPE, and affective load scores were observed after RB compared to PL. There were significant correlations of (i) physical performances and reaction times with (ii) RPE, affective load, and pre- and post-exercise blood glucose levels. Gains in peak and mean power were significantly correlated with reductions in fatigue, anxiety (peak power only), and anger (mean power only). The reduction of reaction times was significantly correlated with decreases in confusion and anger and with increases in vigor. Handgrip force and reaction times were significantly correlated with pre- and post-exercise blood pressures. We conclude that RB ingestion has a positive effect on physical performance and reaction times. This effect is related to ergogenic responses in both psychological (i.e., RPE, affective load, and mood state) and physiological (i.e., blood glucose and blood pressure) domains.

Keywords: caffeine; energy drinks; fatigue; mood state; exercise

---

1. Introduction

Energy drinks (EDs) are beverages that typically contain a mixture of caffeine, taurine, herbal extracts (e.g., guarana, yerba mate, ginseng), vitamins (e.g., riboflavin, niacin, vitamin B-6), glucuronolactone, proprietary blends, and amino acids [1].

They can boost energy, improve alertness and promote wakefulness when performing high-intensity physical exercise [2], and, for this reason, they have become one of the substances most commonly consumed by athletes and other practitioners of physical activity. According to Froiland et al. [3], some 72.9% of U.S. college athletes are ED consumers.

Caffeine-containing EDs have been reported as beneficial in many sporting activities, possibly by enhancing motor unit recruitment.

Del Coso et al. [4,5] showed that the ingestion of 3 mg/kg of caffeine in the form of a commercially available ED increased overall running pace and sprint velocities during a rugby sevens competition. In adolescent basketball players, the same dose increased jump performance with no adverse effect on basketball shooting precision [6].

Del Coso et al. [7] noted that such an ED enhanced ball velocity in the spike test, the mean height of squat and countermovement jumps, and performance on the 15-s rebound jump test and the agility T-test. Furthermore, during a simulated game, players performed successful volleyball actions more frequently (24.6% ± 14.3% vs. 34.3% ± 16.5%, $p < 0.05$) with ingestion of the caffeinated ED rather than the placebo (PL) [7].

Although several studies have investigated the effects of ED on aerobic performance, there is as yet only limited and inconclusive data about their impact on short-term maximal performance [8]. Fukuda et al. [9] reported that the ingestion of supplements containing creatine, or caffeine plus amino acids improved the anaerobic running capacity by 10.8%.

In contrast, Hahn et al. [8] saw no beneficial effects of caffeine-containing ED on vertical jumping and repeated sprinting (i.e., measures of mean and peak anaerobic power). Likewise, Gwacham and Wagner [10] observed no ergogenic effect of caffeine-taurine ED on repeated sprinting (i.e., 6 × 35-s with 10-s rest intervals).

Studies of relationships between caffeine-containing EDs and psychological variables are also inconclusive to date; however, some studies have reported positive effects on subjective alertness, mental focus, energy, and fatigue tolerance [8,11–14].

Alford et al. [11] saw a positive effect on reaction time (a decrease of 88.7 msec). Likewise, Hoffman et al. [12] reported significant improvements in focus (+0.5 arbitrary units, AU) and energy (+0.4 AU) after ingestion of caffeine-containing EDs compared to placebo (PL). Hahn et al. [8] also described a significant reduction of perceived fatigue during repeated sprinting, and Wesnes et al. [15] demonstrated significant improvement in the attentional capacity, vigilance, and numeric and spatial working memory of healthy young adults after ingesting caffeine-containing ED.

However, no significant changes in mood state were seen. In contrast, Petrelli et al. [16] reported significant reductions of anxiety and depression after ingestion of caffeine-containing ED consumption compared to PL.

Physiological responses may also be affected by EDs. Del Coso et al. [17] found that caffeine-containing EDs increased systolic and diastolic blood pressures, although Wesnes et al. [15] did not show any significant change in blood glucose after drinking caffeine-containing EDs.

As yet, it remains unclear whether changes in mood state, blood pressures, and blood glucose levels are related to these ergogenic effects. Thus, the purpose of the present study was to examine relationships between the effects of caffeine-containing ED on (i) short-term maximal performance, (ii) reaction times, and (iii) psychological variables (mood state, rating of perceived exertion (RPE), and affective load) and changes in physiological parameters (i.e., blood pressures and blood glucose levels).

We hypothesized that the ergogenic effects of caffeine-containing EDs on short-term maximal performance and reaction times would be related to positive changes in both psychological factors (mood state, RPE, and affective load) and physiological parameters (blood pressures and blood glucose).

2. Materials and Methods

2.1. Participants Selection: Inclusion and Exclusion Criteria

The sample size was calculated a priori, using procedures suggested by Beck [18] and the software G*Power [19]. Based on the results of Del Coso et al. [4,5], effect sizes were estimated to be 0.62 (medium effect). To reach the desired statistical power and in order to attribute observed differences to factors other than chance alone, a minimum sample of 18 participants was required. To accommodate a possible drop-out of some participants, we recruited a total of 22 healthy and regularly active physical-education male students from various sports disciplines.

Potential participants were initially screened through telephone interviews based on the following inclusion criteria: (i) 18–40 years of age, (ii) body mass index (BMI) less than 25 kg/m^2, and iii) being low (<1.5 g/month [20]) and not regular caffeine users.

Exclusion criteria included: i) diagnosis of any chronic metabolic disease such as type 2 diabetes or cardiovascular disease, ii) diagnosis of an auto-immune disease such as rheumatoid arthritis, lupus, or type 1 diabetes, liver disease and iii) the intake of any medications or dietary supplements known to influence blood glucose concentrations or blood pressures.

The study was conducted according to the declaration of Helsinki and the protocol was fully approved (identification code: 8/16) by the review board "Local Committee of the Laboratory of Biochemistry, CHU Habib Bourguiba, Sfax, Tunisia."

After a thorough explanation of the protocol with responses to all questions, participants signed a written informed consent form.

Subjects were instructed to avoid nicotine, alcohol, dietary supplements, medications, and all other stimulants and to maintain their normal dietary, sleep and physical activity patterns before test sessions.

Caffeine and other caffeinated products (e.g., chocolate, caffeinated gums, caffeine-containing beverages) were avoided for 48 h and food for at least 4 h before testing.

2.2. Experimental Design

A randomized double-blind, placebo-controlled, counterbalanced, crossover design was adopted for this study. The randomized order of testing was determined using free online software (www.randomization.com).

Neither staff nor participants were informed about the names of the two drinks, and blinding was strictly maintained by emphasizing to both staff and participants that both drinks adhered to healthy principles and that each drink was advocated by certain sports medicine experts.

Two familiarization sessions were completed before definitive test sessions in order to eliminate any learning effects on physical performance and reaction time measurements. During the second familiarization session, body mass, and height were recorded.

The experimental design of the present study is pictorially presented in Figure 1.

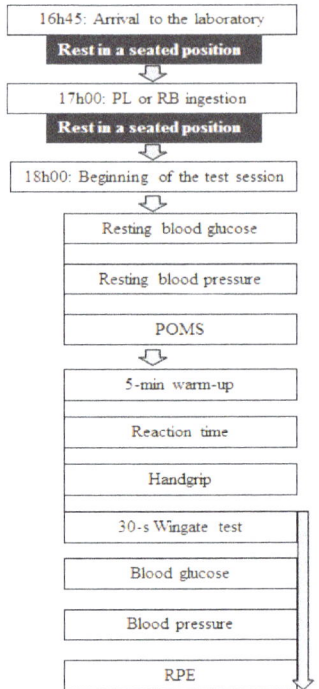

Figure 1. Experimental design. PL = placebo; RB = Red Bull; POMS = profile of mood states; RPE = rating of perceived exertion; HG = handgrip; RT = reaction time.

Each participant visited the laboratory for two formal test sessions, drinking a caffeine-containing ED (RB) and a caffeine and taurine-free beverage drink (PL). All sessions were arranged in the early evening hours to avoid any time of day effects, as suggested by Ammar et al. [21–23]. The two definitive test sessions were separated by an interval of seven days to allow sufficient recovery between tests and to ensure caffeine washout. To avoid identification, two opaque and unmarked cans [24–26] of RB or PL were ingested by each participant (i.e., 500 mL) in the presence of a researcher. The two drinks were similar in volume, texture, and appearance. One can of RB drink (i.e., 250 mL) contained 80 mg of caffeine, 1 g of taurine, 27 g of carbohydrates, 0.6 g of protein, 5 mg of vitamin B6, and 487 kJ of energy. The PL drink was prepared by an agri-food engineer; it did not contain any caffeine or taurine, but comprised carbonated water, carbohydrates, citric acid lemon juice reconstituted from concentrate (1%), supplemented by flavorings of sodium citrate, acesulfame K, sucralose, potassium sorbate and RB flavoring that contains propylene glycol E1520 (0.23 mL). Of note, both the PL and RB drinks were isocaloric.

Beverages were prepared, shaken and chilled in a refrigerator at 14h00 by an investigator who took no part in the test sessions or data analysis, but prepared the alphanumeric code identifying the tested drink. At 17h00, the cooled beverages were served in sealed plastic opaque water bottles and consumed using an opaque straw. Participants were instructed to drink the fluid quickly (within 1 ± 0.5 min) 60 min before their test session and not to discuss or compare tastes or to make any assumption about what they had ingested. The interval of 60 min was chosen as being optimal for a complete caffeine absorption [27] and thus enabling the peaking of caffeine concentration [28].

Subjects were supervised by staff to ensure that they drank the entire quantity of fluid, and no exchange of bottles was allowed. The last standardized meal (i.e., lunch) before the beginning of the test session was taken at 13h00. Temperature and relative humidity of the laboratory were similar over the test sessions, with a temperature of around 22 °C and a relative humidity between 45 and 55%. During each test session (from 18h00), resting blood glucose and blood pressures were measured, and the participants completed the POMS questionnaire.

In order to increase body temperature and thus improve the efficiency of the neuromuscular system [22,29,30], a 5-min treadmill warm-up was performed [20] (Figure 1). After that, the reaction time, the handgrip force and the 30-s Wingate tests were performed. RPE scores, blood glucose, and blood pressures were then measured, and the affective load was calculated. To investigate the effects of RB on the acute physiological and psychological responses to exercise, blood glucose and pressure and RPE measures were collected immediately pre- and post-exercise (Figure 1).

2.3. Blood Glucose and Blood Pressure Measurements

Blood glucose was measured using the electrochemical sensor Rightest GM260 Blood Glucose Monitoring System (Bionime Corporation, Taichung City, Taiwan). The fingertip was pricked with a lancing device, and a specific test strip was soaked with blood and was inserted into the measuring apparatus, with an estimate appearing within 5 s. Systolic blood pressure was measured by the same physician using a stethoscope (Spengler, Germany) and sphygmomanometer (Spengler, Germany). The intra-class correlation coefficient (ICC) and the standard error of the measurement (SEM) showed good reliability for blood glucose pre- (ICC > 0.72, absolute SEM < 0.03) and post-exercise (ICC > 0.71, absolute SEM < 0.04). Similar results were computed for blood pressure pre- (ICC > 0.72, absolute SEM < 0.32) and post-exercise (ICC > 0.67, absolute SEM < 0.38).

2.4. Profile of Mood States (POMS)

The evaluation of mood states was performed using the French language version of the POMS questionnaire. Responses to 65 adjectives (ranging from "Zero" (i.e., not at all) to "Four" (i.e., extremely)) assessed immediate mood states in seven dimensions: tension, depression, anger, vigor, fatigue, confusion, and interpersonal relationships. As previous studies (e.g., [31]) utilized only six parameters of the POMS questionnaire due to large variations affecting the dimension of "interpersonal relationships," this parameter was not included in the analysis. The ICC and SEM showed good reliability for depression (ICC > 0.67, absolute SEM < 1.38), confusion (ICC > 0.68, absolute SEM < 1.39), fatigue (ICC > 0.71, absolute SEM < 1.04), vigor (ICC > 0.67, absolute SEM < 1.42), anger (ICC > 0.66, absolute SEM < 1.37), and tension (ICC > 0.68, absolute SEM < 1.26), The ICC and SEM showed, instead, poor reliability for interpersonal relationships (ICC > 0.1, absolute SEM < 1.95).

2.5. Rating of Perceived Exertion (RPE) and Affective Load

The original Borg RPE scale rates exertion subjectively during or after physical exercise on a 15-point scale ranging from six (extremely light) to twenty (extremely hard). It was used to calculate the affective load; as suggested by Baron et al. [32], the affective load was obtained as the difference between the perceived exertion (negative affective response) and pleasure scores (positive affective response). For example, with an RPE score of six, the negative affective response is zero and the positive affective response is −14. However, if the RPE score rises to 20, the negative affective response is +14 and the positive affective response is zero. The potential affective load thus ranges from −14 to +14. A negative affective load score indicates the dominance of pleasant affective responses and a positive affective load represents the dominance of unpleasant affective responses [33]. RPE and AL. The ICC and the SEM showed good reliability for RPE and AL (ICC > 0.71, absolute SEM < 0.21).

2.6. Reaction Times and Handgrip Strength

A simple visual reaction time test assessed alertness and motor reaction-speed. Subjects responded as quickly as possible to the presentation of a stimulus (the image of a black box) on a computer screen (15" LCD). When this appears, the participant should press the index finger on a computer key.

The signal appeared in random order within 1–10-s time intervals. Each participant was allowed ten attempts and the mean reaction time was calculated, using React! V0.9 software.

Handgrip strength was recorded by a dynamometer (T.K.K. 5401; Takei, Tokyo, Japan). The maximal handgrip force was determined for the dominant hand. Participants exerted their maximal strength for 4–5-s. With the hand hanging downwards, the dynamometer was held freely and without support. Three attempts were allowed with 1-min rest intervals, and the largest value was recorded. The ICC and the SEM showed excellent reliability for both reaction time (ICC > 0.89, absolute SEM < 0.14) and handgrip strength (ICC > 0.92, absolute SEM < 0.67) measurements.

2.7. Wingate Test

A calibrated mechanically-braked cycle ergometer (Monark 894; Stockholm, Sweden) interfaced with a microcomputer was utilized for the 30-s Wingate test. Subjects pedaled as fast as possible for 30-s against a constant load calculated according to the participant's body mass (i.e., 8.7%). After maintaining a constant ~60 rpm speed for 4–6-s against minimal resistance, the selected load was applied. The participant sat on the cycle throughout and was strongly encouraged to maximize pedaling rates and to maintain a high speed. Peak and mean power (i.e., the average power output after 30-s) were recorded. The fatigue index was calculated as follows:

$$\text{Fatigue index (\%)} = (\text{peak power} - \text{minimal power})/\text{peak power} \times 100 \qquad (1)$$

The ICC and the SEM showed excellent reliability for peak power (ICC > 0.98, absolute SEM < 0.21), mean power (ICC > 0.98, absolute SEM < 0.23) and fatigue index (ICC > 0.76, absolute SEM < 1.99).

2.8. Statistical Analysis

Results for all parameters are presented as mean ± standard deviation (SD). Data analyses were carried out using the commercial software "Statistical Package for Social Sciences" SPSS v21.0 software (SPSS Inc., Chicago, IL) and Microsoft Excel 2010 (Microsoft Corp., Redmont, WA, USA).

To determine whether two familiarization sessions had been sufficient to remove any learning effects, the intra-class correlation coefficient (ICC) and the standard error of the measurement (SEM) were calculated for all parameters. ICC values over 0.75 were considered as evidence of excellent reproducibility, ICC values between 0.4 and 0.75 were considered as good reproducibility and ICC values less than 0.4 were considered as poor reproducibility.

All parameters met parametric assumptions on the basis of the Shapiro-Wilk's test. Student's t-test was used to compare RB and PL and RB with the exception of blood glucose and blood pressures. The effect size (ES) was calculated according to the formula of Glass and magnitudes were interpreted using the Cohen scale: ES < 0.2 was considered as small, ES around 0.5 was considered as medium and ES > 0.8 was considered as large. The mean confidence interval (CI) was determined at 95%.

For blood glucose and blood pressure, a two-way analysis of variance (ANOVA) (2 (Drink) × 2 (Exercise)) was utilized. When a significant main effect or interaction was detected, pair-wise comparisons were assessed using the Bonferroni test in order to ensure protection against multiple comparisons. The Δ-change induced by the drinks (i.e., the difference between PL and RB) was calculated as follow:

$$\Delta\text{-change drink} = \text{RB} - \text{PL} \qquad (2)$$

The Δ-change associated with the exercise bout (i.e., the difference between pre- and post-Wingate) was calculated as follow:

$$\Delta\text{-change exercise} = \text{POST} - \text{PRE} \qquad (3)$$

To assess the relationships between (i) physical and performance and (ii) psychological, physiological, and reaction time parameters, Bland–Altman correlations were used. The significant difference was set at an alpha level of $p \leq 0.05$ throughout, except in those cases in which multiple

3. Results

3.1. Participant Characteristics

Over the study, three participants were unable to complete all test sessions due to muscle pain or injury (Figure 2). Thus, 19 participants (age: 21.2 ± 1.2 years; height: 1.76 ± 0.8 m; body-mass: 76.6 ± 12.6 kg) completed all test sessions (Figure 2).

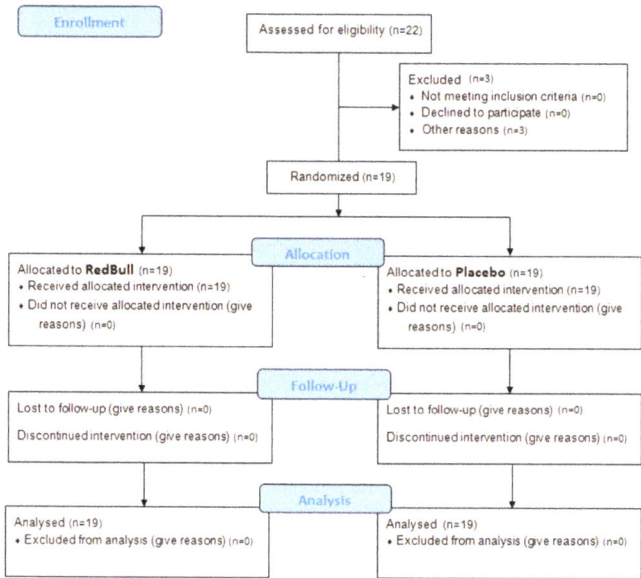

Figure 2. CONSORT flow chart-trial of the study protocol.

3.2. Physical Performance and Reaction Times

Physical parameters and reaction time recorded during the RB and PL conditions are presented in Table 1.

Table 1. Confidence intervals (CI), Δ-change and mean and standard deviations (SD) of peak and mean power and the fatigue index registered during the Wingate test, handgrip force, and reaction times recorded during the Red Bull (RB) and placebo (PL) conditions.

Parameters	PL		RB		Δ-Change
	Mean ± SD	CI	Mean ± SD	CI	
Peak power (W·kg^{-1})	10.5 ± 1.5	9.8–11.2	11.4 ± 0.9	11.0–11.9	0.93 *
Mean power (W·kg^{-1})	8.1 ± 1.0	7.65–8.63	9.01 ± 0.92	8.56–9.46	0.87 **
Fatigue index (%)	47.9 ± 8.1	44.0–51.8	49.1 ± 4.8	46.8–51.4	1.21
Hand grip force (kg)	55.5 ± 2.7	54.18–57.03	58.2 ± 2.4	56.8–59.4	2.69 **
Reaction time (s)	0.36 ± 0.05	0.34–0.39	0.28 ± 0.02	0.27–0.29	−0.08 ***

*, **, ***: Significant difference between RB and PL at $p < 0.05$, $p < 0.01$ and $p < 0.001$ respectively.

Statistical analysis showed a significant improvement for peak power ($t = -2.33$; $p = 0.0250$), mean power ($t = -2.74$; $p = 0.0093$), and hand grip force ($t = -3.21$; $p = 0.0027$) between PL and RB and there was a significant reduction in the reaction time ($t = 5.94$; $p < 0.0005$) with RB ingestion as compared to PL, but there was no significant difference of fatigue index between the two drink conditions ($t = -0.56$; $p = 0.5775$).

3.3. Blood Glucose and Blood Pressures

Blood glucose levels recorded pre- and post-exercise are presented in Figure 3.

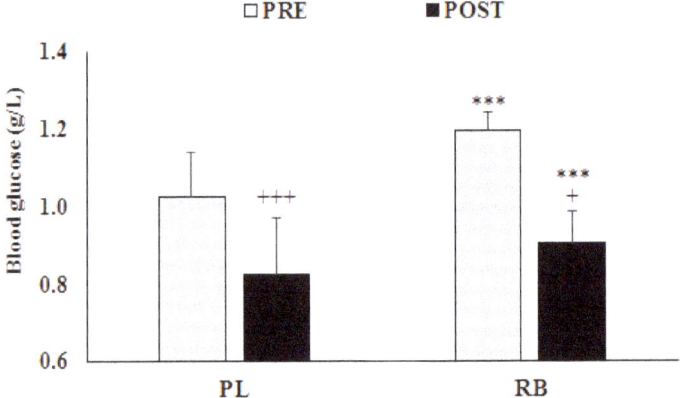

Figure 3. Evolution of blood glucose levels (mean ± SD) from pre- to post-exercise during the placebo (PL) and the Red Bull (RB) sessions. ***: Significant differences compared to PL at $p < 0.001$. +, +++: Significant difference compared to pre-exercise at $p < 0.05$ and $p < 0.001$ respectively.

There were significant main effects for Drink (F = 36.75; $\eta_p^2 = 0.67$; $p < 0.0005$) and Exercise (F = 76.94; $\eta_p^2 = 0.81$; $p < 0.0005$), and the interaction Drink × Exercise was also significant (F = 8.96; $\eta_p^2 = 0.33$; $p = 0.0077$). Post-hoc testing showed that blood glucose was significantly lower after rather than before exercise in both conditions ($p < 0.0005$ for PL and for RB), with a greater reduction during RB than in the PL condition (Δ-change: −0.29 g/L vs. −0.20 g/L). However, post-hoc testing revealed significant increases of blood glucose with RB in comparison to PL, both pre- ($p < 0.0005$) and post-exercise ($p = 0.0105$), with greater gains before rather than after exercise (Δ-change: 0.17 g/L vs. 0.08 g/L).

Blood pressures before and after exercise are presented in Figure 4.

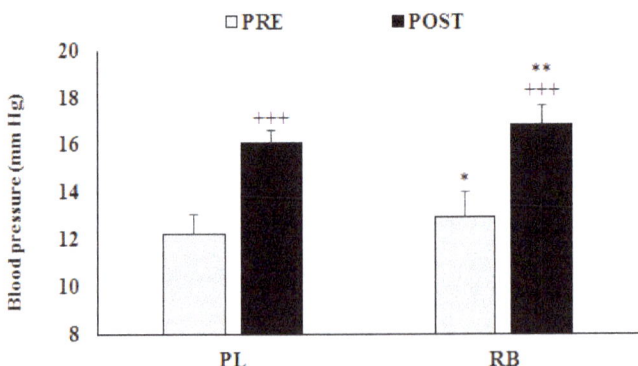

Figure 4. Evolution of blood pressure (Mean ± SD) between pre- and post-exercise during the placebo (PL) and the red bull (RB) sessions. *, **: Significant difference compare to PL at $p < 0.05$ and $p < 0.01$ respectively. +++: Significant difference compared to pre-exercise at $p < 0.001$.

There were significant main effects for Drink (F = 34.30; η_p^2 = 0.65; p < 0.0005) and Exercise (F = 216.49; η_p^2 = 0.92; p < 0.0005), but the interaction Drink × Exercise was not significant (F = 0.02; η_p^2 = 0.001; p = 0.9005). Post-hoc testing showed significantly higher values of blood pressure after than before exercise in both conditions (p < 0.0005). Moreover, post-hoc tests revealed significant greater blood pressure with RB in comparison to PL at both pre- (p = 0.0120) and post-exercise (p = 0.0080).

3.4. Ratings of Perceived Exertion (RPE), Affective Load and Profile of Mood States (POMS)

POMS parameters, affective load and RPE during PL and RB conditions are presented in Table 2.

Table 2. Confidence interval (CI), Δ-change and mean and standard deviation (SD) for individual Profile of Mood State parameters (i.e., depression, confusion, fatigue, vigor, anger, and anxiety) and ratings of perceived exertion (RPE) recorded during the red bull (RB) and placebo (PL) conditions.

POMS Parameter/RPE	PL		BE		Δ-Change (AU) Induced by RB
	Mean ± SD	CI	Mean ± SD	CI	
Depression (AU)	6.1 ± 5.1	3.6–8.5	4.8 ± 2.2	3.8–5.9	−1.2
Confusion (AU)	7.3 ± 6.0	4.4–10.2	4.2 ± 2.0	3.2–5.1	−3.1 *
Fatigue (AU)	13.8 ± 2.1	12.9–14.8	12.7 ± 2.1	11.7–13.8	−1.1 *
Vigor (AU)	14.7 ± 5.8	12.0–17.5	18.2 ± 4.2	16.1–20.2	3.4 *
Anger (AU)	4.8 ± 3.2	3.2–6.3	3.4 ± 3.2	1.9–5.0	−14.*
Anxiety (AU)	10.8 ± 5.3	8.2–13.3	8.3 ± 2.9	6.9–9.7	−2.5
RPE (AU)	17.5 ± 1.3	16.9–18.2	15.9 ± 1.1	15.4–16.4	−17 ***
Affective load (AU)	9.1 ± 2.6	7.8–10.3	5.8 ± 2.1	4.8–6.8	−3.3 ***

*, ***: Significant difference between RB and PL at p < 0.05 and p < 0.001 respectively.

Although no significant difference between the two drinks conditions was reported for depression (t = 1.07; p = 0.2952) and anxiety (t = 1.94; p = 0.0675), RB was associated with a significant reduction in scores for confusion (t = 2.32; p = 0.0322), fatigue (t = 2.34; p = 0.0305), anger (t = 2.43; p = 0.0258), RPE (t = 4.30; p = 0.0001), and affective load (t = 4.77; p = 0.0001). In contrast, vigor increased significantly (t = −2.63; p = 0.0167) with RB.

3.5. Correlations between the Recorded Parameters

Peak power was significantly correlated with RPE (r = −0.48; p = 0.0322), affective load (r = −0.48; p = 0.0322), pre- (r = 0.59; p < 0.01) and post-exercise (r = 0.65; p = 0.0019) levels of blood glucose, and scores for fatigue (r = −0.50; p = 0.0230) and anxiety (r = −0.50; p = 0.0244). Mean power was also significantly correlated with RPE (r = −0.64; p = 0.0023), affective load (r = −0.64; p = 0.0023), pre- (r = 0.68; p = 0.0009) and post-exercise (r = 0.69; p = 0.0007) blood glucose levels, pre-exercise blood pressure (r = −0.50; p = 0.0233) and scores for fatigue (r = −0.55; p = 0.0113) and anger (r = −0.54; p = 0.0148). However, no significant correlations were observed between fatigue index and blood glucose, blood pressure POMS scores, affective load, or RPE. Handgrip force was significantly correlated with RPE (r = −0.60 p = 0.0049), affective load (r = −0.60; p = 0.0049), pre- (r = 0.78; p < 0.0005) and post-exercise (r = 0.57; p = 0.0082) blood glucose and pre- (r = 0.62; p = 0.0037) and post-exercise (r = 0.54; p = 0.0139) blood pressures. Reaction time was significantly correlated with RPE (r = 0.72; p < 0.0005), affective load (r = 0.72; p < 0.0005), pre- (r = 0.57; p = 0.0080) and post-exercise (r = 0.48; p = 0.0290) blood glucose, pre- (r = −0.73; p < 0.0005) and post-exercise (r = −0.72; p < 0.0005) blood pressures and POMS scores for confusion (r = 0.46; p = 0.0387), vigor (r = −0.62; p = 0.0035), and anger (r = 0.46; p = 0.0393).

4. Discussion

The main findings from the present study were that RB increases peak power (+0.93 W·kg^{-1}) and mean power (+0.87 W·kg^{-1}) during the 30-s Wingate test, and handgrip force (+2.69 kg), also speeding the reaction time (−0.08 s). Additionally, physiological responses to exercise (i.e., blood glucose and blood pressure) are increased and the RB increases vigor with reduction of ratings for depression, confusion, fatigue, anger, anxiety, RPE, and affective load.

In agreement with the present results, Alford et al. [11] reported that RB had a positive effect on short-term maximal performance during the Wingate test. Forbes et al. [34] also found that RB tended to a positive (but not significant effect) on peak and mean power during three consecutive Wingate tests. The latter authors also reported significant increases in total repetitions over three sets of bench press exercises.

In the present study, increases of peak and mean power during the 30-s Wingate test were significantly correlated with decreases in RPE, affective load, and scores for fatigue, anxiety (for peak power only), and anger (for mean power only). Increases in handgrip force were also related to decreases of RPE and affective load. A previous study also reported that the handgrip force was greater after caffeinated-ED than after PL [7,35]. In agreement with the present study' results, Hahn et al. [8] reported significant reductions in fatigue scores when performing a repeated-sprint exercise. However, they did not show any improvement in performance during the repeated sprinting. From the present results, the increases in short-term maximal performances induced by RB could be explained by a reduced perception of exertion and fatigue. Increases are also related to a reduction of affective load, a change of perceptions in that part of the brain responsible for pacing strategy during physical exercise.

Pacing regulates energy expenditures during exercise. Better short-term maximal performance after RB ingestion reflects higher energy expenditures, as shown by the higher pre- and post-exercise blood glucose concentrations during the RB session and by the greater decreases of blood sugar from before to after exercise (−0.29 g/L vs. −0.20 g/L in PL).

Lim et al. [36] showed that in people who do not normally consume caffeine, taurine ingestion is detrimental to maximal voluntary muscle power and both maximal isometric and isokinetic peak torque, whereas taurine ingestion in caffeine-deprived caffeine consumers improves maximal voluntary muscle power but has no effect on other aspects of contractile performance.

Graham et al. [37] showed that the beneficial effects of caffeine ingestion on short-term maximal performance were related to muscle fat oxidation and better glycogen sparing capacity. A recent meta-analysis by Grgic [38] and by Grgic et al. [39] concluded that caffeine ingestion may increase both peak and mean power output during the Wingate test. In an umbrella review of 21 published meta-analyses, Grgic et al. [40] concluded that caffeine ingestion improved a broad range of exercise performance measures such as muscle strength, muscle endurance, anaerobic power, and aerobic endurance. Mechanisms explaining such findings include an increased Ca^{2+} release from the sarcoplasmic reticulum, which may lead to an increase in tetanic tension, and the alterations that caffeine might have on the neuromuscular transmission [41]. In an animal study, it has been shown that caffeine may enhance Ca^{2+} release from the sarcoplasmic reticulum and improve motor unit recruitment by inhibiting the action of adenosine on the central nervous system [42]. Glucose is an important metabolic substrate responsible for most of the energy release during anaerobic exercise. Thus, the pre- and post-exercise increases of blood glucose could, in part, explain the improvement of short-term maximal performance.

In support of these hypotheses, the present results demonstrated a significant correlation between peak and mean power during the 30-s Wingate test and the pre- and post-exercise glucose. Also, it has been reported that glucose increases are related to an improvement in cognitive performance [43]. In this context, the present study showed significant correlations between pre- and post-exercise blood glucose and reaction time. Alford et al. [11] also reported significant improvements in choice reaction time, memory, and concentration (i.e., the number of correct cancellations) after RB ingestion compared to the PL condition. These authors concluded that RB ingestion improved alertness. This same conclusion is supported by Mets et al. [44], who showed that RB ingestion improved driving performance and reduced driver sleepiness. The present study indicated a significant correlation between peak and mean power during the Wingate test and negative components of mood state (i.e., anxiety and anger).

Lara et al. [45] also reported a significant improvement in the short-term maximal performance of swimmers and a significant reduction in anxiety scores after ED consumption.

The present study demonstrated a significant correlation between (i) reaction time and (ii) positive (i.e., vigor) and negative (i.e., confusion and anger) components of mood state. Therefore, the enhancement of reaction time could be explained in part by a reduction of confusion and anger and an improvement of vigor. These findings are supported by Wesnes et al. [15] who suggested that cognitive performance increased with the improvement of positive and a reduction of negative components of mood state. On the other hand, as previously reported by Del Coso et al. [4,5] and Abian-Vicen et al. [6] some subjects do not seem to respond to the ergogenic effects of caffeine-containing ED. In the present study, four participants could be classified as non- responders in terms of their performance on the Wingate test; although their performance of the handgrip and reaction time tests did improve after RB ingestion compared to the PL.

Limitations

One limitation when interpreting this research is that the commercially-prepared ED evaluated contained several potentially ergogenic ingredients, including compounds such as caffeine, carbohydrates, and taurine while the PL control drink did not include these substances. Therefore, it was not possible to identify the specific influence of any one of these several active ingredients on performance. Future studies should focus on the specific influence of individual active ingredients.

Another limitation inherent to the present study is that the participants were not regular caffeine users and, then, results could not be generalized to people who do regularly consume caffeine. Also, the fact that no-baseline (i.e., before RB or PL consumption) measurement was performed represents another shortcoming of the present investigation.

No immediate adverse effects were seen from the RB, but a more deliberate search for negative consequences of caffeine ingestion, such as an increase of speed at the expense of skills, would seem justified. Another limitation of the present study is that enrolled subjects were all male. Future studies using female or mixed-gender samples are warranted.

Further, the effectiveness of subject blinding was not tested by post-study debriefing. This is of some importance, because outcomes may be influenced if a participant recognizes that one of the beverages provided contains caffeine [46]. Tallis et al. [47] underlined that the psychological effects of "expectancy" and "belief" could have a significant impact on performance. Therefore, future studies should use a double-blind design and assess the effectiveness of the blinding.

5. Conclusions

The present study has demonstrated that cognitive (i.e., reaction time) and short-term maximal (i.e., handgrip and Wingate) performances are improved after RB ingestion. Further, ingestion of this ED increases physiological responses to the 30-s Wingate test, with increases of pre- and post-exercise blood glucose and blood pressures. Further RB consumption reduces negative effects on mood state (i.e., decreased scores for depression, confusion, fatigue, anger, and anxiety) and enhances the positive components of mood state (i.e., vigor), with favorable changes of RPE and affective load, thus leading to improvements in physical performance.

Gains of physical performance after RB consumption reflect changes in blood glucose and blood pressure. Cognitive gains (i.e., a speeding of reaction time) are related to both psychological (i.e., a reduction of confusion, anger, and RPE and an increase of vigor) and physiological responses (i.e., changes in blood glucose and blood pressure) ergogenic changes.

Author Contributions: Conceptualization, H.C. and K.T.; methodology, H.C., K.T., A.A., and N.L.B.; software, A.A.; validation, H.C., K.T., and N.L.B.; formal analysis, A.A. and N.L.B.; investigation, H.C., K.T., A.A., and N.L.B.; resources, N.L.B.; data curation, A.A.; writing—original draft preparation, H.C., K.T., and A.A.; writing—review and editing, N.L.B. and R.J.S.; visualization, N.L.B.; supervision, H.C.; project administration, N.L.B.; funding acquisition, N.L.B.

Funding: This research received no external funding.

Conflicts of Interest: The authors declare no conflict of interest.

References

1. Higgins, J.P.; Babu, K.; Deuster, P.A.; Shearer, J. Energy drinks: A contemporary issues paper. *Curr. Sports Med. Rep.* **2018**, *17*, 65–72. [CrossRef]
2. Jacobson, B.H.; Hester, G.M.; Palmer, T.B.; Williams, K.; Pope, Z.K.; Sellers, J.H.; Conchola, E.C.; Woolsey, C.; Estrada, C. Effect of energy drink consumption on power and velocity of selected sport performance activities. *J. Strength Cond. Res.* **2018**, *32*, 1613–1618. [CrossRef] [PubMed]
3. Froiland, K.; Koszewski, W.; Hingst, J.; Kopecky, L. Nutritional supplement use among college athletes and their sources of information. *Int. J. Sport. Nutr. Exerc. Metab.* **2004**, *14*, 104–120. [CrossRef]
4. Del Coso, J.; Portillo, J.; Muñoz, G.; Abián-Vicén, J.; Gonzalez-Millán, C.; Muñoz-Guerra, J. Caffeine containing energy drink improves sprint performance during an international rugby sevens competition. *Amino Acids* **2013**, *44*, 1511–1519. [CrossRef] [PubMed]
5. Del Coso, J.; Ramirez, J.A.; Muñoz, G.; Portillo, J.; Gonzalez-Millán, C.; Muñoz, V.; Barbero-Álvarez, J.C.; Muñoz-Guerra, J. Caffeine containing energy drink improves physical performance of elite rugby players during a simulated match. *Appl. Physiol. Nutr. Metab.* **2013**, *38*, 368–374. [CrossRef]
6. Abian-Vicen, J.; Puente, C.; Salinero, J.J.; González-Millán, C.; Areces, F.; Muñoz, G.; Muñoz-Guerra, J.; Del Coso, J. A caffeinated energy drink improves jump performance in adolescent basketball players. *Amino Acids* **2014**, *46*, 1333–1341. [CrossRef]
7. Del Coso, J.; Pérez-López, A.; Abian-Vicen, L.; Salinero, J.J.; Lara, B.; Valadés, D. Enhancing physical performance in male volleyball players with a caffeine-containing energy drink. *Int. J. Sports Physiol. Perform.* **2014**, *9*, 1013–1018. [CrossRef]
8. Hahn, C.J.; Jagim, A.R.; Camic, C.L.; Andre, M.J. Acute Effects of a Caffeine-Containing Supplement on Anaerobic Power and Subjective Measurements of Fatigue in Recreationally Active Men. *J. Strength Cond. Res.* **2018**, *32*, 1029–1035. [CrossRef] [PubMed]
9. Fukuda, D.; Smith, A.; Kendall, K.; Stout, J. The possible combinatory effects of acute consumption of caffeine, creatine, and amino acids on the improvement of anaerobic running performance in humans. *Nutr. Res.* **2010**, *30*, 607–614. [CrossRef]
10. Gwacham, N.; Wagner, D.R. Acute effects of a caffeine-taurine energy drink on repeated sprint performance of American college football players. *Int. J. Sport Nutr. Exerc. Metab.* **2012**, *22*, 109–116. [CrossRef]
11. Alford, C.; Cox, H.; Wescott, R. The effects of red bull energy drink on human performance and mood. *Amino Acids* **2001**, *21*, 139–150. [CrossRef]
12. Hoffman, J.; Kang, J.; Ratamess, N.; Hoffman, M.; Tranchina, C.; Faigenbaum, A. Examination of a pre-exercise, high energy supplement on exercise performance. *J. Int. Soc. Sports Nutr.* **2009**, *6*, 1–8. [CrossRef]
13. Brunyé, T.; Mahoney, C.; Lieberman, H.; Taylor, H. Caffeine modulates attention network function. *Brain Cogn.* **2010**, *72*, 181–188. [CrossRef]
14. Jagim, A.; Jones, M.; Wright, G.; Antoine, C.; Kovacs, A.; Oliver, J. The acute effects of multi-ingredient pre-workout ingestion on strength performance, lower body power, and anaerobic capacity. *J. Int. Soc. Sports Nutr.* **2016**, *13*, 1–10. [CrossRef]
15. Wesnes, K.A.; Brooker, H.; Watson, A.W.; Bal, W.; Okello, E. Effects of the Red Bull energy drink on cognitive function and mood in healthy young volunteers. *J. Psychopharmacol.* **2017**, *31*, 211–221. [CrossRef] [PubMed]
16. Petrelli, F.; Grappasonni, I.; Evangelista, D.; Pompei, P.; Broglia, G.; Cioffi, P.; Kracmarova, L.; Scuri, S. Mental and physical effects of energy drinks consumption in an Italian young people group: a pilot study. *J. Prev. Med. Hyg.* **2018**, *59*, E80–E87. [PubMed]
17. Del Coso, J.; Salinero, J.J.; González-Millán, C.; Abián-Vicén, J.; Pérez-González, B. Dose response effects of a caffeine-containing energy drink on muscle performance: a repeated measures design. *J. Int. Soc. Sports Nutr.* **2012**, *9*, 21. [CrossRef]
18. Beck, T.W. The importance of a priori sample size estimation in strength and conditioning research. *J. Strength. Cond. Res.* **2013**, *27*, 2323–2337. [CrossRef]
19. Faul, F.; Erdfelder, E.; Lang, A.G.; Buchner, A.G. Power 3: A flexible statistical power analysis program for the social, behavioral, and biomedical sciences. *Behav. Res. Methods.* **2007**, *39*, 175–191. [CrossRef]

20. Prins, P.J.; Goss, F.L.; Nagle, E.F.; Beals, K.; Robertson, R.J.; Lovalekar, M.T.; Welton, G.L. Energy Drinks Improve Five-Kilometer Running Performance in Recreational Endurance Runners. *J. Strength. Cond. Res.* **2016**, *30*, 2979–2990. [CrossRef]
21. Ammar, A.; Chtourou, H.; Hammouda, O.; Trabelsi, K.; Chiboub, J.; Turki, M.; AbdelKarim, O.; El Abed, K.; Ben Ali, M.; Hoekelmann, A.; Souissi, N. Acute and delayed responses of C-reactive protein, malondialdehyde and antioxidant markers after resistance training session in elite weightlifters: Effect of Time of day. *Chronobiol. Int.* **2015**, *32*, 1211–1222. [CrossRef]
22. Ammar, A.; Chtourou, H.; Souissi, N. Effect of time-of-day on biochemical markers in response to physical exercise. *J. Strength. Cond. Res.* **2017**, *31*, 272–282. [CrossRef] [PubMed]
23. Ammar, A.; Chtourou, H.; Hammouda, O.; Turki, M.; Ayedi, F.; Kallel, C.; AbdelKarim, O.; Hoekelmann, A.; Souissi, N. Relationship between biomarkers of muscle damage and redox status in response to a weightlifting training session: effect of time-of-day. *Physiol. Int.* **2016**, *103*, 243–261. [CrossRef]
24. Ammar, A.; Turki, M.; Hammouda, O.; Chtourou, H.; Trabelsi, K.; Bouaziz, M.; Abdelkarim, O.; Hoekelmann, A.; Ayadi, F.; Souissi, N.; Bailey, S.J.; Driss, T.; Yaich, S. Effects of Pomegranate Juice Supplementation on Oxidative Stress Biomarkers Following Weightlifting Exercise. *Nutrients* **2017**, *9*, 819. [CrossRef]
25. Ammar, A.; Bailey, S.J.; Chtourou, H.; Trabelsi, K.; Turki, M.; Hökelmann, A.; Souissi, N. Effects of pomegranate supplementation on exercise performance and post-exercise recovery: A systematic review. *Br. J. Nutr.* **2018**, *20*, 1201–1216. [CrossRef]
26. Ammar, A.; Turki, M.; Chtourou, H.; Hammouda, O.; Trabelsi, K.; Kallel, C.; Abdelkarim, O.; Hoekelmann, A.; Bouaziz, M.; Ayadi, F.; Driss, T.; Souissi, N. Pomegranate Supplementation Accelerates Recovery of Muscle Damage and Soreness and Inflammatory Markers after a Weightlifting Training Session. *PLoS ONE* **2016**, *11*, e0160305. [CrossRef]
27. Armstrong, L.E. Caffeine, body fluid-electrolyte balance, and exercise performance. *Int. J. Sport Nutr. Exerc. Metab.* **2002**, *12*, 189–206. [CrossRef] [PubMed]
28. Graham, T.E. Caffeine and exercise: metabolism, endurance and performance. *Sports Med.* **2001**, *31*, 785–807. [CrossRef] [PubMed]
29. Joch, W.; Uckert, S. Il riscaldamento ed i suoi effetti. *Scuola Dello Sport Italie.* **2001**, *20*, 49–54.
30. Ammar, A.; Chtourou, H.; Trabelsi, K.; Padulo, J.; Turki, M.; El Abed, K.; Hoekelmann, A.; Hakim, A. Temporal specificity of training: intra-day effects on biochemical responses and Olympic-Weightlifting performances. *J. Sports Sci.* **2015**, *33*, 358–368. [CrossRef]
31. Yeun, E.J.; Shin-Park, K.K. Verification of the profile of mood states-brief: Cross-cultural analysis. *J. Clin. Psychol.* **2006**, *62*, 1173–1180. [CrossRef]
32. Baron, B.; Moullan, F.; Deruelle, F.; Noakes, T.D. The role of emotions on pacing strategies and performance in middle and long duration sport events. *Br. J. Sports Med.* **2011**, *45*, 511–517. [CrossRef] [PubMed]
33. Abel, A.; Baron, B.; Grappe, F.; Francaux, M. Effect of environmental feedbacks on pacing strategy and affective load during a self-paced 30 min cycling time trial. *J. Sports Sci.* **2018**, *18*, 1–7.
34. Forbes, S.C.; Candow, D.G.; Little, J.P.; Magnus, C.; Chilibeck, P.D. Effect of Red Bull energy drink on repeated Wingate cycle performance and bench-press muscle endurance. *Int. J. Sport Nutr. Exerc. Metab.* **2007**, *17*, 433–444. [CrossRef]
35. Astley, C.; Souza, D.B.; Polito, M.D. Acute Specific Effects of Caffeine-containing Energy Drink on Different Physical Performances in Resistance-trained Men. *Int. J. Exerc. Sci.* **2018**, *11*, 260–268.
36. Lim, Z.X.; Singh, A.; Leow, Z.Z.X.; Arthur, P.G.; Fournier, P.A. The Effect of Acute Taurine Ingestion on Human Maximal Voluntary Muscle Contraction. *Med. Sci. Sports Exerc.* **2018**, *50*, 344–352. [CrossRef] [PubMed]
37. Graham, T.E.; Battram, D.S.; Dela, F.; El-Sohemy, A.; Thong, F.S. Does caffeine alter muscle carbohydrate and fat metabolism during exercise? *Appl. Physiol. Nutr. Metab.* **2008**, *33*, 1311–1318. [CrossRef]
38. Grgic, J. Caffeine ingestion enhances Wingate performance: a meta-analysis. *Eur. J. Sport Sci.* **2018**, *18*, 219–225. [CrossRef] [PubMed]
39. Grgic, J.; Trexler, E.T.; Lazinica, B.; Pedisic, Z. Effects of caffeine intake on muscle strength and power: A systematic review and meta-analysis. *J. Int. Soc. Sports Nutr.* **2018**, *15*, 11. [CrossRef]

40. Grgic, J.; Grgic, I.; Pickering, C.; Schoenfeld, B.J.; Bishop, D.J.; Pedisic, Z. Wake up and smell the coffee: Caffeine supplementation and exercise performance—An umbrella review of 21 published meta-analyses. *Br. J. Sports Med.* **2019**. [CrossRef] [PubMed]
41. Davis, J.K.; Green, J.M. Caffeine and anaerobic performance: Ergogenic value and mechanisms of action. *Sports Med.* **2009**, *39*, 813–832. [CrossRef] [PubMed]
42. Davis, J.M.; Zhao, Z.; Stock, H.S.; Mehl, K.A.; Buggy, J.; Hand, G.A. Central nervous system effects of caffeine and adenosine on fatigue. *Am. J. Physiol. Regul. Integr. Comp. Physiol.* **2003**, *284*, R399–R404. [CrossRef] [PubMed]
43. Benton, D.; Owens, D.S. Blood glucose and human memory. *Psychopharmacology* **1993**, *113*, 83–88. [CrossRef] [PubMed]
44. Mets, M.A.; Ketzer, S.; Blom, C.; van Gerven, M.H.; van Willigenburg, G.M.; Olivier, B.; Verster, J.C. Positive effects of Red Bull® Energy Drink on driving performance during prolonged driving. *Psychopharmacology* **2011**, *214*, 737–745. [CrossRef] [PubMed]
45. Lara, B.; Gonzalez-Millán, C.; Salinero, J.J.; Abian-Vicen, J.; Areces, F.; Barbero-Alvarez, J.C.; Muñoz, V.; Portillo, L.J.; Gonzalez-Rave, J.M.; Del Coso, J. Caffeine containing energy drink improves physical performance in female soccer players. *Amino Acids.* **2014**, *46*, 1385–1392. [CrossRef] [PubMed]
46. Saunders, B.; de Oliveira, L.F.; da Silva, R.P.; de Salles Painelli, V.; Gonçalves, L.S.; Yamaguchi, G.; Mutti, T.; Maciel, E.; Roschel, H.; Artioli, G.G.; Gualano, B. Placebo in sports nutrition: A proof-of-principle study involving caffeine supplementation. *Scand. J. Med. Sci. Sports.* **2017**, *27*, 1240–1247. [CrossRef]
47. Tallis, J.; Muhammad, B.; Islam, M.; Duncan, M.J. Placebo effects of caffeine on maximal voluntary concentric force of the knee flexors and extensors. *Muscle Nerve.* **2016**, *54*, 479–486. [CrossRef] [PubMed]

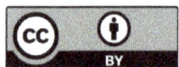

© 2019 by the authors. Licensee MDPI, Basel, Switzerland. This article is an open access article distributed under the terms and conditions of the Creative Commons Attribution (CC BY) license (http://creativecommons.org/licenses/by/4.0/).

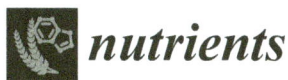

Communication

Challenging the Myth of Non-Response to the Ergogenic Effects of Caffeine Ingestion on Exercise Performance

Juan Del Coso *, Beatriz Lara, Carlos Ruiz-Moreno and Juan José Salinero

Exercise Physiology Laboratory, Camilo José Cela University, 28692 Madrid, Spain; blara@ucjc.edu (B.L.); cruizm@ucjc.edu (C.R.-M.); jjsalinero@ucjc.edu (J.J.S.)
* Correspondence: jdelcoso@ucjc.edu; Tel.: +34-918-153-131

Received: 7 March 2019; Accepted: 27 March 2019; Published: 29 March 2019

Abstract: The ergogenicity of caffeine on several exercise and sport situations is well-established. However, the extent of the ergogenic response to acute caffeine ingestion might greatly vary among individuals despite using the same dosage and timing. The existence of one or several individuals that obtained minimal ergogenic effects or even slightly ergolytic effects after caffeine intake (i.e., non-responders) has been reported in several previous investigations. Nevertheless, the concept non-responding to caffeine, in terms of physical performance, relies on investigations based on the measurement of one performance variable obtained once. Recently it has been suggested that correct identification of the individual ergogenic effect induced by caffeine intake requires the repeated measurement of physical performance in identical caffeine–placebo comparisons. In this communication, we present data from an investigation where the ergogenic effect of acute caffeine intake (3 mg/kg) was measured eight times over a placebo in the same individuals and under the same conditions by an incremental cycling test to volitional fatigue and an adapted version of the Wingate cycling test. The ergogenic response to caffeine varied from 9% to 1% among individuals, but all participants increased both cycling power in the incremental test and Wingate mean power at least three to eight times out of eight the caffeine–placebo comparisons. These data expand the suggestion of a minimal occurrence of caffeine non-responders because it shows that all individuals responded to caffeine when caffeine is compared to a placebo on multiple and repeated testing sessions.

Keywords: individual responses; responders; exercise performance; ergogenic aids

1. Introduction

2018 has been a prolific year for the publication of manuscripts aimed at explaining the causes of the interindividual variations for the ergogenic response of caffeine ingestion on exercise performance. Particularly, we read with interest the reviews by Southward et al. [1] and Fulton et al. [2] and the letter by Grgic [3], published in *Nutrients* in 2018, because they offered new insights towards unveiling the causes of the variability on physiological responses to caffeine. With this communication, we want to expand the understanding about why some individuals obtain less ergogenic benefits after the ingestion of a moderate dose of caffeine than others, and perhaps it will help to dispel the myth/concept of non-responders to caffeine, at least when referring to exercise performance.

2. Individual Responses to Ergogenic Effects of Caffeine Ingestion

The utility of caffeine to increase physical performance in several exercise and sport situations is well-established and has been recently confirmed by systematic reviews and meta-analyses [4–7]. In addition, the use of caffeine or caffeinated products before competition is high, especially in individual sports or athletes of sports with an aerobic-like nature [8]. However, a small number of investigations have shown that the extent of the ergogenic response(s) to acute caffeine ingestion might greatly vary among individuals ([9–11] and the analysis of several investigations in [3]). These latter investigations have used cross-over and randomized experimental designs where the intake of a moderate dose of caffeine (1–6 mg/kg) is compared to a placebo condition in a group of individuals. Interestingly, these investigations indicated that, despite caffeine having produced an increase in physical performance as a group mean, one or several individuals obtained minimal ergogenic effects or even slightly ergolytic effects after caffeine intake despite being under the same experimental protocol. These individuals are frequently categorized as non-responders to the ergogenic effects of caffeine [12] and the causes for the lack of a positive physical response to caffeine have been associated to genetic (CYP1A2 and ADORA2A polymorphisms) and environmental factors, such as tolerance developed by chronic caffeine use and inappropriate timing and dose of administration or training status [13,14].

3. The Concept of Non-Responding to Caffeine Based on One Caffeine–Placebo Comparison

Recently, Pickering and Kiely [13] and Grgic [3] have criticized the concept non-responding to caffeine, in terms of physical performance, because this notion mostly relies on investigations based on the measurement of one performance variable obtained once. This experimental methodology to assess individual responses to caffeine ingestion might produce erroneous inferences because an individual does not always respond to caffeine to the same extent in all forms of exercise testing [9,15]. In addition, the reliability of the exercise test also needs to be considered when extrapolating conclusions regarding possible non-responses to the performance-enhancing effects of acute caffeine intake [3]. In fact, investigations where the ergogenic response to caffeine was explored by using the results of more than one physical performance test have shown that one participant might be categorized as a responder and a non-responder to caffeine at the same time due to his/her different outcomes in the different performance tests [9,15]. Pickering and Kiely [13] and Grgic [3] concur in suggesting that correct identification of the individual ergogenic effect induced by caffeine intake requires the repeated measurement of physical performance in identical caffeine–placebo comparisons. As suggested by Grgic [3], one of the following options can be selected to assess the individual ergogenic effect induced by caffeine: (1) multiple exercise tests with the same dose of caffeine or, (2) multiple doses of caffeine with the same exercise test, or (3) using a more complex protocol that combines repeated assessments of physical performance on different days using the same exercise test and dose of caffeine. If this is the case, most of the previous investigations on the study of individual responses to ergogenic effects of caffeine might not be methodologically correct because the categorization has been mainly based on one caffeine–placebo comparison.

4. Repeated Testing of the Ergogenic Effect of Caffeine Ingestion Measured on Two Exercise Tests

We have recently published an investigation where the ergogenic effect of caffeine (3 mg/kg) was measured eight times over a placebo in the same individuals by using two physical performance tests: an incremental cycling test to volitional fatigue (25 W/minutes) and an adapted version of the Wingate cycling test [16]. The performance measurements were accompanied by the measurement of resting blood pressure, in addition to other physiological variables. The investigation was aimed at determining the time course of tolerance to the performance benefits of caffeine, and 11 participants ingested 3 mg/kg/day of caffeine, or a placebo, for 20 consecutive days. It is important to indicate that all participants were light caffeine consumers and refrained from all sources of dietary caffeine for the month before the onset of the experiment to eliminate the effect of habituation to caffeine (which represents another possible source of error when assessing individual responses). The caffeine–placebo comparisons were made after 1, 4, 6, 8, 13, 15, 18, and 20 days of consecutive caffeine or placebo ingestion while the order of the 20-day treatments was randomized. The coefficient of variation of the exercise tests and of the arterial blood pressure measurement were calculated by using the values obtained in the 20-day placebo treatment. A complete description of methods and standardizations can be found in the publication of this experiment [16].

Because the tolerance to the ergogenic effect of caffeine was not completed after 20 days of consecutive ingestion, we have performed a sub-analysis for this communication to present the individual responses to acute caffeine intake in each of the eight identical caffeine–placebo comparisons. Figure 1 presents individual box-and-whisker plots for changes induced by caffeine intake, over the ingestion of a placebo, on cycling power obtained during the incremental test (Wmax) and mean cycling power obtained during the 15-second Wingate test. Figure 1 is a clear example of the interindividual variability in response to caffeine ingestion, with diverse caffeine-induced ergogenicity observed among individuals. Figure 1 has been organized in a ergogenicity-decrescent manner from left to right, with the participant showing the highest response to the ergogenic effects of caffeine at the left (subject 1 = 9.0 ± 3.6% and 2.3 ± 1.4% for Wmax and Wingate cycling power, respectively) and the individual with the lowest response at the right (subject 11 = 0.6 ± 6.3% and 1.6 ± 4.2% for Wmax and Wingate cycling power, respectively). Furthermore, Figure 1 also shows the intraindividual variability for the ergogenic effects of caffeine on both exercise performance tests. This figure disputes the notion of non-responding to the ergogenic effect of caffeine because all of the 11 included participants improved performance following caffeine ingestion, in either the graded exercise test or the Wingate test, in at least three testing occasions (with the magnitude of improvements exceeding the coefficient of variation for each test). These data expand the suggestion of a minimal occurrence of non-responders [3] because it shows that all individuals responded to caffeine, to an extent above the random error of the performance tests, when a repeated caffeine–placebo testing protocol was used to assess individual responses to caffeine. Thus, in the opinion of the authors of this manuscript, the concept of non-responders to the ergogenic effects of caffeine should be revisited.

Figure 2 offers further insights on this topic because it presents individual data on caffeine-induced changes on resting systolic and diastolic blood pressure, measured before exercise, which is a variable also employed to categorize individual responses to acute caffeine ingestion [17]. As it happens with the ergogenic effect of caffeine, the outcomes of caffeine on blood pressure had great inter- and intraindividual variability. However, the participants with the highest responses to the cardiovascular effects of caffeine were the ones with the lowest response to the ergogenic effects of caffeine (with the exception of subject 5). To further explore this relationship, Figure 3 associates ergogenic and cardiovascular responses to caffeine ingestion. Interestingly, changes induced by caffeine intake in both systolic and diastolic blood pressures were negatively related to caffeine ergogenicity in both cycling performance tests. Briefly, this would mean that the individual with a high response to the cardiovascular effects of caffeine would be less prone to obtain ergogenic benefits from this substance. Although the mechanism behind this association is not evident from the current analysis, the association between high cardiovascular response to caffeine and decreased performance effects of caffeine has support in the literature. Wardle et al. [18] found that high cardiovascular responders to a 200-mg dose of caffeine decreased their willingness to exert an effort, a negative outcome that was not present in low cardiovascular responders to caffeine. This information might suggest that the cardiovascular and performance effects of caffeine might be incompatible and implies that high and low responders to the ergogenic effect of caffeine may exhibit divergent blood pressure response following acute caffeine ingestion. However, given the overall low sample number of the current study, this is an area that merits future research. If we can pinpoint that simple measurements such as blood pressure responses to caffeine ingestion are related to the magnitude of improvements in performance, this information may be of considerable practical importance for coaches and athletes when determining an optimal approach to caffeine supplementation.

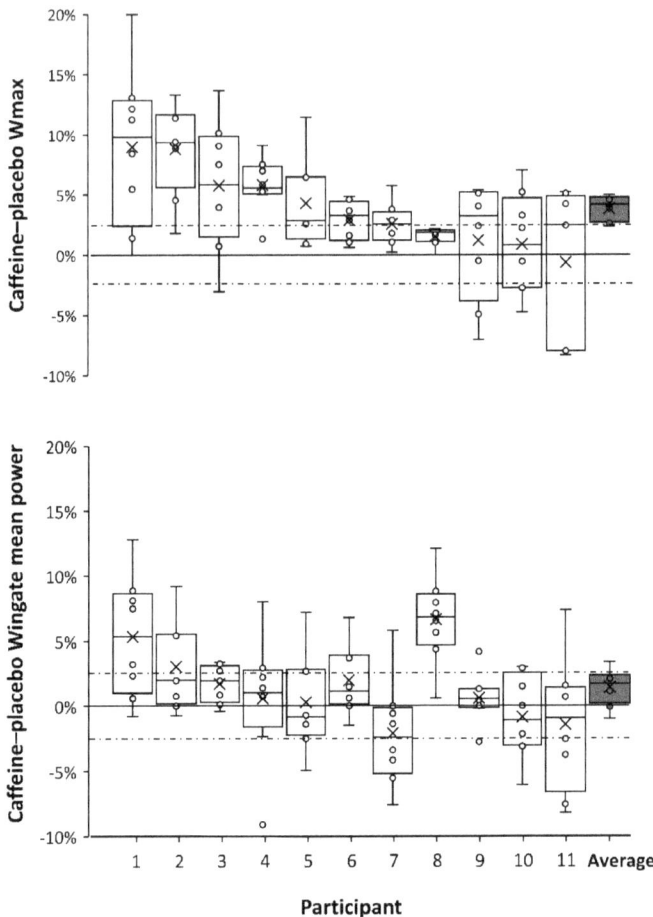

Figure 1. Box-and-whisker plots for the ergogenic effects of 3 mg/kg of caffeine on cycling power during a graded exercise test (upper panel) and during a 15-second Wingate test (lower panel). Caffeine was compared to a placebo on eight different occasions and each plot represents the results of these eight caffeine–placebo comparisons for each participant. "Average" represents the mean values for all 11 participants. The cross depicts the mean value for each individual while the lower, middle, and upper lines of the box represent the 25%, 50%, and 75% percentile for each individual. Whiskers represent the lowest and highest values (range). The black dashed line represents the natural variation of the graded exercise test ($\pm$ 2.4%) and the 15-second Wingate test ($\pm$ 2.7%) measured during the placebo treatment.

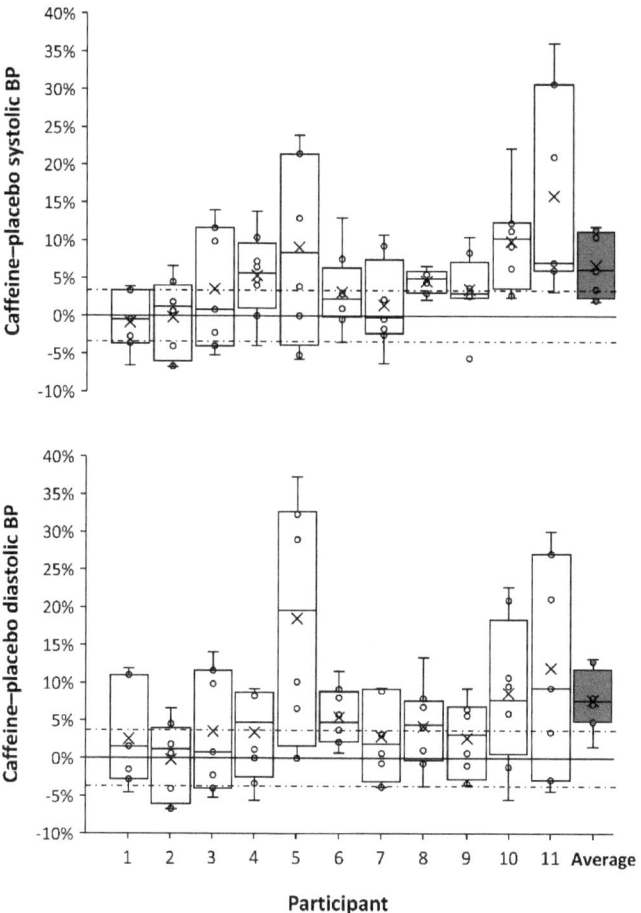

Figure 2. Box-and-whisker plots for the effects of 3 mg/kg of caffeine on resting systolic (upper panel) and diastolic (lower panel) blood pressure (BP). Caffeine was compared to a placebo on eight different occasions and each plot represents the results of these eight caffeine–placebo comparisons for each participant. "Average" represents the mean values for all 11 participants. The cross depicts the mean value for each individual while the lower, middle, and upper lines of the box represent the 25%, 50%, and 75% percentile for each individual. Whiskers represent the lowest and highest values (range). The black dashed line represents the natural variation of the systolic (± 3.3%) and diastolic blood pressure (± 3.8%) measured during the placebo treatment.

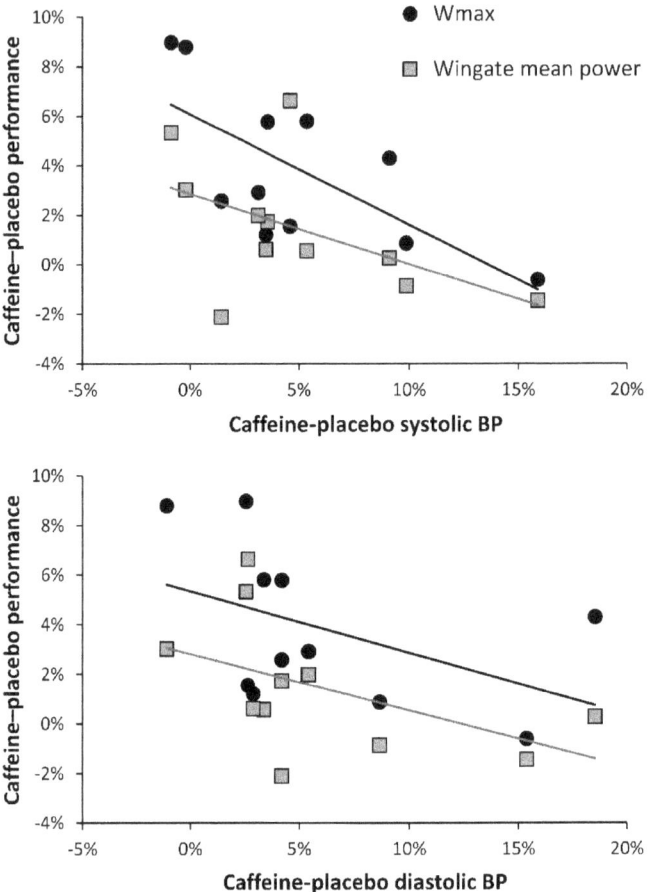

Figure 3. Relationships between the ergogenic effect of caffeine and systolic (upper panel) and diastolic (lower panel) blood pressure (BP). The ergogenic effect of caffeine was obtained by measuring peak cycling power during a graded exercise test (Wmax) and during a 15-second Wingate test. Caffeine was compared to a placebo on eight different occasions and each dot represents an average of these eight caffeine–placebo comparisons for each participant.

5. Conclusions

In conclusion, the data provided in this communication do not dispute the existence of a great interindividual variability to the ergogenic effects of caffeine ingestion, nor the genetic, environmental, or epigenetic causes associated to this variability. However, this analysis suggests that all individuals, to some extent, positively respond to the acute ingestion of 3 mg/kg of caffeine, while the magnitude of the ergogenic effect might be the result of the totality of consequences induced by caffeine ingestion on the human body. In this respect, this communication suggests that the individuals with a high response to the cardiovascular effects of caffeine would be less prone to obtaining ergogenic benefits from this stimulant. Caffeine ergogenicity might be subject to genetic influence, but future investigations on this topic should assess the individual ergogenic response to caffeine by using different forms of exercise testing and/or by using well-standardized caffeine–placebo comparisons on multiple, repeated testing sessions. In the point of view of the authors, this repeated measurement of the ergogenic effect of caffeine would help to reduce the equivocal findings of previous investigations on genetic variations [2]. From a practical perspective, the adjustment of appropriate dosage, timing, and form of administration of caffeine for an athlete might require several examinations in which physical performance and side-effects of caffeine should be measured and registered over a control situation. Gathering conclusions about the ergogenic effect of caffeine in one individual solely based on the results from one performance test might induce erroneous conclusions in both scientific and sport settings. The use of multiple, repeated comparisons between a potentially active substance vs. a placebo might also be recommended when investigating the individual ergogenic responses to other ergogenic substances/supplements.

Author Contributions: Conceptualization: J.D.C., B.L., C.R.-M., and J.J.S.; methodology: J.D.C., B.L., C.R.-M., and J.J.S.; writing—original draft preparation: J.D.C.; writing—review and editing: B.L., C.R.-M., and J.J.S.; supervision: J.D.C.; project administration: J.D.C.

Funding: This investigation did not receive any funding.

Acknowledgments: The authors of this investigation want to acknowledge the effort of all the laboratory personnel of the Doping Control Laboratory in Madrid that participated in the measurement of the urine samples that made this investigation possible.

Conflicts of Interest: The authors declare no conflict of interest.

References

1. Southward, K.; Rutherfurd-Markwick, K.; Badenhorst, C.; Ali, A. The Role of Genetics in Moderating the Inter-Individual Differences in the Ergogenicity of Caffeine. *Nutrients* **2018**, *10*. [CrossRef] [PubMed]
2. Fulton, J.L.; Dinas, P.C.; Carrillo, A.E.; Edsall, J.R.; Ryan, E.J. Impact of Genetic Variability on Physiological Responses to Caffeine in Humans: A Systematic Review. *Nutrients* **2018**, *10*. [CrossRef] [PubMed]
3. Grgic, J. Are There Non-Responders to the Ergogenic Effects of Caffeine Ingestion on Exercise Performance? *Nutrients* **2018**, *10*. [CrossRef] [PubMed]
4. Salinero, J.J.; Lara, B.; Del Coso, J. Effects of acute ingestion of caffeine on team sports performance: A systematic review and meta-analysis. *Res. Sports Med.* **2018**, 1–19. [CrossRef] [PubMed]
5. Souza, D.B.; Del Coso, J.; Casonatto, J.; Polito, M.D. Acute effects of caffeine-containing energy drinks on physical performance: A systematic review and meta-analysis. *Eur. J. Nutr.* **2017**, *56*, 13–27. [CrossRef] [PubMed]
6. Southward, K.; Rutherfurd-Markwick, K.J.; Ali, A. The Effect of Acute Caffeine Ingestion on Endurance Performance: A Systematic Review and Meta-Analysis. *Sports Med.* **2018**, *48*, 1913–1928. [CrossRef] [PubMed]
7. Grgic, J.; Trexler, E.T.; Lazinica, B.; Pedisic, Z. Effects of caffeine intake on muscle strength and power: A systematic review and meta-analysis. *J. Int. Soc. Sports Nutr.* **2018**, *15*, 11. [CrossRef] [PubMed]
8. Aguilar-Navarro, M.; Munoz, G.; Salinero, J.J.; Munoz-Guerra, J.; Fernandez-Alvarez, M.; Plata, M.D M.; Del Coso, J. Urine Caffeine Concentration in Doping Control Samples from 2004 to 2015. *Nutrients* **2019**, *11*. [CrossRef] [PubMed]
9. Lara, B.; Ruiz-Vicente, D.; Areces, F.; Abian-Vicen, J.; Salinero, J.J.; Gonzalez-Millan, C.; Gallo-Salazar, C.; Del Coso, J. Acute consumption of a caffeinated energy drink enhances aspects of performance in sprint swimmers. *Br. J. Nutr.* **2015**, *114*, 908–914. [CrossRef] [PubMed]
10. Jenkins, N.T.; Trilk, J.L.; Singhal, A.; O'Connor, P.J.; Cureton, K.J. Ergogenic effects of low doses of caffeine on cycling performance. *Int. J. Sport. Nutr. Exerc. Metab.* **2008**, *18*, 328–342. [CrossRef] [PubMed]
11. Puente, C.; Abian-Vicen, J.; Del Coso, J.; Lara, B.; Salinero, J.J. The CYP1A2 -163C>A polymorphism does not alter the effects of caffeine on basketball performance. *PLoS ONE* **2018**, *13*, e0195943. [CrossRef] [PubMed]
12. Salinero, J.J.; Lara, B.; Ruiz-Vicente, D.; Areces, F.; Puente-Torres, C.; Gallo-Salazar, C.; Pascual, T.; Del Coso, J. CYP1A2 Genotype Variations Do Not Modify the Benefits and Drawbacks of Caffeine during Exercise: A Pilot Study. *Nutrients* **2017**, *9*. [CrossRef] [PubMed]
13. Pickering, C.; Kiely, J. Are the Current Guidelines on Caffeine Use in Sport Optimal for Everyone? Inter-individual Variation in Caffeine Ergogenicity, and a Move Towards Personalised Sports Nutrition. *Sports Med.* **2018**, *48*, 7–16. [CrossRef] [PubMed]

14. Pickering, C. Caffeine, CYP1A2 genotype, and sports performance: is timing important? *Ir. J. Med. Sci.* **2018**. [CrossRef]
15. Grgic, J.; Mikulic, P. Caffeine ingestion acutely enhances muscular strength and power but not muscular endurance in resistance-trained men. *Eur. J. Sport Sci.* **2017**, *17*, 1029–1036. [CrossRef]
16. Lara, B.; Ruiz-Moreno, C.; Salinero, J.J.; Del Coso, J. Time course of tolerance to the performance benefits of caffeine. *PLoS ONE* **2019**, *14*, e0210275. [CrossRef]
17. Apostolidis, A.; Mougios, V.; Smilios, I.; Rodosthenous, J.; Hadjicharalambous, M. Caffeine Supplementation: Ergogenic in Both High and Low Caffeine Responders. *Int. J. Sports Physiol. Perform.* **2018**, 1–25. [CrossRef] [PubMed]
18. Wardle, M.C.; Treadway, M.T.; de Wit, H. Caffeine increases psychomotor performance on the effort expenditure for rewards task. *Pharmacol. Biochem. Behav.* **2012**, *102*, 526–531. [CrossRef]

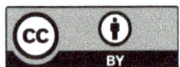

© 2019 by the authors. Licensee MDPI, Basel, Switzerland. This article is an open access article distributed under the terms and conditions of the Creative Commons Attribution (CC BY) license (http://creativecommons.org/licenses/by/4.0/).

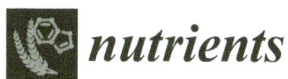

Article

Caffeine Increased Muscle Endurance Performance Despite Reduced Cortical Activation and Unchanged Neuromuscular Efficiency and Corticomuscular Coherence

Paulo Estevão Franco-Alvarenga [1,2], Cayque Brietzke [1], Raul Canestri [1], Márcio Fagundes Goethel [1], Bruno Ferreira Viana [1,3] and Flávio Oliveira Pires [1,*]

1. Exercise Psychophysiology Research Group, School of Arts, Sciences and Humanities, University of São Paulo, São Paulo 03828-000, Brazil
2. Physical Education, Estácio de Sá University, Resende, Rio de Janeiro 27515-010, Brazil
3. Rehabilitation Sciences Graduate Program, Augusto Motta University Center, Rio de Janeiro 21041-010, Brazil
* Correspondence: piresfo@usp.br; Tel.: +55-11-2648-0118

Received: 6 July 2019; Accepted: 26 August 2019; Published: 15 October 2019

Abstract: The central and peripheral effects of caffeine remain debatable. We verified whether increases in endurance performance after caffeine ingestion occurred together with changes in primary motor cortex (MC) and prefrontal cortex (PFC) activation, neuromuscular efficiency (NME), and electroencephalography–electromyography coherence (EEG–EMG coherence). Twelve participants performed a time-to-task failure isometric contraction at 70% of the maximal voluntary contraction after ingesting 5 mg/kg of caffeine (CAF) or placebo (PLA), in a crossover and counterbalanced design. MC (Cz) and PFC (Fp1) EEG alpha wave and vastus lateralis (VL) muscle EMG were recorded throughout the exercise. EEG–EMG coherence was calculated through the magnitude squared coherence analysis in MC EEG gamma-wave (CI > 0.0058). Moreover, NME was obtained as the force–VL EMG ratio. When compared to PLA, CAF improved the time to task failure ($p = 0.003$, d = 0.75), but reduced activation in MC and PFC throughout the exercise ($p = 0.027$, d = 1.01 and $p = 0.045$, d = 0.95, respectively). Neither NME ($p = 0.802$, d = 0.34) nor EEG–EMG coherence ($p = 0.628$, d = 0.21) was different between CAF and PLA. The results suggest that CAF improved muscular performance through a modified central nervous system (CNS) response rather than through alterations in peripheral muscle or central–peripheral coupling.

Keywords: fatigue; placebo; ergogenic; EEG–EMG coherence

1. Introduction

Caffeine is one of the most widely ergogenic aids traditionally used to improve physical performance in different exercise scenarios [1,2] such as team sports [3], cycling exercise [4,5], and muscular function tests [6–8]. However, the underlying mechanism of caffeine ingestion on either whole-body or muscular endurance exercise performance is still controversial, as it involves central and peripheral hypotheses such as alterations in central nervous system (CNS) and skeletal muscles, respectively. It has been well known that caffeine inhibits A1 adenosine receptor and postsynaptic A2a receptor in CNS [9,10] and muscles [7,8], thereby, improving spinal and supraspinal excitability and altering cortical and muscular activation during exercise. Nevertheless, it is still debatable whether caffeine improves endurance performance through coupled or uncoupled alterations in both central and peripheral sites.

Results of studies using micromolar doses of caffeine suggest that alterations in CNS are the likely mechanism of the caffeine effects on endurance performance. Studies have shown an increased spinal and supraspinal excitability with caffeine [11,12], thus justifying the increased muscular endurance performance as measured as the time to task failure at a submaximal target force [13]. Interestingly, an earlier study observed that caffeine ingestion (6 mg·kg^{-1} of body mass) reduced the motor-related cortical potential at the vertex during a submaximal isometric knee extension. The authors concluded that caffeine decreased the magnitude of excitatory inputs from frontal and primary motor cortex (MC) areas necessary to produce a given force, likely due to an enhanced spinal and supraspinal excitability [14]. Based on these arguments, one may expect that less activation in MC and frontal cortex areas would be required to sustain a target force after caffeine ingestion, thus improving the muscular endurance capacity as measured by time to task failure. Unfortunately, that study used a closed-loop isometric exercise (i.e., 4 × 10 muscle contractions), so that time-to-task failure measures were not provided. Moreover, motor-related cortical potential measure may be indicative of readiness (i.e., excitability) rather than activation, thus cortical electroencephalography (EEG) measures throughout a time-to-task failure exercise may be insightful for this proposal. In fact, an earlier study found a reduced cortical EEG alpha wave after caffeine ingestion at rest [15] so that a study exploring the cortical EEG alpha wave during exercise is yet to be provided.

On the other hand, studies have suggested that caffeine may also improve endurance exercise performance through an enhanced muscular function. For example, an earlier study had observed that caffeine increased tetanic force stimulated at 20 Hz but not at 40 Hz [7]. Additionally, another study verified that caffeine (6 mg·kg^{-1} of body mass) increased biceps brachii electromyography (EMG) and maximal isokinetic force of elbow flexion at different angular velocities [8]. Somehow, caffeine may have also improved neuromuscular efficiency as caffeine ingestion increased muscle fiber conduction velocity. Consequently, beyond the reduced cortical activation one may argue that caffeine ingestion improves muscular endurance capacity through an ameliorated neuromuscular efficiency. However, evidence that caffeine may improve muscular endurance (i.e., time to task failure) together with a reduced cortical activation and increased neuromuscular efficiency has yet to be provided in a single study design.

There is a paucity of studies simultaneously investigating the caffeine effects on both central and peripheral responses to a muscular endurance performance. For example, an earlier study verified that the increased maximal voluntary force during maximal knee extensions after caffeine ingestion was associated with alterations in central more than in peripheral responses [16]. In contrast, a recent study observed that improved single-leg knee extension performance after caffeine ingestion was associated with ameliorated central and peripheral fatigue indexes [12]. Therefore, studies simultaneously investigating central and peripheral responses to caffeine ingestion during muscular endurance performance are insightful to reveal the importance of central and peripheral effects of caffeine.

In a central vs. peripheral fatigue scenario, it is still unknown whether caffeine improves muscular endurance performance through a coupled alteration in central and peripheral locations, as one may argue that caffeine could improve exercise performance through independent effects on cortical and muscle responses. Analysis of the strength of corticomuscular coupling during a time-to-task failure protocol may be helpful to understand how caffeine affects the link of information being processed in these two different locations [17]. In this regard, analysis of the EEG–EMG linear dependency in time and frequency domains indicates the neuronal synchronicity between cortical and muscle activation [18], so that EEG–EMG coherence during a time-to-task failure protocol may provide insights into caffeine effects on corticomuscular coupling and fatigue. Unfortunately, possible caffeine effects on fatigue and EEG–EMG coherence relationship remain uninvestigated.

The present study verified whether increases in endurance performance after caffeine ingestion occurred together with changes in cortical activation, neuromuscular efficiency, and EEG–EMG coherence. Based on independent results, we hypothesized that caffeine ingestion would reduce cortical activation and increase neuromuscular efficiency, thereby increasing the time to task failure during single-leg knee extension protocol. Additionally, a likely improved coherence between central (i.e., MC EEG) and peripheral sites was expected with caffeine ingestion.

2. Materials and Methods

2.1. Participants

A sample size of 10 participants was determined, having a significance level of 5%, a power >0.95, and an effect size (ES) >0.8 (G-Power software, version 3.1., Dusseldorf, Germany). However, we expected a 20% dropout so that 12 participants volunteered to participate in this study. Thus, recreationally trained cyclists (34.3 ± 6.2 years old; 179.3 ± 5.1 cm; 77.6 ± 6.8 kg), non-smokers and free from cardiovascular, visual, auditory, and cognitive disorders were recruited. Briefly, three were non-consumers (≤40 mg of caffeine per day), five were occasional consumers (≤250 mg of caffeine per day), and four were daily consumers of caffeine (250 < consumption < 572 mg of caffeine per day), according to classification proposed elsewhere [1,19]. Importantly, caffeine has been suggested as an ergogenic aid capable of improving endurance performance, regardless of habitual caffeine consumption [5,20]. They were oriented to avoid consumption of coffee or any stimulant (energy drink, etc.) and alcoholic beverages, as well as intense exercise for 48 h preceding the sessions. Experimental procedures, risks, and benefits were explained before collecting their written consent form signature. The procedures were previously approved by a local Ethics Committee (Process: 63787816.1.0000.5390) from the University of São Paulo and performed according to the Declaration of Helsinki.

2.2. Study Design

The design of the present study involved five sessions. During the sessions 1 and 2, participants were familiarized with instruments and procedures of knee isometric extension (IC) and EMG and EEG measures. Moreover, participants performed three maximal voluntary contractions (MVC) and a submaximal IC to task failure set at 70% MVC. These procedures were repeated during session 2, and the force attained in MVC was adopted to determine the IC intensity (i.e., 70% MVC) used in the following sessions. Session 3, baseline trial (CON): Participants performed a baseline IC to task failure with no supplementation; sessions 4 and 5, supplementation trials: Participants performed a submaximal IC exercise ~45 min after caffeine (CAF) or placebo (PLA) ingestion. Sessions 1, 2, and 3 were performed in sequential order, as we were interested in properly familiarizing participants with procedures before assessing EEG, muscular efficiency, and EEG–EMG coherency in baseline submaximal IC. Then, we performed sessions 4 and 5 in a double-blinded, counterbalanced order as we intended to investigate central and peripheral responses to IC exercise after caffeine ingestion. Therefore, the baseline session was used as a familiarization when assessing physiological responses to a "natural" non-supplemented IC exercise. The study was finished within 30 days. The sessions were interspersed by a 3–7 day washout period, being performed at the same time of the day in a controlled environment (~24 °C and 50%–60% humidity). This experimental setup was part of an umbrella research project that studied caffeine effects on several psychophysiological responses to different exercise modes. Importantly, experimental procedures used in other parts of the umbrella project that have been already published [4] are unlikely to influence the outcomes measured in the present study [20]. Hence, with the exception of the ingested substance, all experimental trials (CON, CAF, and PLA) were conducted under identical and controlled conditions, thus ensuring the reliability of the present study.

2.3. Caffeine and Placebo Ingestion

Participants ingested 5 mg·kg^{-1} of body mass of caffeine 45 min before the submaximal IC to task failure. This is in accordance with recommendations of the International Society of Sports Nutrition (ISSN) for caffeine ingestion [1], suggesting that 3–6 mg·kg^{-1} of body mass of caffeine significantly improves endurance performance when ingested from 45 to 60 min before the exercise bout [1]. Caffeine and placebo were manipulated in capsules of the same size, color, and smell so that participants and the researcher directly involved in data sampling were unaware about the substance ingested. Participants received a capsule containing CAF or PLA (lubricant, magnesium stearate, and magnesium silicate) in a typical double-blind trial, having 50% chance of ingesting the actual active or placebo substance. The blinding efficacy was checked after the participants finished their participation.

2.4. MVC and Isometric Contraction to Task Failure

Initially, participants were accommodated in a custom-built single-leg knee extension chair attached to a cell load (EMG System®, São José dos Campos, Brazil) to measure a force of 2 kHz frequency, having their hips and knees at 90° and 60° from the horizontal axis, respectively. Their chest and hips were carefully fixed in order to avoid accessory movements. After familiarizing with the MVC and IC protocols in session 1, participants repeated them in session 2. Moreover, in session 2 participants performed three sets of three MVC (interspersed by a 3 min interval) in order to assess the highest peak force value between them and subsequently determine the submaximal IC workload. The IC protocol consisted of performing an isometric knee extension to task failure at 70% MVC. Therefore, after a warm-up consisting of unloaded squats (two sets of 15 repetitions with 1 min interval between sets), participants sat on the chair which was individually adjusted. They were oriented to maintain the force corresponding to 70% MVC (±5% variation) by using a visual feedback on a computer screen. The task failure was identified as the inability to maintain the target force after three verbal encouragements [21]. Measures of force (expressed as kgf), EEG, and EMG were recorded throughout the submaximal IC.

2.5. Measures and Instruments

2.5.1. Electroencephalography (EEG)

Activation in MC and PFC was continuously obtained through an EEG unit (Emsa®, EEG BNT 36, TiEEG, Rio de Janeiro, Brazil) at Cz and Fp1 position, respectively, according to the international EEG 10–20 system [22]. These positions were ensured according to frontal and sagittal planes, referenced to the mastoid. The EEG was recorded at a 600 Hz sampling frequency, through active electrodes (Ag–AgCl) with resistance ~5 KΩ. After exfoliation and cleaning, electrodes were fixed with a conductive gel, adhesive tape, and medical strips. The EEG signal was recorded during a 3 min baseline before CAF or PLA ingestion (when participants were completely calm) as well as throughout the submaximal IC. They were oriented to avoid head and trunk movements during baseline and exercise phases.

An EEG signal with amplitude >100 µV was considered as an artifact (n = 1–2, depending on the moment of the experimental setup) and removed from analysis [23]. In baseline EEG data, data recorded during the first and last 30 s of a 180 s time window were removed (to avoid noise associated with the increased expectation of the start and stop of EEG sampling) and a fast-Fourier transformation calculated the total power spectral density (tPSD) within 8–13 Hz (alpha wave) over the most steady (i.e., lowest standard deviation (SD)) 30 s time window. In exercise EEG data, a fast-Fourier transformation calculated the tPSD within the alpha wave over the last 2 s of every 25% of the submaximal IC duration (i.e., 25%, 50%, 75%, and 100%), thereafter the exercise EEG data were expressed as a percentage of the baseline. Importantly, we used the EEG alpha wave to indicate activation as this EEG frequency is suggested to reflect an increased number of neurons coherently activated [24] as indicated by the increase in inhibited neurons–to–disinhibited neurons relationship [25]. In this regard, an increased alpha wave may indicate a cooperative-synchronized behavior of a large number of activated neurons [25]. All EEG analyses were performed through an algorithm in Matlab® environment.

2.5.2. Neuromuscular Efficiency (NME)

Initially, participants had their skin shaved, exfoliated, and cleaned with isopropyl alcohol to reduce the skin impedance. Thereafter, a bipolar electrode was placed over the belly of the vastus lateralis muscle (VL) according to the probable muscle fiber orientation. The EMG signal was recorded throughout the submaximal IC through an EMG unit (EMG System, São José dos Campos, Brazil) at a 2 kHz sample rate (gain 1000) with a recursive fourth-order Butterworth bandpass filter (cutoff frequencies between 20 and 500 Hz), before calculating the root-mean-square value (RMS) of the EMG signal. All EEG data collection followed the Surface Electromyography for the Non-Invasive Assessment of Muscles standards [26].

The neuromuscular efficiency (NME) was obtained as the force–EMG RMS ratio of the EMG burst over the last 2 s of every 25% of the submaximal IC duration, as proposed elsewhere [27]. Importantly, as a reduction in NME is expected as fatigue progresses, indicating that more motor units have been recruited to produce the same force, NME has been suggested as a peripheral fatigue index [27]. Hence, to obtain the NME, we also filtered force data through a recursive fourth-order Butterworth low-pass filter, having a cutoff frequency determined by residual analysis at 7 Hz, before normalizing force data by body mass. Thereafter, the NME index (expressed as arbitrary units) was calculated as the integral of the force–EMG RMS relationship over a 250 ms time window with a 249.5 ms overlap (Equation (1)).

$$NME = \sum_{i}^{i+1} \int \frac{Force_{(i)}}{\sqrt{1/500 \cdot \left(x_i^2 + x_{i+1}^2 + \ldots + x_{i+499}^2\right)_{(i)}}} \tag{1}$$

2.5.3. EEG–EMG Coherence

Initially, we checked through a 95% confidence interval (CI) calculation which EEG spectral wave from MC (Cz position) revealed coherence with VL EMG signal, as suggested elsewhere [28]:

$$CL = 1 - 0.05^{1/n-1} \tag{2}$$

where n is the number of windows used for spectral estimation. Given the varied time to task failure, the number of windows was not the same for all spectral estimates.

Afterward, we computed the power spectral of the rectified EMG and EEG gamma wave (30–50 Hz) through Welch's method, having a 50% overlapped Hamming window with 512 samples in each section. Only active data (i.e., between onset and offset of each trial) were used to calculate the power spectral, and the magnitude squared coherence between EEG and EMG (expressed as arbitrary units) was then obtained:

$$coh_{c1,c2}(f) = \frac{|S_{c1c2}(f)|^2}{S_{c1c1}(f) \cdot S_{c2c2}(f)} \tag{3}$$

where Sc_1c_1 and Sc_2c_2 are the auto-spectra of each signal; Sc_1c_2 is the cross-spectra. Accordingly, EEG–EMG coherence data were calculated at each 25% of the submaximal IC duration.

2.5.4. Statistical analyses

Results were reported as mean and standard deviation (±SD). Firstly, one-way ANOVA (Bonferroni as a post hoc) was used to compare muscle endurance performance (expressed as time to task failure in submaximal IC) in baseline, CAF, and PLA conditions. Additionally, we also expressed endurance performance as a percentage of alteration from the baseline session, thus comparing CAF and PLA trough a paired T-test. Secondly, MC and PFC activation (indicated by EEG alpha wave), NME, and EEG–EMG coherence responses to submaximal IC between CAF and PLA conditions were compared at every 25% of the total exercise duration through a 4 × 2 mixed model, having time (25%, 50%, 75%, and 100%) and ingestion (CAF vs. PLA) as fixed factors and participants as the random one. The AIC index (Akaike's information criterion) determined the covariance matrix that best fitted to the dataset (homogeneous and heterogeneous compound symmetric, first-order auto-regressive, auto-regressive moving average, and Toeplitz), while Bonferroni test was used in multiple comparisons.

We reported the post hoc ES analysis (expressed as d-Cohen) as a qualitative analysis approach, so that ES was interpreted as small (<0.2), moderate (0.2–0.6), large (0.6–1.2), very large (1.2–2.0), and extremely large (>2.0), as suggested elsewhere [29]. Results were significant when $p < 0.05$.

3. Results

3.1. Baseline Session and Blinding Efficacy

Participants attained a task failure in 28.5 ± 16.4 s in baseline session. In order to check the blinding of manipulation, participants were asked to guess which substance they thought they ingested in each session. In total, nine participants correctly identified CAF (and consequently PLA) ingestion, while three did not. Participants reported no adverse effects from caffeine ingestion.

3.2. Caffeine Effects on Muscle Performance

A condition main effect was found (F = 8.489; $p = 0.002$; d = 1.242 very large ES) so that the absolute time to task failure was greater in CAF than in PLA (0.007) and baseline (0.006). When expressed as a percentage of alteration from baseline session, CAF (33.5 ± 14.2 s; (95% CI = 23.9, 40.2), 9.1% ± 36.4% from baseline) further improved muscular endurance performance (t = 3.993, $p = 0.003$, d = 0.75 large ES) when compared to PLA ingestion (25.8 ± 10.6 s; (95% CI = 18.6, 30.8), −7.7% ± 25.1% from baseline) (Figure 1).

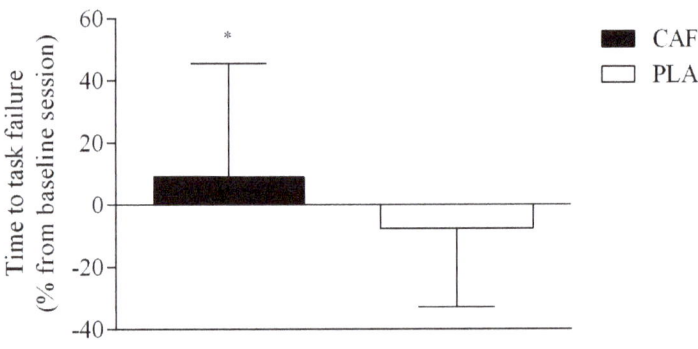

Figure 1. Changes in time to task failure during submaximal isometric contraction after caffeine (CAF) and placebo (PLA) ingestion. * Indicates significantly different from PLA ($p = 0.003$). Data are reported as mean ± standard deviation (SD).

3.3. Caffeine Effects on Central and Peripheral Indexes

Regarding MC activation, EEG Cz activity was significantly reduced (F = 5.654, $p = 0.027$, d = 1.01 large ES) when compared to PLA. Furthermore, a moment main effect was observed as MC activation increased throughout the exercise (F = 3.767, $p = 0.025$, d = 0.83 very large ES). In contrast, no ingestion by moment interaction effects were found (F = 2.462, $p = 0.125$, d = 0.67 large ES). Accordingly, an ingestion main effect (F = 4.925, $p = 0.045$, d = 0.946 large ES) as well as a moment main effect (F = 10.360, $p = 0.001$, d = 1.37, very large ES) was observed in PFC activation, as CAF reduced the EEG Fp1 activity when compared to PLA, although PFC activation has increased throughout the submaximal

IC exercise. Moreover, no ingestion by moment interaction effects was found (F = 1.280, p = 0.343, d = 0.48, moderate ES). Figure 2 shows these EEG results.

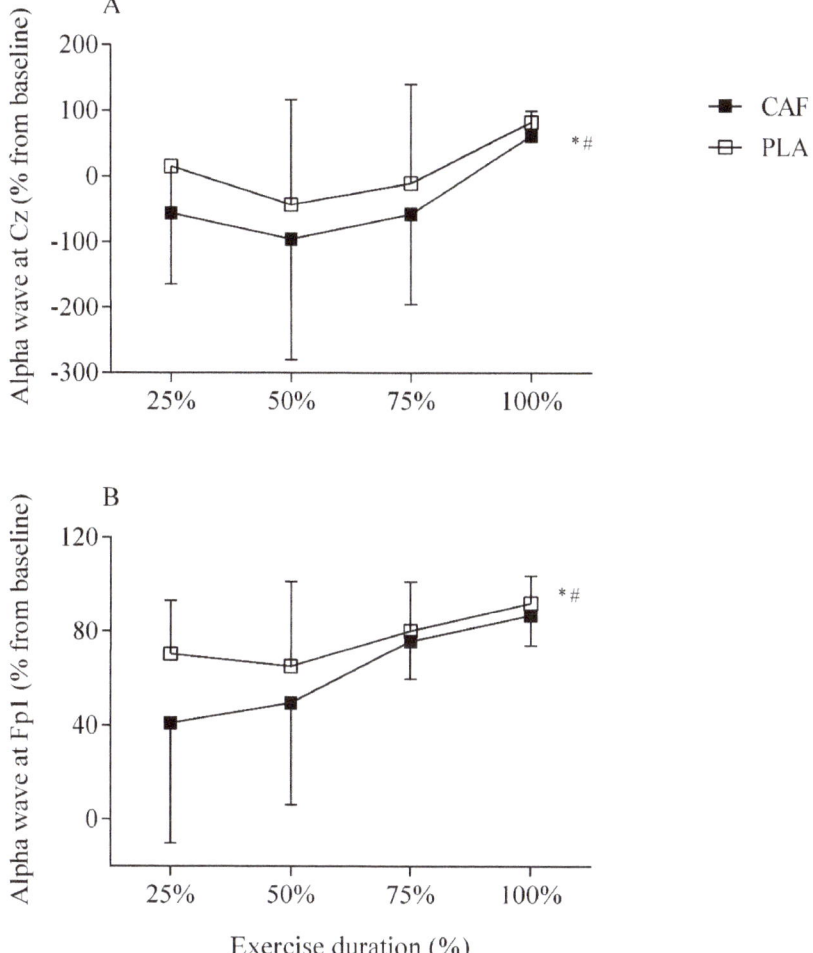

Figure 2. Electroencephalography (EEG) alpha wave recorded at Cz (**A**) and Fp1 (**B**) positions during isometric contraction in CAF (filled square) and PLA (open square) sessions. * Indicates condition main effect in Cz ($p = 0.027$) and PFC ($p = 0.045$). # indicates moment main effect in Cz ($p = 0.000$) and Fp1 ($p = 0.001$). Data are reported as mean ± SD.

Regarding the NME results, caffeine ingestion was ineffective in improving VL muscle efficiency when compared to PLA (F = 0.065, p = 0.802, d = 0.34 moderate ES). However, a moment main effect was detected as NME changed throughout the exercise (F = 7.97, p < 0.001, d = 1.20 very large ES). Additionally, no ingestion by moment interaction effect was observed (F = 0.006, p = 1.00, d = 0.02 small ES). Figure 3 depicts these results.

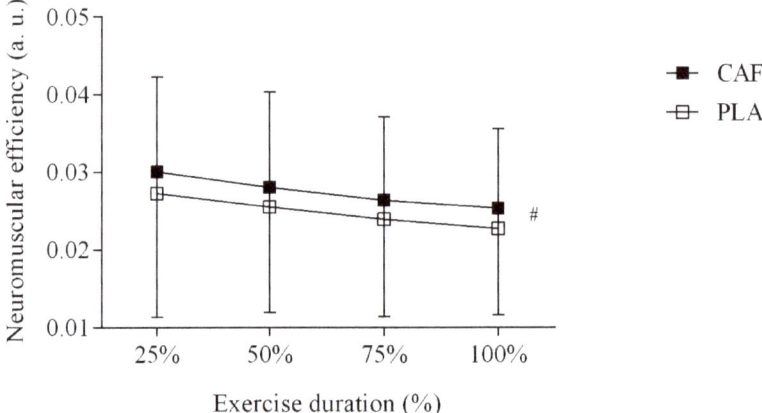

Figure 3. Changes in neuromuscular efficiency (NME) of vastus lateralis muscle during isometric contraction in caffeine (CAF) and placebo (PLA) sessions. # Is moment main effect ($p = 0.000$). Data are reported as mean ± SD.

Previous analysis revealed that EEG–EMG coherence was significant (CI > 0.0058) in EEG gamma wave, as shown by spectrograms (Figure 4). We observed that neither CAF session ($F = 0.240$, $p = 0.628$, $d = 0.21$ moderate ES) nor moment main effect ($F = 0.437$, $p = 0.727$, $d = 0.28$ moderate ES) changed EEG–EMG coherence. Accordingly, we did not observe ingestion by moment interaction effects ($F = 0.522$, $p = 0.670$, $d = 0.35$ moderate ES) in EEG–EMG coherence, as shown in Figure 5. Table 1 presents mean (±SD) and 95% confidence interval (95% CI) values of dependent variables.

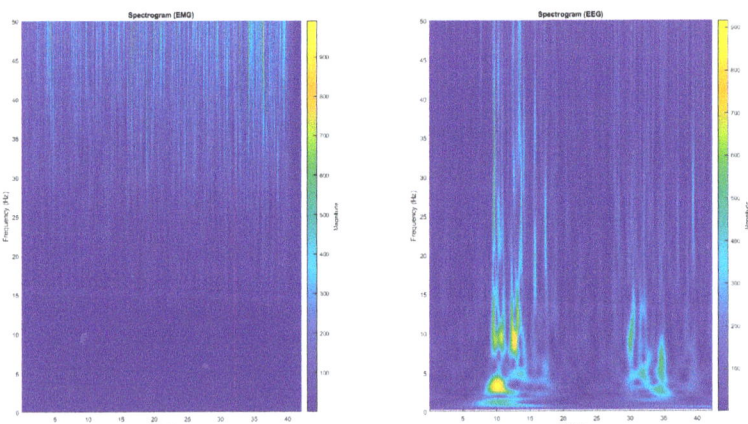

Figure 4. Spectrogram of EEG gamma wave at Cz position and vastus lateralis electromyography (EMG).

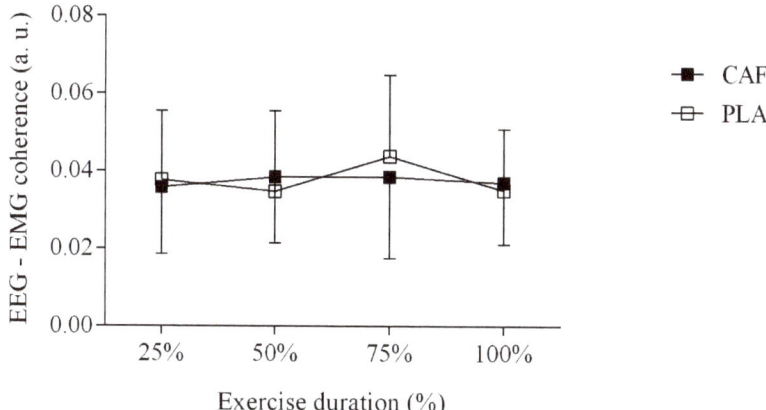

Figure 5. EEG–EMG coherence in CAF (filled square) and PLA (open square) sessions. Data are reported as mean ± SD.

Table 1. Mean (±SD) and 95% confidence interval (95% CI) for dependent variables.

Ingestion	Dependent Variable	25%	50%	75%	100%
				Time of Exercise	
CAF	Prefrontal EEG	40.9 ± 54.0	49.4 ± 43.2	75.7 ± 16.0	86.7 ± 12.9
	95% CI	(−507.5–245.1)	(−60.2–93.6)	(−187.8–80.2)	(−366.9–274.2)
	Motor Cortex EEG	−311.8 ± 634.7	−95.6 ± 184.4	−99.9 ± 197.1	33.1 ± 75.2
	95% CI	(−176.6–62.6)	(−216.1–19.1)	(−185.7–46.1)	(22.2–88.3)
	NME	0.03 ± 0.01	0.02 ± 0.01	0.02 ± 0.01	0.03 ± 0.01
	95% CI	(0.01–0.04)	(0.01–0.04)	(0.01–0.03)	(0.01–0.03)
	EEG–EMG Coherence	0.06 ± 0.05	0.04 ± 0.02	0.04 ± 0.02	0.06 ± 0.06
	95% CI	(0.02–0.06)	(0.02–0.05)	(0.02–0.03)	(0.02–0.06)
PLA	Prefrontal EEG	70.2 ± 22.9	64.9 ± 36.3	80.1 ± 21.1	92.1 ± 11.6
	95% CI	(45.2–96.8)	(2.7–84.3)	(33.1–104.3)	(81.6–102.3)
	Motor Cortex EEG	−27.0 ± 148.9	−80.7 ± 191.9	−10.3 ± 150.3	66.2 ± 57.5
	95% CI	(57.0–88.6)	(−165.7–79.6)	(−109.1–121.1)	(66.4–107.4)
	NME	0.03 ± 0.01	0.02 ± 0.01	0.02 ± 0.01	0.02 ± 0.01
	95% CI	(0.01–0.06)	(0.01–0.05)	(0.01–0.04)	(0.01–0.04)
	EEG–EMG Coherence	0.06 ± 0.06	0.04 ± 0.03	0.09 ± 0.09	0.05 ± 0.05
	95% CI	(0.02–0.06)	(0.02–0.06)	(0.03–0.08)	(0.02–0.06)

NME—neuromuscular efficiency; EEG—electroencephalography; EMG—electromyography; CAF—caffeine; PLA—placebo.

4. Discussion

The present study aimed to verify whether an increased time to task failure with CAF ingestion would be followed by changes in cortical activation, neuromuscular efficiency, and EEG–EMG coherence during a single-leg knee extension exercise. Our findings showed that caffeine improved endurance performance, despite a reduced activation in both PFC and MC and unaltered neuromuscular efficiency and EEG–EMG coherence. These results suggested that caffeine ingestion improved muscular endurance performance through located modifications in the CNS rather than alterations in peripheral muscle. Importantly, this is the first study showing that caffeine effects on CNS were uncoupled from peripheral responses.

Different studies have indicated that caffeine effects on A1 adenosine receptor and postsynaptic A2a receptor in CNS are the most likely mechanism underlying improvements in endurance performance [9,10,30]. We hypothesized that caffeine may improve muscular endurance performance in a time to task failure regardless of a reduced activation in PFC and MC as reported elsewhere [15].

Although the increase in PFC and MC activity was a main exercise effect, there was a reduced PFC and MC activation throughout the submaximal IC protocol in the CAF session. A likely explanation of this reduced cortical activation during exercise is an increased CNS excitability with caffeine ingestion, as suggested [10] and confirmed elsewhere [11]. Caffeine has been suggested to increase both the corticospinal [31] and spinal excitability [11], thereby, leading to less excitatory input from frontal to vertex areas as well as from vertex to peripheral muscles, when generating the same force or power output [14,30]. Although we have not measured CNS excitability responses in the present study, the fact that participants maintained the same force requiring less PFC and MC activation throughout most of the submaximal IC exercise may be suggestive of an increased CNS excitability after caffeine ingestion. Thus, as a result of the lower cortical activation necessary to produce a given force, participants may have been capable of further increasing the time to task failure in the CAF session. Interestingly, one may argue that a likely increased spinal and corticospinal excitability promoted by caffeine ingestion extended the time to reach a "cortical activation limit", as both PFC and MC activation were lower in CAF than PLA from the beginning to 50% and 75% of the exercise duration, respectively, matching a "maximal cortical activation" (as recorded in the PLA session) only at 100% of the IC exercise. However, this suggestion must be interpreted with caution, as this argument is based on visual more than statistical analysis.

Despite the decreased NME as a main exercise effect, caffeine was ineffective in improving muscle efficiency during submaximal IC exercise, so that the improved muscular endurance performance in the CAF session cannot be related to peripheral responses. Controversial results of caffeine ingestion on peripheral responses have been reported. For example, some have found positive caffeine effects either on calcium release from the sarcoplasmic reticulum [32,33] or muscle fiber conduction velocity [8], thereby supporting the notion of a caffeine ergogenic effect on peripheral muscles. However, others have failed to find positive caffeine effects on peripheral muscle indexes such as a peripheral silent period [31] or M-wave [7], suggesting that sarcolemma excitability and tubule T propagation are unaffected by caffeine. In the present study, we observed that caffeine ingestion was ineffective in enhancing neuromuscular efficiency calculated as the force–EMG RMS ratio, thus, indirectly suggesting no caffeine effects on muscle properties. Such an ineffectiveness of caffeine in improving peripheral responses may be related to the muscle contraction stimulation frequency of the submaximal IC exercise, as it has been proposed that caffeine changes muscle properties through alterations in calcium release rather than through potassium accumulation [33]. Thus, assuming that calcium metabolism is associated with force losses mainly in frequencies <20–30 Hz [7,34,35] and that our submaximal IC exercise required a muscle contraction frequency mostly higher than 50 Hz [36], perhaps caffeine ingestion is ineffective in improving key muscular properties enhance muscle endurance performance during submaximal IC. Somehow, the fact that coherence analysis indicated a significant coupling between gamma wave EEG (30–50 Hz) and EMG may reinforce this argument.

Despite studies proposing EEG–EMG coherence analysis as a tool to investigate the corticomuscular coupling between motor cortex and pooled motor units [37–39], only a few have been designed to investigate the EEG–EMG coherence and fatigue relationship [18,39]. Coherence, defined as a spectral power covariance between signals from different origins, may provide an estimation of the corticomuscular coupling [39] signals. In a muscle fatigue scenario, EEG–EMG coherence is expected to decrease as exercise progresses, thus suggesting a corticomuscular desynchronization with fatigue [18]. Unexpectedly, we found no main exercise effects on EEG–EMG coherence. Perhaps, the fact that we used a constant rather than an intermittent muscle contraction during submaximal IC can be related to this unaltered coherence during exercise [38], given the less-complex muscle recruitment strategy in this mode of contraction [40,41]. Importantly, the present study was the first to provide evidence that caffeine ingestion maintained the corticomuscular coupling between the motor cortex and pooled motor units in submaximal IC exercise, despite reductions in MC activation and increased muscle endurance. Somehow, the likely increase in corticospinal and spinal excitability in the CAF session [30] may have been associated with a longer sustained force output despite the reduced MC activation, as the signal from MC areas remained coupled with the signal at pooled motor units, even though the progressive fatigue in the CAF session.

5. Methodological Aspects, Strength, and Limitations

Beta and gamma waves have been suggested for EEG–EMG coherence analysis of isometric and isotonic muscle contractions, respectively [38,40]. An earlier coherence study observed a greater EEG gamma wave coherence with EMG signal in isometric knee extension, although both EEG beta and gamma frequencies were significantly coherent with EMG [38]. In the present study, we first verified which EEG waves from MC would best reveal coherence with peripheral muscle during IC exercise. In contrast to earlier results [38,40], we found significant coherence in EEG gamma wave during isometric exercise. Perhaps, the fact that our participants had to sustain a target force throughout the exercise until the task failure, while fatigue progressed, may have induced an increase in the median frequency of the motor command to peripheral muscles, thus shifting the coherence toward higher EEG frequencies such as the gamma wave. Additionally, the fact that our participants had to focus on visual feedback on the screen (i.e., horizontal lines delimiting the target force) during the submaximal IC exercise may have also led to a shift toward higher EEG frequencies, as EEG–EMG coherence can occur at higher EEG frequencies when individuals modulate the target force through visual feedback [41].

Importantly, results of the check of blinding efficacy challenged the use of traditional placebo-controlled clinical trials, as suggested elsewhere [42]. Agreeing with previous results [43], we observed that nine out of 12 participants correctly guessed when caffeine was ingested, despite using a typical double-blind, placebo-controlled design. Therefore, one may argue that some of the endurance performance improvements in CAF session may have been potentiated by the expectation of ingesting caffeine, as a recent study verified that placebo perceived as caffeine improved cycling performance as much as caffeine [44]. As recently recommended, future research must take caffeine expectancies into account when investigating caffeine effects on performance [42].

Although we have included participants with different caffeine habituation in the present study, responsiveness and habituation were seemingly not an issue in the present results, as a recent study by Del Coso et al. [20] observed that different individuals responded to caffeine ingestion improving aerobic and anaerobic cycling performance from 9% to 1% across multiple testing sessions and Wilk et al. [45] found ergogenic effects of caffeine ingestion in athletes habitually using caffeine. Moreover, a well-controlled study by Goncalves et al. [5] verified that habitual caffeine consumption did not influence its potential ergogenic effect. Therefore, together these studies reinforce the notion that caffeine consumption habituation had no impact on results of the present study.

Only a few studies have simultaneously investigated central and peripheral effects of caffeine on exercise performance, mainly in a well-controlled design [12,16]. In this regard, the present study contributes to the improvement of the available literature as we showed that caffeine potentiated muscular endurance performance through central rather than through peripheral effects. Importantly, this is the first study showing that caffeine effects on CNS were uncoupled with muscle responses, as we found no effects of caffeine ingestion on corticomuscular coupling. This may be of value for exercise performance and clinical scenarios, as one may want to focus on CNS alterations without altering CNS–muscle coupling or muscle responses. However, an obvious limitation is that caffeine may play a role in multiple physiological responses beyond the electrophysiological ones investigated in the present study, thus caution is needed when inferring caffeine effects on other physiological responses such as tissue oxygenation and cell metabolism.

6. Conclusions

Results of the present study showed that caffeine improved muscle endurance performance, regardless of reductions in both PFC and MC activation and unaltered neuromuscular efficiency and EEG–EMG coherence. These results may suggest that caffeine ingestion improved performance in isometric contraction through a modified CNS response rather than through alterations in peripheral muscle or central–peripheral coupling.

Author Contributions: All authors contributed to conceiving the study and its design (P.E.F.-A., C.B., R.C., M.F.G., B.F.V. and F.O.P.), collecting data (P.E.F.-A., C.B., and R.C.), analyzing data (P.E.F.-A., M.F.G., R.C., and F.O.P.) writing (P.E.F.-A., M.F.G., B.F.V., and F.O.P.), and reviewing the manuscript (P.E.F.-A., M.F.G., B.F.V., and F.O.P).

Funding: P.E.F.A., C.B., R.C., and M.F.G. are grateful to CAPES for their scholarships (#001) and F.O.P. is grateful to CNPq-Brazil for his researcher scholarship (#307072/2016-9). This study was supported by FAPESP-Brazil (#2016/16496-3).

Conflicts of Interest: The authors declare that the research was conducted in the absence of any commercial or financial relationships that could be construed as a potential conflict of interest.

References

1. Goldstein, E.R.; Ziegenfuss, T.; Kalman, D.; Kreider, R.; Campbell, B.; Wilborn, C.; Taylor, L.; Willoughby, D.; Stout, J.; Graves, B.S.; et al. International society of sports nutrition position stand: Caffeine and performance. *J. Int. Soc. Sport. Nutr.* **2010**, *7*, 5. [CrossRef]
2. Sökmen, B.; Armstrong, L.E.; Kraemer, W.J.; Casa, D.J.; Dias, J.C.; Judelson, D.A.; Maresh, C.M. Caffeine use in sports: Considerations for the athlete. *J. Strength Cond. Res.* **2008**, *22*, 978–986. [CrossRef]
3. Mielgo-Ayuso, J.; Calleja-Gonzalez, J.; Del Coso, J.; Urdampilleta, A.; León-Guereño, P.; Fernández-Lázaro, D. Caffeine supplementation and physical performance, muscle damage and perception of fatigue in soccer players: A systematic review. *Nutrients* **2019**, *11*, 440. [CrossRef]
4. Franco-Alvarenga, P.E.; Brietzke, C.; Canestri, R.; Goethel, M.F.; Hettinga, F.; Santos, T.M.; Pires, F.O. Caffeine improved cycling trial performance in mentally fatigued cyclists, regardless of alterations in prefrontal cortex activation. *Physiol. Behav.* **2019**, *204*, 41–48. [CrossRef]
5. Goncalves, L.S.; Painelli, V.S.; Yamaguchi, G.; de Oliveira, L.F.; Saunders, B.; da Silva, R.P.; Maciel, E.; Artioli, G.G.; Roschel, H.; Gualano, B. Dispelling the myth that habitual caffeine consumption influences the performance response to acute caffeine supplementation. *J. Appl. Physiol.* **2017**. [CrossRef]
6. Grgic, J.; Trexler, E.T.; Lazinica, B.; Pedisic, Z. Effects of caffeine intake on muscle strength and power: A systematic review and meta-analysis. *J. Int. Soc. Sports Nutr.* **2018**, *15*, 11. [CrossRef]
7. Tarnopolsky, M.; Cupido, C. Caffeine potentiates low frequency skeletal muscle force in habitual and nonhabitual caffeine consumers. *J. Appl. Physiol.* **2000**, *89*, 1719–1724. [CrossRef]
8. Bazzucchi, I.; Felici, F.; Montini, M.; Figura, F.; Sacchetti, M. Caffeine improves neuromuscular function during maximal dynamic exercise. *Muscle Nerve* **2011**, *43*, 839–844. [CrossRef]
9. Davis, J.M.; Zhao, Z.; Stock, H.S.; Mehl, K.A.; Buggy, J.; Hand, G.A. Central nervous system effects of caffeine and adenosine on fatigue. *Am. J. Physiol. Regul. Integr. Comp. Physiol.* **2003**, *284*, CR399–CR404. [CrossRef]
10. Kalmar, J.M. The influence of caffeine on voluntary muscle activation. *Med. Sci. Sports Exerc.* **2005**, *37*, 2113–2119. [CrossRef]
11. Walton, C.; Kalmar, J.; Cafarelli, E. Caffeine increases spinal excitability in humans. *Muscle Nerve* **2003**, *28*, 359–364. [CrossRef]
12. Bowtell, J.L.; Mohr, M.; Fulford, J.; Jackman, S.R.; Ermidis, G.; Krustrup, P.; Mileva, K.N. Improved exercise tolerance with caffeine is associated with modulation of both peripheral and central neural processes in human participants. *Front. Nutr.* **2018**, *5*, 6. [CrossRef]
13. Plaskett, C.J.; Cafarelli, E. Caffeine increases endurance and attenuates force sensation during submaximal isometric contractions. *J. Appl. Physiol.* **2001**, *91*, 1535–1544. [CrossRef]
14. de Morree, H.M.; Klein, C.; Marcora, S.M. Cortical substrates of the effects of caffeine and time-on-task on perception of effort. *J. Appl. Physiol.* **2014**, *117*, 1514–1523. [CrossRef]
15. Deslandes, A.; Veiga, H.; Cagy, M.; Fiszman, A.; Piedade, R.; Ribeiro, P. Quantitative electroencephalography (qEEG) to discriminate primary degenerative dementia from major depressive disorder (depression). *Arq. Neuropsiquiatr.* **2004**, *62*, 44–50. [CrossRef]
16. Behrens, M.; Mau-Moeller, A.; Weippert, M.; Fuhrmann, J.; Wegner, K.; Skripitz, R.; Bader, R.; Bruhn, S. Caffeine-induced increase in voluntary activation and strength of the quadriceps muscle during isometric, concentric and eccentric contractions. *Sci. Rep.* **2015**, *5*, 10209. [CrossRef]

17. Grosse, P.; Cassidy, M.J.; Brown, P. EEG-EMG, MEG-EMG and EMG-EMG frequency analysis: Physiological principles and clinical applications. *Clin. Neurophysiol.* **2002**, *113*, 1523–1531. [CrossRef]
18. Tuncel, D.; Dizibuyuk, A.; Kiymik, M.K. Time frequency based coherence analysis between EEG and EMG activities in fatigue duration. *J. Med. Syst.* **2010**, *34*, 131–138. [CrossRef]
19. Fitt, E.; Pell, D.; Cole, D. Assessing caffeine intake in the United Kingdom diet. *Food Chem.* **2013**, *140*, 421–426. [CrossRef]
20. Del Coso, J.; Lara, B.; Ruiz-Moreno, C.; Salinero, J.J. Challenging the myth of non-response to the ergogenic effects of caffeine ingestion on exercise performance. *Nutrients* **2019**, *11*, 732. [CrossRef]
21. Mau-Moeller, A.; Jacksteit, R.; Jackszis, M.; Feldhege, F.; Weippert, M.; Mittelmeier, W.; Bader, R.; Skripitz, R.; Behrens, M. Neuromuscular function of the quadriceps muscle during isometric maximal, submaximal and submaximal fatiguing voluntary contractions in knee osteoarthrosis patients. *PLoS ONE* **2017**, *12*, e0176976. [CrossRef]
22. Pfurtscheller, G.; Lopes da Silva, F.H. Event-related EEG/MEG synchronization and desynchronization: Basic principles. *Clin. Neurophysiol.* **1999**, *110*, 1842–1857. [CrossRef]
23. Maurits, N. *From Neurology to Methodology and Back an Introduction to Clinical Neuroengineering*; Springer: London, UK, 2011; ISBN 9781461411314.
24. Uusberg, A.; Uibo, H.; Kreegipuu, K.; Allik, J. EEG alpha and cortical inhibition in affective attention. *Int. J. Psychophysiol.* **2013**, *89*, 26–36. [CrossRef]
25. von Stein, A.; Sarnthein, J. Different frequencies for different scales of cortical integration: From local gamma to long range alpha/theta synchronization. *Int. J. Psychophysiol.* **2000**, *38*, 301–313. [CrossRef]
26. Hermens, H.J.; Freriks, B.; Disselhorst-Klug, C.; Rau, G. Development of recommendations for SEMG sensors and sensor placement procedures. *J. Electromyogr. Kinesiol.* **2000**, *10*, 361–374. [CrossRef]
27. Deschenes, M.R.; Giles, J.A.; McCoy, R.W.; Volek, J.S.; Gomez, A.L.; Kraemer, W.J. Neural factors account for strength decrements observed after short-term muscle unloading. *Am. J. Physiol. Regul. Integr. Comp. Physiol.* **2002**, *282*, R578–R583. [CrossRef]
28. Rosenberg, J.R.; Amjad, A.M.; Breeze, P.; Brillinger, D.R.; Halliday, D.M. The Fourier approach to the identification of functional coupling between neuronal spike trains. *Prog. Biophys. Mol. Biol.* **1989**, *53*, 1–31. [CrossRef]
29. Hopkins, W.G.; Marshall, S.W.; Batterham, A.M.; Hanin, J. Progressive statistics for studies in sports medicine and exercise science. *Med. Sci. Sport. Exerc.* **2009**, *41*, 3–13. [CrossRef]
30. Kalmar, J.M.; Cafarelli, E. Caffeine: A valuable tool to study central fatigue in humans? *Exerc. Sport Sci. Rev.* **2004**, *32*, 143–147. [CrossRef]
31. Cerqueira, V.; de Mendonça, A.; Minez, A.; Dias, A.R.; de Carvalho, M. Does caffeine modify corticomotor excitability? *Neurophysiol. Clin.* **2006**, *36*, 219–226. [CrossRef]
32. Fiege, M.; Wappler, F.; Weisshorn, R.; Ulrich Gerbershagen, M.; Steinfath, M.; Schulte Esch, J. Results of contracture tests with halothane, caffeine, and ryanodine depend on different malignant hyperthermia-associated ryanodine receptor gene mutations. *Anesthesiology* **2002**, *97*, 345–350. [CrossRef]
33. Tarnopolsky, M.A. Effect of caffeine on the neuromuscular system—potential as an ergogenic aid. *Appl. Physiol. Nutr. Metab.* **2008**, *33*, 1284–1289. [CrossRef]
34. Westerblad, H.; Duty, S.; Allen, D.G. Intracellular calcium concentration during low-frequency fatigue in isolated single fibers of mouse skeletal muscle. *J. Appl. Physiol.* **1993**, *75*, 382–388. [CrossRef]
35. de Lima, F.D.R.; Brietzke, C.; Franco-Alvarenga, P.E.; Asano, R.Y.; Viana, B.F.; Santos, T.M.; Pires, F.O. Traditional models of fatigue and physical performance. *J. Phys. Educ.* **2018**, *29*.
36. Pincivero, D.M.; Campy, R.M.; Salfetnikov, Y.; Bright, A.; Coelho, A.J. Influence of contraction intensity, muscle, and gender on median frequency of the quadriceps femoris. *J. Appl. Physiol.* **2001**, *90*, 804–810. [CrossRef]
37. Enders, H.; Nigg, B.M. Measuring human locomotor control using EMG and EEG: Current knowledge, limitations and future considerations. *Eur. J. Sport Sci.* **2016**, *16*, 416–426. [CrossRef]
38. Gwin, J.T.; Ferris, D.P. Beta- and gamma-range human lower limb corticomuscular coherence. *Front. Hum. Neurosci.* **2012**. [CrossRef]
39. Qi, Y.; Siemionow, V.; Wanxiang, Y.; Sahgal, V.; Yue, G.H. Single-Trial EEG-EMG coherence analysis reveals muscle fatigue-related progressive alterations in corticomuscular coupling. *IEEE Trans. Neural Syst. Rehabil. Eng.* **2010**, *18*, 97–106.

40. Yang, Q.; Fang, Y.; Sun, C.-K.; Siemionow, V.; Ranganathan, V.K.; Khoshknabi, D.; Davis, M.P.; Walsh, D.; Sahgal, V.; Yue, G.H. Weakening of functional corticomuscular coupling during muscle fatigue. *Brain Res.* **2009**, *1250*, 101–112. [CrossRef]
41. Omlor, W.; Patino, L.; Hepp-Reymond, M.-C.; Kristeva, R. Gamma-range corticomuscular coherence during dynamic force output. *Neuroimage* **2007**, *34*, 1191–1198. [CrossRef]
42. Shabir, A.; Hooton, A.; Tallis, J.; Higgins, F.M. The influence of caffeine expectancies on sport, exercise, and cognitive performance. *Nutrients* **2018**, *10*, 1528. [CrossRef]
43. Saunders, B.; de Oliveira, L.F.; da Silva, R.P.; de Salles Painelli, V.; Goncalves, L.S.; Yamaguchi, G.; Mutti, T.; Maciel, E.; Roschel, H.; Artioli, G.G.; et al. Placebo in sports nutrition: A proof-of-principle study involving caffeine supplementation. *Scand. J. Med. Sci. Sport.* **2016**, *27*. [CrossRef]
44. Pires, F.O.; Anjos, C.A.S.D.o.s.; Covolan, R.J.M.; Fontes, E.B.; Noakes, T.D.; Gibson, A.S.C.; Magalhães, F.H.; Ugrinowitsch, C. Caffeine and placebo improved maximal exercise performance despite unchanged motor cortex activation and greater prefrontal cortex deoxygenation. *Front. Physiol.* **2018**, *9*, 1144. [CrossRef]
45. Wilk, M.; Filip, A.; Krzysztofik, M.; Maszczyk, A.; Zajac, A. The acute effect of various doses of caffeine on power output and velocity during the bench press exercise among athletes habitually using caffeine. *Nutrients* **2019**, *11*, 1465. [CrossRef]

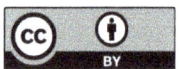

© 2019 by the authors. Licensee MDPI, Basel, Switzerland. This article is an open access article distributed under the terms and conditions of the Creative Commons Attribution (CC BY) license (http://creativecommons.org/licenses/by/4.0/).

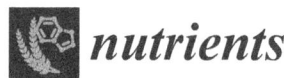

Article

The Influence of Caffeine Expectancies on Simulated Soccer Performance in Recreational Individuals

Akbar Shabir [1], Andy Hooton [1], George Spencer [1], Mitch Storey [1], Olivia Ensor [1], Laura Sandford [1], Jason Tallis [2], Bryan Saunders [3] and Matthew F. Higgins [1,*]

1. Human Sciences Research Centre, University of Derby, Kedleston Road, Derby DE22 1GB, UK; a.shabir2@derby.ac.uk (A.S.); a.hooton@derby.ac.uk (A.H.); g.spencer5@derby.ac.uk (G.S.); m.storey2@unimail.derby.ac.uk (M.S.); o.ensor1@unimail.derby.ac.uk (O.E.); l.sandford1@unimail.derby.ac.uk (L.S.)
2. Centre for Applie and Biological and Exercise Sciences, Coventry University, Priory Street, Coventry CV1 5FB, UK; ab0289@coventry.ac.uk
3. Applied Physiology and Nutrition Research Group, School of Physical Education and Sport, Rheumatology Division, College of Medicine FMUSP, University of Sao Paulo, Sao Paulo, SP 05508-030, Brazil; drbryansaunders@outlook.com
* Correspondence: m.higgins@derby.ac.uk

Received: 28 July 2019; Accepted: 23 September 2019; Published: 25 September 2019

Abstract: Caffeine (CAF) has been reported to improve various facets associated with successful soccer play, including gross motor skill performance, endurance capacity and cognition. These benefits are primarily attributed to pharmacological mechanisms. However, evidence assessing CAF's overall effects on soccer performance are sparse with no studies accounting for CAF's potential psychological impact. Therefore, the aim of this study was to assess CAF's psychological vs. pharmacological influence on various facets of simulated soccer performance. Utilising a double-dissociation design, eight male recreational soccer players (age: 22 ± 5 years, body mass: 78 ± 16 kg, height: 178 ± 6 cm) consumed CAF (3 mg/kg/body mass) or placebo (PLA) capsules, 60 min prior to performing the Loughborough Intermittent Shuttle Test (LIST) interspersed with a collection of ratings of perceived exertion (RPE), blood glucose and lactate, heart rate and performing the Loughborough Soccer Passing Test (LSPT). Whole-body dynamic reaction time (DRT) was assessed pre- and post- LIST, and endurance capacity (T_{LIM}) post, time-matched LIST. Statistical analysis was performed using IBM SPSS (v24) whilst subjective perceptions were explored using template analysis. Mean T_{LIM} was greatest ($p < 0.001$) for synergism (given CAF/told CAF) (672 ± 132 s) vs. placebo (given PLA/told PLA) (533 ± 79 s). However, when isolated, T_{LIM} was greater ($p = 0.012$) for CAF psychology (given PLA/told CAF) (623 ± 117 s) vs. pharmacology (given CAF/told PLA) (578 ± 99 s), potentially, via reduced RPE. Although DRT performance was greater ($p = 0.024$) post-ingestion (+5 hits) and post-exercise (+7 hits) for pharmacology vs. placebo, psychology and synergism appeared to improve LSPT performance vs. pharmacology. Interestingly, positive perceptions during psychology inhibited LSPT and DRT performance via potential CAF over-reliance, with the opposite occurring following negative perceptions. The benefits associated with CAF expectancies may better suit tasks that entail lesser cognitive-/skill-specific attributes but greater gross motor function and this is likely due to reduced RPE. In isolation, these effects appear greater vs. CAF pharmacology. However, an additive benefit may be observed after combining expectancy with CAF pharmacology (i.e., synergism).

Keywords: sport; exercise; expectancy; belief; perceptions; placebo effect

1. Introduction

Caffeine (CAF) is the most frequently used psychoactive substance in sport, and has been observed to improve various exercise modalities that may benefit soccer performance including: strength and power output [1,2] endurance capacity [3–5] and gross motor skill performance [6–8]. Caffeine's ergogenic effects are typically observed with oral doses between 3–9 mg/kg/body mass (BM), with its most commonly associated mechanism ascribed to the blockade of adenosine receptor sites and subsequent central nervous stimulation [9,10].

Caffeine's stimulatory properties may improve soccer performance by ameliorating physical and/or cognitive fatigue, which has been observed to reduce the total distance ran (~5%–10%) and frequency of sprints (~3%–4%) between the first and second half of games [11–16]. Associatively, the majority of goals conceded are also within the latter stages of halves [17], specifically, between min 30–45 (18%) and 75–90 (23%) whereby physical and/or cognitive fatigue has likely peaked. In contrast, the least goals are conceded within min 0–15 (12%) and 45–60 (16%) when physical and/or cognitive fatigue is at its lowest or has been somewhat replenished during the half-time interval. However, studies directly assessing CAF's influence on soccer performance remain scarce and those that have done so almost exclusively attribute any benefits to pharmacological mechanisms [3,4,6–8].

Shabir et al. [18] indicate the psychological permutations (e.g., changes in motivation, perceptual exertion, belief, mood states, etc.) associated with expectancy of oral caffeine consumption may influence sport, exercise and/or cognitive performance comparably or to a greater extent vs. CAF pharmacology [19,20]. Expectancy effects of varying magnitude were observed across 13/17 studies. Moreover, studies assessing sport and exercise performance were always influenced by expectancies. These effects were facilitated by various mechanisms including the perception of mild side effects and augmented physiological arousal [21–23], changes in mood states [21,24], reductions in perceived effort [22,25] and changes in motivation [21,26]. Moreover, in contrast to adenosine receptor sensitivity, expectancies/beliefs may be trained and/or manipulated, further enhancing any ergogenic experience. However, at present the influence of CAF expectancies remain generally unaccounted for across sport and exercise performance with no soccer-specific studies accounting for any potential effects. However, CAF supplementation in recreational sport is commonly achieved via off-the-shelf products (e.g., coffee, energy drinks etc.) many of which entail low CAF doses (likely lower than 3 mg/kg/BM in most cases), thus CAF-induced benefits here may already originate from expectancy rather than pharmacology. Furthermore, expectancies have been found to enhance attributes that may facilitate improvements in soccer performance, including lower limb strength/power output [19,21,22,25,27], endurance capacity [19,27–29], concentration [30], memory [31] and attentional focus [32]. Expectancies could also ameliorate the quality of exercise recovery, training, and preparation for sports competitions which may be impaired following CAF consumption prior to late evening games due to changes in melatonin production and molecular oscillations [33]. Moreover, regular CAF dosing (such as that which might be expected across the course of a season in soccer) may result in a reduced pharmacological effect due to habituation to CAF's central effects [34–36] and this may be overcome if expectancy elicits an effect.

In order to validly compare CAF's psychological vs. pharmacological influence on sport and exercise performance, participant beliefs should be intentionally manipulated in accordance with the experimental purpose. This reduces the discrepancy of individuals guessing which supplement they have ingested that if uncontrolled might cause overlaps between pharmacology and psychology, making it difficult to delineate the individual effects of these properties. The double-dissociation design is considered most suitable here [18] and includes four groups representing a placebo (given placebo (PLA)/told PLA (GP/TP)) and the pharmacological (given CAF/told PLA (GC/TP)), psychological (given PLA/told CAF (GP/TC)) and synergistic effect(s) of CAF (given CAF/told CAF (GC/TC)) on the dependent variable(s) assessed.

Thus, the novelty and purpose of this study was to explore CAF's psychological vs. pharmacological impact on measures of simulated soccer performance (e.g., skill proficiency, dynamic reaction time (DRT), and endurance capacity) and perceptual states, prior to, during and following intermittent exercise replicating the metabolic demands of a 90-min soccer game [37]. We hypothesised, in comparison to a placebo (i.e., given placebo/told placebo), CAF's isolated psychological and/or pharmacological impetus would improve all facets of soccer performance to a greater extent. Moreover, synergism of CAF psychology and pharmacology would instigate the greatest benefit, although CAF psychology would prove of greater efficacy vs. CAF pharmacology and any improvements would be driven by enhanced perceptions.

2. Methods

2.1. Participants

After obtaining institutional ethical approval (ethics code—39-1617-ASs), participants were emailed an information sheet including all relevant study specific information which was confirmed verbally before informed consent was provided. Participants were required to be healthy, non-smoking, recreational male soccer players, between 18–40 years old. Subsequently, eight male participants (age: 22 ± 5 years, body mass: 78 ± 16 kg, height: 178 ± 6 cm) completed this study. This sample size is similar to previous studies exploring the influence of CAF expectancies on sport and exercise performance [21]. Recreational participation was defined as involvement in soccer specific activities (e.g., 5, 8 and/or 11 aside soccer games) at an amateur standard for 1.5 h per week, across at least 6 months. Although habitual CAF consumption was not confirmed, beliefs regarding CAF ergogenicity were explored at various time points (Section 2.8).

2.2. Pre-Experimental Procedures

Participants completed physical activity readiness (PAR-Q) and blood-screening questionnaires prior to participation. Participants were required to avoid strenuous exercise and alcohol 24 h, and CAF 12 h, prior to all exercise trials [38–40]. All participants verbally confirmed that they were not using ergogenic aids at the onset of this study and were prohibited to do so during participation. Participants attended trials 2 h post-prandial and were asked to maintain the same diet 24 h prior. This was recorded via self-reported food diaries and checked visually (e.g., food items included within diet logs were examined and compared to logs obtained during previous trials to ensure replication) whilst participants also verbally confirmed the aforementioned prior to each session. To avoid the confounding influence of changes in macronutrient and/or energy availability, significant importance was placed on consuming the same meal prior to each session. Dependent on the time of trials, an ideal breakfast/lunch plan was outlined to assist participants replicating their diets. Subsequently, all participants replicated their diets prior to each experimental trial. Each participants' trials commenced at the same time of day to avoid the influence of circadian changes on exercise performance [41].

2.3. VO_{2MAX} and Brief Familiarisation

This study entailed a within-subjects, counterbalanced, double-blind, double dissociation, mixed methods design. Participants attended the laboratory on 6 separate occasions, with trials separated by at least 48 h recovery. Trial one (T1) involved ascertaining an estimate of maximal oxygen uptake (VO_{2MAX}) via a 20 m progressive shuttle run test [42] similar to that used in Nicholas et al. [37], and familiarisation of the main experimental protocols adopted. Briefly, after 5 min seated rest, heart rate (HR; F1 Polar Heart Rate Monitor, Polar, Kempele, Finland) was telemetrically recorded, and a finger prick capillary blood sample was taken to later assess blood lactate BLa and glucose BG concentrations (Biosen C_line, EKF Diagnostic, Magdeburg, Germany). Blood was collected into a 20 µL sodium heparinised capillary tube (EKF diagnostics, Cardiff, United Kingdom) which was then added to a 1 mL Eppendorf tube and mixed well before being placed into the Biosen C-Line for analysis. The shuttle run test involved 20 m running bouts between two cones at increasingly fast speeds until volitional exhaustion. This was controlled by auditory beeps (20M Bleep Test; Version 2.1; developer: Adam Howard, United Kingdom, London, 2016) using a smart phone device connected to a large portable speaker. Volitional exhaustion was defined as an inability to reach two consecutive cones in the allotted time, or via voluntary stoppage. To stimulate maximum effort, participants were provided consistent verbal encouragement. Upon completion, HR, blood sampling, both as previously described and ratings of perceived exertion (RPE; 6–20 category scale [43]) were recorded. From this, running speeds corresponding to 55% and 95% VO_{2MAX} were calculated for subsequent use during the Loughborough Intermittent Shuttle Test (LIST) [37].

Following a further 45-min seated rest, participants completed familiarisation and a baseline session measuring DRT (see Section 2.6), before performing the Loughborough Soccer Passing Test (LSPT) as described in McGregor et al. [44]. Two consecutive 15 min bouts of LIST (e.g., repeated sequences of: 3 × walking, 1 × sprint, 3 × cruising (55% VO_{2MAX}) and 3 × jogging (95% VO_{2MAX}); Part A) were then performed, with each bout followed by recording RPE and HR, blood sampling and completion of the LSPT, prior to 3 min rest (N.B. bouts of LIST across all trials were followed by similar measurements). All bouts pertaining to part A were controlled using a LIST sequencer software package (Nottingham Trent University, Nottingham, Clifton, England). Part B (T_{LIM}) (only relevant to trials 2 to 6, inclusive) was controlled manually using an online tone generator [45] and involved 20 m running bouts at 55% and 95% VO_{2MAX} until volitional exhaustion. Following completion of both 15 min LIST bouts, a second session measuring DRT was performed before participants left the laboratory.

2.4. Full Familiarisation and Experimental Trials

An outline of the main methodological practices implemented during full familiarisation (T2) and experimental trials (T3–T6), can be found in Figure 1. Trials lasted approximately 4 h. Briefly, following 5 min seated rest, HR and a blood sample were taken to measure BLa and BG concentrations. Mood states were subsequently assessed using the Brunel Mood Scale (BRUMS; Section 2.7) [46]. Individuals then performed the LSPT, before familiarisation and a baseline session measuring DRT. This was followed by administration of 1/4 treatments (Section 2.5). Treatments were consumed within 5 min of a 60 min seated ingestion period [10], where participants rested quietly in a semi-supine position. Following this all baseline parameters were reassessed. After completing the LSPT, individuals then rested for 3 min before performing 3 consecutive bouts of the LIST. A 15 min break replicating the half-time interval during soccer games was implemented prior to bouts 4, and 5, followed by part B of the LIST. All measures following LIST were recorded for a final time, as were DRT and completion of the BRUMS.

During the full familiarisation session water intake was measured and replicated during experimental trials. Furthermore, at the start of familiarisation and experimental trials 1 and 3, participants completed the CAF expectancies questionnaire (Section 2.8) ((CaffEQ): 47) which aimed to assess habituated expectancies and whether expectancies changed between trials. Additionally, using a Dictaphone (Section 2.9), individuals recorded a short verbal description of their experiences at the end of experimental trials 2 and 4.

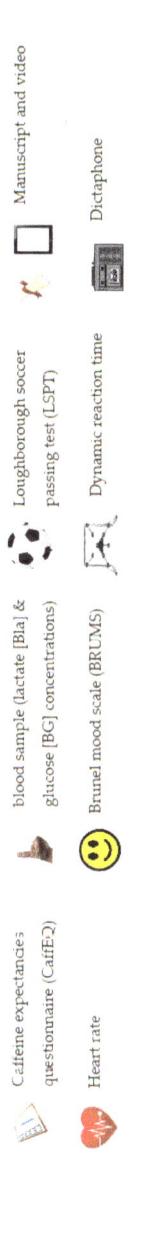

Figure 1. Experimental protocol outline for trials 2–6. Legend (N.B: Caffeine expectancies questionnaire (CaffEQ) and Dictaphone only utilised during trials 2, 3 and 5 and trials 4 and 6, respectively). (PLA = placebo; CAF = caffeine; RPE = ratings of perceived exertion [43]; LIST = Loughborough Intermittent Shuttle Test; CaffEQ = caffeine expectancies questionnaire [50].

2.5. Treatments

Treatments involved oral consumption of visually identical PLA (3 mg/kg/BM cornflower) or CAF (3 mg/kg/BM) capsules and were always administered by a member of the technical support team who was otherwise uninvolved during data collection. We adopted the lowest typical ergogenic dose of CAF [10], as Goldstein et al. [5] observed no differences in sport and exercise performance between low to moderate (3–6 mg/kg/BM) doses. Furthermore, greater doses may induce debilitative side effects and, therefore, override CAF ergogenicity, for some individuals [47]. To facilitate expectancies for CAF ergogenicity a manuscript and brief video [48] highlighting CAF's benefits on exercise performance were used for told CAF conditions. Contrastingly, the manuscript used during told PLA conditions was designed to invoke a neutral effect, whilst the video [49] was standardised to have minimal impact on perceptual states, or influence information relayed during told CAF conditions. These manuscripts/videos were re-administered within the first 5 min of the half-time interval. As such four treatments were administered across experimental trials: (1) placebo (given PLA/told PLA), (2) pharmacology (given CAF/told PLA), (3) psychology (given PLA/told CAF) and (4) synergism (given CAF/told CAF).

2.6. Dynamic Reaction Time (DRT)

Whole body dynamic reaction time was measured using the BATAK Pro (Quotronics Limited, Surrey, UK) and is considered an important component across various soccer skills including tackling and shooting [51,52]. Individuals were required to hit as many randomly illuminated targets as possible, within 60 s (s). To our knowledge there is currently no familiarisation data regarding DRT using the BATAK Pro; therefore, we adopted a comparable protocol to the Sport Vision Trainer which is validated in assessment of reliability and repeatability pertaining to hand–eye co-ordination [53]. The mean deviation in DRT scores were within ~1–2 hits across all experimental trials, suggesting participants were appropriately familiarised to this protocol. All experimental data is reported as the average of 2 × 60 s attempts (defined as one session), with each attempt separated by 1 min of seated recovery.

2.7. Brunel Mood Scale (BRUMS)

The BRUMS assessed participant mood states. The BRUMS consists of 24 items equally arranged into six subscales (anger, confusion, depression, fatigue, tension and vigour), and like all other perceptual measures employed, its purpose was explained, and demonstrated prior to use. Participants were required to rate each item on a subscale of 'not at all' to 'extremely' with each rating entailing a corresponding numerical, arbitrary unit (AU) (0 = not at all, 1 = a little, 2 = moderately, 3 = quite a bit, 4 = extremely). The sum of responses for each subscale was subsequently divided by 4 to provide a final score. The BRUMS has high reliability and validity, with details of its development and validation found in Terry et al. [54].

2.8. Caffeine Expectancies Questionnaire (CaffEQ)

The CaffEQ is a 47-item self-report questionnaire which assesses habituated expectancies across a range of subscales related to caffeine expectancies including: withdrawal/dependence, energy/work enhancement, social/mood enhancement, appetite suppression, physical performance enhancement, anxiety/negative physical effects, and sleep disturbances. The CaffEQ involved choosing a vehicle that best described individuals most commonly used CAF source(s). If participants were naive to CAF use, they were advised to base responses on their expectancies. Each item was evaluated on a scale of 'very unlikely' to 'very likely' with each rating ascribed a numerical value (0 = very unlikely, 1 = unlikely, 2 = a little unlikely, 3 = a little likely, 4 = likely, 5 = very likely) which was later analysed to provide a score for each corresponding sub scale. The CaffEQ represents good, internal consistency (0.88–0.96) and construct validity (0.80–0.94) [50].

2.9. Dictaphone

Using a standardised neutral script, participants were encouraged to record a verbal description (lasting up to 5 min) comparing their experiences at the end of experimental trials 2 and 4. Information reminding what perceived treatment participants had consumed was provided within an A4 sheet of paper which was folded to uphold confidentiality from the lead researcher. Specific importance was placed on individuals remaining honest and there being no right/wrong answer(s). Participants were instructed only to commence recording once they understood what was expected from them and not to share any information with the research team. Participants were then provided an opportunity to ask any questions before being left alone for recording to commence. A member of the technical support team later collected the Dictaphone. These recordings were only made available to the lead researcher following completion of data collection.

2.10. Qualitative Analysis

Following auditory transcription of Dictaphone logs, written data was explored by means of template analysis [55]. Template analysis provides flexible use of theoretical underpinnings from both content analysis [56] and grounded theory [57]. To facilitate template analysis, each transcription was explored thematically, in line with the phases outlined in Braun and Clarke [58]. The subsequent findings were, therefore, relative to the researcher's interpretation of subjective quotes. Once a list of codes had been compiled for each participant, these were linked/and or differentiated to create themes. Moreover, in line with Jackson [59], the following three practices were implemented to enhance trustworthiness [60] and credibility [61] during analysis:

(1) An in-depth description of the data collection and analysis procedure.
(2) Involvement of A.H and M.F.H in guiding the qualitative process, by making implicit enquiries to the lead researcher (A.S) about the data collection/analysis procedure. This assisted in minimising biases, whilst improving the clarity of interpretations.
(3) Brainstorming of pre-existing ideologies associated with the phenomenon in question to ensure the researcher was cognisant of their own inherent beliefs and their influence upon the identification of codes, themes, and/or concepts [59,62].

Participant identity was protected by use of pseudonyms. However, to provide greater meaning to the qualitative findings, names were used as opposed to numbers.

2.11. Statistical Analysis

Quantitative statistical analysis was completed using IBM SPSS (v25 IBM Corp, Armonk, New York, NY, USA). For all data, normality (via Shapiro-Wilk's test) and homogeneity of variance/sphericity (via Mauchly's test) was checked. If sphericity was violated or data was non-normally distributed, degrees of freedom were corrected using Greenhouse–Geisser values or the appropriate non-parametric test was selected [63]. Confidence intervals were explored using least significant difference (LSD) (none) over Bonferroni corrections to minimise the potential of missing meaningful effects. The Bonferroni correction aims to reduce the chance of type 1 errors but subsequently increases the likelihood of type 2 errors and may be regarded a conservative approach that is better suited to experiments that have no clear hypothesis [64]. For analysis of variance (ANOVA, i.e., repeated measures) main effects and interactions, the effect size (ES) is reported as the partial η^2 value. Otherwise, the ES (Cohens d) was calculated using the difference in means divided by the pooled standard deviation (SD) of the compared values for normally distributed data [65], and $Z/\sqrt{n}$ for non-normally distributed data [66]. Data is presented as mean ± standard deviation unless otherwise stated. The statistical threshold was set at $p \leq 0.05$ [67,68].

3. Results

3.1. Endurance Capacity (T_{LIM})

There were no order effects for T_{LIM} ($p = 0.485$). A main effect for treatment was observed ($p < 0.001$; $F = 23.638$; $\eta^2 = 0.772$). Mean T_{LIM} was greatest ($p < 0.001$) for synergism (672 ± 132 s) vs. placebo (533 ± 79 s) (Figure 2). However, when isolated, T_{LIM} was greater ($p = 0.012$; ES = 0.4) for psychology (623 ± 117 s) vs. pharmacology (578 ± 99 s) with all participants running longer for psychology (Figure 2).

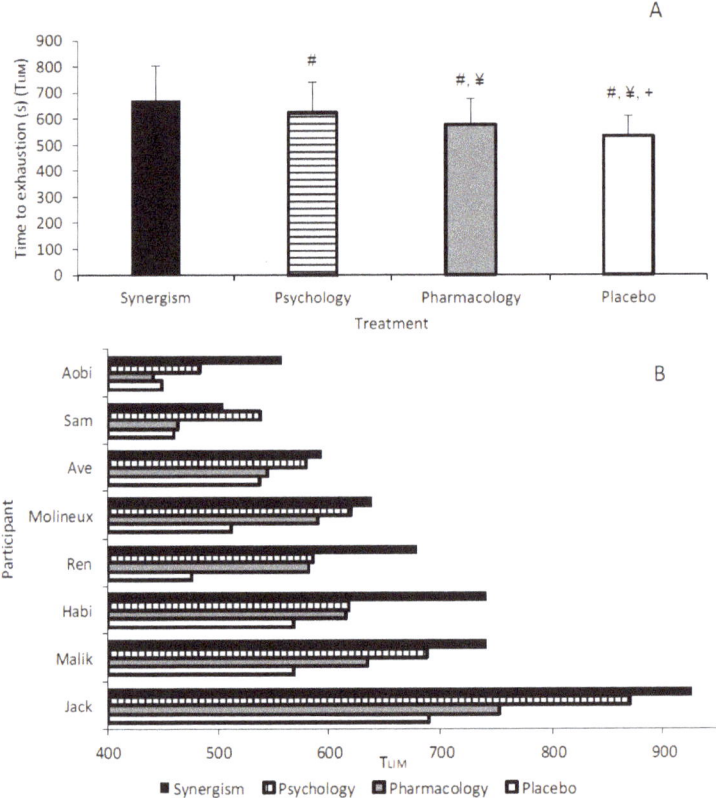

Figure 2. Endurance capacity (TLIM) scores (s). (**A**) Mean T_{LIM} (s) across treatments (#, ¥ and + denotes significantly lower vs. synergism, psychology and pharmacology, respectively); (**B**) subjective T_{LIM} across treatments.

Although main effects were observed for RPE, HR, BLa and BG across time (i.e., greater scores were observed for T_{LIM} vs. time matched exercise (isotime) (bouts of LIST)) with the exception of HR, no treatment or interaction effects were observed. However, when these measures at post-exercise were divided by each minute of T_{LIM}, a trend of reduction was observed for synergism followed by psychology, pharmacology and placebo (Tables 1 and 2).

Table 1. Post-exercise ratings of perceived exertion (RPE) divided by T_{LIM} per min (exercise termination across treatments advocated by *).

Treatment	1 min	2 min	3 min	4 min	5 min	6 min	7 min	Post-Exercise (Placebo)	Post-Exercise (Pharmacology)	Post-Exercise (Psychology)	Post-Exercise (Synergism)
Synergism	2	3	5	6	8	10	11	14	15	17	18*
Psychology	2	3	5	7	9	10	12	15	16	18*	-
Pharmacology	2	4	6	8	10	11	13	17	18*	-	-
Placebo	2	4	6	8	10	12	14	18*	-	-	-

Table 2. Post-exercise heart rate (HR), BLa and BG divided by T_{LIM} per min (exercise termination across treatments advocated by *).

Treatment	Post-Exercise (Placebo)	Post-Exercise (Pharmacology)	Post-Exercise (Psychology)	Post-Exercise (Synergism)
	Heart Rate (HR; bpm^{-1})			
Synergism	147	159	172	185*
Psychology	160	173	187*	-
Pharmacology	172	186*	-	-
Placebo	184*	-	-	-
	Blood Lactate (BLa; mmol/L)			
Synergism	6.8	7.3	7.9	8.5*
Psychology	7.4	7.9	8.6*	-
Pharmacology	8.4	9.0*	-	-
Placebo	8.6*	-	-	-
	Blood Glucose (BG; mmol/L)			
Synergism	3.5	3.8	4.1	4.4*
Psychology	3.4	3.7	4.0*	-
Pharmacology	3.8	4.1*	-	-
Placebo	4.0*	-	-	-

3.2. Dynamic Reaction Time (DRT)

No treatment x time interaction was observed ($p = 0.759$; $F = 0.561$; $\eta^2 = 0.074$) but main effects were detected for treatment ($p = 0.024$; $F = 3.854$; $\eta^2 = 0.355$) and time ($p < 0.001$; $F = 20.802$; $\eta^2 = 0.748$). Fatigue appeared to debilitate DRT performance ($p < 0.05$), with a mean reduction of between 4 to 7 hits following T_{LIM} vs.

Baseline and 5 to 9 hits vs. post-ingestion. However, pharmacology ameliorated this decline by 2 to 4 hits vs. all treatments. Individuals also achieved 5 hits more at post-ingestion ($p = 0.05$; ES = 0.5) and 7 hits more following T_{LIM} ($p = 0.008$; ES = 0.5), for pharmacology vs. placebo (Figure 3).

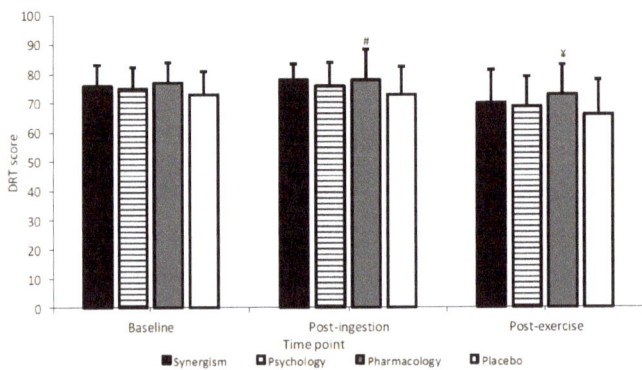

Figure 3. Mean dynamic reaction time (DRT) across treatments and time (# and ¥ denotes significantly greater difference vs. placebo).

3.3. Loughborough Soccer Passing Test (LSPT)

No interaction or main effects were observed across any LSPT parameter. However, time taken to complete LSPT following isotime exercise was fastest for placebo (70 ± 3 s) followed by synergism and psychology (74 ± 1 s) which were 2 s faster vs. pharmacology (76 ± 2 s) (Figure 4).

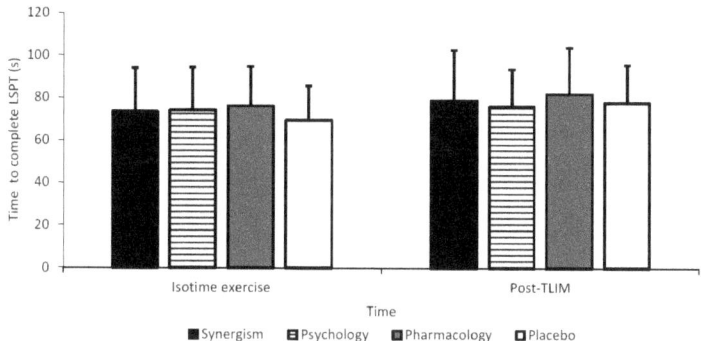

Figure 4. Time taken to complete the Loughborough Soccer Passing Test (LSPT) across treatments and time.

3.4. Heart Rate

No treatment x time interaction was observed for HR ($p = 0.053$; $F = 1.613$; $\eta^2 = 0.187$), however main effects for treatment ($p = 0.033$; $F = 5.359$; $\eta^2 = 0.434$) and time ($p < 0.001$; $F = 1495.447$; $\eta^2 = 0.995$) showed greater overall HR for given PLA vs. CAF conditions and greater HR with increasing time.

3.5. Blood Variables

No treatment x time interaction or main effect for treatment was observed for BLa and BG. However, a main effect of time was detected for BLa ($p < 0.001$; $F = 147.898$; $\eta^2 = 0.967$) and BG ($p = 0.009$; $F = 3.281$; $\eta^2 = 0.396$) with BLa greater with increasing time, whilst BG was reduced.

3.6. BRUMS

No treatment x time interaction or main effect for treatment was observed for any BRUMS subscale. However, a main effect of time was detected for fatigue ($p < 0.001$; $F = 51.501$; $\eta^2 = 0.880$) and vigour ($p = 0.04$; $F = 14.587$; $\eta^2 = 0.646$). Generally, fatigue was greater with time, whilst vigour was reduced.

3.7. CaffEQ

Participant responses regarding caffeine expectancies entailed six independent modes of CAF consumption, with only Aobi representing more than one (Table 3).

Table 3. Beverage chosen during caffeine expectancies questionnaire (CaffEQ) responses.

Participant	Responses Based on
1-Jack	Caffeine in general
2-Malik	Energy drinks
3-Habi	Soft drinks
4-Ren	Energy drinks
5-Molineux	Other (not specified)
6-Ave	Caffeine in general
7-Sam	Energy drinks
8-Aobi	Coffee, soft drinks and tea

No mean differences were observed between trials 1 and 3 across any CaffEQ subscales irrespective of the treatment administered. However, following subjective analysis various differences were observed across trials (Table 4).

Table 4. Subjective CaffEQ scores across trials 1 and 3, alteration in expectancy type denoted by *. (i.e., 1 = unlikely, 2 = a little unlikely, 3 = a little likely, 4 = likely, 5 = very likely). T1 and T3 = trials 1 and 3.

Participant	Withdrawal		Energy		Mood Enhancement		Appetite Suppression		Physical Performance Enhancement		Anxiety/Negative Physical Effects		Sleep Disturbances	
	T1	T3	T1	T3	T1	T3	T1	T3	T1	T3	T1	T3	T1	T3
Jack	2	2	3	3	3	3	2	2	3	3	2	1	1	1
Malik	0	0	2	2	1	1	0	0	1	1	0	0	1	1
Habi	0	0	0	0	0	0	0	0	0	0	0	0	0	0
Ren	3	2*	4	4	4	3	3	2*	4	4	1	3*	3	3
Molineux	2	3*	2	3*	1	2	2	3*	3	3	2	3*	1	2
Ave	0	1	2	2	1	1	0	3*	2	3*	0	1	0	2*
Sam	1	0	3	2*	1	1	0	1	2	3*	0	0	0	0
Aobi	2	1	3	3	2	2	2	2	2	3*	3	2*	3	2*

4. Qualitative Findings

Following template analysis, 5 areas of discussion became prominent (general perceptions, DRT, LSPT, T_{LIM} and LIST; Table 5). Although the success of expectancy manipulation was not explicity confirmed, no participants correctly guessed the deception employed. Moreover, during Dictaphone use, Habi, Ren, Ave and Aobi referred to treatments as they were administered (i.e., told CAF/PLA), whilst Malik, Jack, Sam and Molineux referred to at least 2/4 treatments. Thus, it appeared participants believed the deception employed.

Table 5. Themes and supporting statements across areas of discussion.

Themes	Supporting Statements
General Perceptions	
Expectancies facilitated perceptions	• Aobi—'I felt like I needed the lift that day and you could definitely feel like the caffeine (trial—psychology) had an impact on me' (greater mood and energy, and lowered fatigue perception vs. told PLA treatments).
	• Ren—'Compared to the two placebo trials, after the ingestion period (synergism), I almost immediately felt more alert, more active, more confident, and more energetic'. Synergism also reduced fatigue perception during LIST, vs. told PLA treatments.
	• Ave—Had 'a bit more energy' for synergism vs. told PLA conditions.
Told PLA treatments had minimal effect	• Aobi—Told PLA conditions induced neutral expectancies and/or a lack of 'psychological effect' and 'didn't really do much'
	• Ren—'I didn't feel it had any effect on the (sic), obviously knowing it's a placebo, both placebos (told PLA treatments), I expect what you're expected to feel'
	• Ave, Molineux and Habi indicated no differences between treatments.
Dynamic reaction time (DRT)	
Expectancies > told PLA treatments	• Ren—Expected 'to feel fatigued and slower' during told PLA treatments prior to measurement of post-exercise DRT, whilst feeling quicker during synergism.
	• Molineux and Aobi felt 'more alert' for psychology vs. placebo
	• Aobi—Psychology improved 'reaction times' on a day when he 'wasn't really feeling up to it'.
	• Ave—Told CAF conditions 'really helped', with synergism resulting in 'a lot less misses' and better performance vs. all other treatments
	• Aobi—Felt more familiarised to complete DRT, however this was augmented by 'the burst from the caffeine' during synergism.
LSPT and T_{LIM}	
Synergism > all other Treatments	• Ave and Ren—Synergism improved LSPT vs. pharmacology Due to increased speed. Ren also felt he 'was getting worse, getting a few more mistakes, missing the targets more' during pharmacology.
	• Aobi and Molineux were able to give more due to reduced fatigue perception for synergism vs. told PLA treatments, during T_{LIM}.
	• Ave—Synergism improved T_{LIM} vs. placebo due to reduced fatigue perception associated with 'the caffeine'. However, 'struggled' more during psychology.

Table 5. Cont.

	General Perceptions
Themes	Supporting Statements
	LIST
Debilitative psychology	• Malik put everything into LIST bout 1, and subsequently felt 'fatigued' and a 'lack of motivation' for psychology vs. told placebo treatments
	• Ren—perceived greater cardiovascular and leg fatigue during psychology vs. pharmacology.
	• Ave—felt tired during psychology but attributed this to a 'lack of sleep' and not the treatment.
	• Ave and Molineux—no 'improvement' for psychology vs. placebo.

PLA = placebo; LIST = Loughborough Intermittent Shuttle Test; CAF = caffeine; LSPT = Loughborough Soccer Passing Test.

5. Discussion

Through implementation of a double-dissociation design, this study is the first to compare CAF's pharmacological vs. psychological impact on various facets of simulated soccer performance. Although all treatments enhanced T_{LIM} vs. placebo, synergism resulted in the greatest improvements. However, when isolated, psychology improved T_{LIM} by 7% (~45 s) vs. pharmacology with all participants displaying improvements for psychology. These findings indicate CAF expectancy is an important contributor to the performance-enhancing benefit(s) of CAF. In relation to tasks involving a greater cognitive influence, pharmacology improved post-exercise DRT performance vs. all other treatments, whilst told CAF conditions improved the time taken to complete LSPT vs. pharmacology. Hence, CAF may be an effective nutritional supplement to evoke improved exercise performance. In some cases such benefits may occur with only the belief that CAF has been consumed and these effects may be greater vs. CAF's pharmacology impetus. However, an additive effect may be observed after combining expectancy with CAF pharmacology [18].

Irrespective of the ingested treatment, expectancies improved T_{LIM} with psychology and synergism resulting in 90 and 95 s improvements vs. placebo and pharmacology, respectively. Using a double-dissociation model, only two other studies have explored the influence of CAF expectancies on T_{LIM}, albeit during cycle ergometer based maximal incremental tests. Brietzke et al. [28] found synergism and psychology resulted in ~19% (~75 s) and ~17% (~68 s) improvements in endurance capacity vs. a control (i.e., no treatment administered; (CON)), whereas Pires et al. [29] observed ~15% (63 s) and ~17% (71 s) improvements vs. CON. Both studies utilised 6 mg/kg/BM CAF capsules, and recreationally active participants. Pires et al. [29] showed rectus femoris activation and pre-frontal cortex deoxygenation were augmented across both CAF treatments, vs. CON. The latter effect is associated with antagonism of A_1 and A_{2A} adenosine receptors, and subsequent corticospinal excitability. Moreover, whilst Brietzke et al. [28] observed similar RPE for synergism and psychology, magnitude-based inferences indicated 75% probability of a beneficial effect for both conditions vs. CON. Comparably, we observed similar RPE across treatments following T_{LIM}. However, when RPE was divided by T_{LIM}, a trend of reduction was observed for synergism, followed by psychology, pharmacology and placebo. A similar trend was also observed for HR, BLa and BG. Hence, T_{LIM} performance was likely facilitated by lowered cardiovascular, hematological and/or perceptual strain, which appeared greater influenced by CAF expectancies vs. pharmacology. In support, Benedetti et al. [69] advocate that expectancies could influence changes in physiological processes associated with perceptual, motor, and homeostatic relevance. Furthermore, the psychobiological model of endurance performance posits that interventions designed to reduce perceptual exertion and/or enhance motivation may improve exercise tolerance [70,71]. Indeed, placebos have been observed to increase frontal alpha asymmetry and associated positive affect appraisal of effort perception, when described as ergogenic aids [72]. It is also plausible that perceptual exertion and/or motivation may share an inverse relationship [73], though subjective motivation was not directly assessed here. In contrast to the current study, the aforementioned studies were performed single-blind (i.e., potentially influenced by experimenter bias), whilst subjective perceptions were unexplored which are important in advocating CAF's mechanisms of action [18].

Pharmacology resulted in five and seven score improvements during measurement of DRT, at post-ingestion and post-exercise, respectively, vs. placebo. Synergism also improved DRT at post-ingestion by 5 scores vs. placebo, thus CAF possibly facilitated augmented performance via central effects [74]. Moreover, the decline in DRT performance observed at post-exercise vs. baseline and post-ingestion was also ameliorated during pharmacology, with scores 2 to 4 and 2 to 3 hits greater vs. all other conditions. In contrast, Oei and Hartley [31] detected comparable performance on a self-designed sustained attention task for given CAF (~143 mg) (2.57 s) and told CAF (2.47 s) treatments. Moreover, similar findings were observed on the Bakan vigilance task for psychology, placebo and pharmacology (200 mg) [38]. The difference in results between the present study and the aforementioned studies may relate to the differences in tasks employed. Caffeine initiates excitability at the supraspinal level which may improve gross motor function (i.e., agility, reaction time, whole body movement) before, during and after sports activities [3,75–77]. In contrast, expectancy effects may be overestimated during the performance of simple reaction tests due to inhibition of fine motor skills associated with CAF over arousal and impaired cognitions [78].

Although the time taken to complete the LSPT declined over time, psychology and synergism appeared to mediate this following time matched exercise and T_{LIM}, vs. pharmacology. These results were likely due to expectancies for CAF ergogenicity as performance was comparable for synergism and psychology. Gant et al. [62] reported CAF (3.7 mg/kg/BM) improved LSPT performance by 1.5 s following isotime exercise vs. CON, in 15 amateur male soccer players. Comparatively, Foskett et al. [7] observed a 2.3 s reduction for CAF (6 mg/kg/BM) vs. CON, across 12 university soccer players. Although neither study explored CAF's psychological impact, Foskett et al. [7] found 4 individuals correctly, and 3 incorrectly, identified CAF trials with 5 declining to comment. Thus, although disparate, expectancies likely influenced these findings and this issue may be associated with a lack of double-dissociation design whereby expectancies were uncontrolled [18]. Moreover, expectancy effects are likely individually (based on belief and concurrent level of motivation), temporally and experientially modulated further highlighting the need to explore subjective perceptions. These issues may have also persisted in Gant et al. [79], although were not explored.

The changes in BG and BLa with increasing exercise intensity are likely causal and concomitant to augmented glucose metabolism associated with greater energy output and metabolite accumulation [80,81]. Furthermore, similar effects were observed for HR and are likely associated with a greater cellular requirement for oxygen and nutrients (e.g., glucose) and removal of metabolites and carbon dioxide [82]. Moreover, the 2 to 4 bpm^{-1} between-treatment variances in HR were likely physiologically negligible, especially as HR following isotime exercise was comparable across treatments (~164 bpm^{-1}). These findings correlate with BRUMS, whereby fatigue increased and vigour decreased across time.

5.1. Qualitative Implications

5.1.1. T_{LIM}

The qualitative implications associated with T_{LIM} highlight the individualistic nature of subjective perceptions. However, told CAF treatments always facilitated greater or comparable T_{LIM} vs. told PLA and this was irrespective of whether perceptions for CAF ergogenicity were positive or negative [73]. For example, psychology was considered detrimental for Ren, yet T_{LIM} was comparable vs. pharmacology. Interestingly, Ren displayed expectancies for negative physical effects/anxiety but also performance enhancements on the CaffEQ, hence a relationship between these expectancies is plausible. Comparably, Ave documented significant fatigue perception across psychology and pharmacology, nonetheless T_{LIM} for psychology was comparable to synergism but 30 s greater vs. pharmacology. Molineux perceived minimal differences across treatments, though told CAF conditions performed comparably but ≥ 30 s vs. pharmacology. In contrast, Malik and Habi displayed limited expectancies across the CaffEQ, yet Malik felt psychology was the worst trial, whilst Habi indicated no differences. Interestingly, T_{LIM} was improved (53 s) or comparable vs. pharmacology, for Malik and Habi respectively. Thus, expectation of CAF consumption appeared to be the greatest mediating factor here. Furthermore, these findings are likely influenced by neutral expectancies and/or a lack of perceived effect for told PLA conditions. However, although the aforementioned was not confirmed, participants referred to treatments as they were administered (i.e., told CAF/PLA) and none guessed the deception employed.

5.1.2. DRT and LSPT

The themes associated with DRT and LSPT appeared unrelated to performance outcomes. Instead, our findings indicate negative perceptions associated with CAF may invoke a greater cognitive impetus associated with alertness, concentration and technique which is otherwise impaired following positive perceptions due to CAF over reliance [23,26]. For example, for DRT, Aobi indicated psychology improved 'reaction times' on a day when he 'wasn't really feeling up to it'; however, 7 and 14 score reductions were observed vs. placebo at post-ingestion and post-exercise. Moreover, 'the burst from the caffeine' during synergism was also perceived to improve DRT, yet scores were comparable to placebo and 5 less vs. pharmacology, at post-ingestion. In contrast, Ren perceived greater fatigue for psychology vs. synergism, yet post-exercise DRT was 8 and 11 hits greater vs. synergism and placebo. Comparably, time to complete the LSPT was fastest for psychology vs. all other conditions after Malik felt the treatment impaired concentration, balance, motivation and technique. Opposingly, Aobi felt psychology was facilitative, yet LSPT performance was 7 to 12 s slower vs. all other conditions. This notion is supported by Tallis et al. [26] who propose an inverse relationship between expectations and motivation, with too positive an expectation resulting in reductions in conscious effort due to over confidence. We speculate similarly low expectancies associated with placebo may have driven improvements in LSPT due to increased conscious effort. However, greater clarity is required here, as limited subjective information was ascertained regarding placebo, following template analysis.

Although positive expectancies following psychology enhanced motivation, Harrell and Juliano [23] observed slower reaction times and less hits on the rapid visual information processing task vs. told impair conditions. Moreover, pharmacology appeared to improve performance vs. all treatments, irrespective of expectancies. Thus, much like the inverted U-hypothesis proposed by Yerkes and Dodson [83], expectations may need to be modulated to an optimal point for the greatest benefits and this point might differ individually (based on belief and concurrent level of motivation), temporally and experientially [18]. Given the potential difficulty in achieving this and the multi-faceted demands of soccer and other team sports activities, CAF expectancies might not be appropriate here given the potential for over-reliance with respect to cognitive-based tasks. Alternatively, CAF expectancies may better suit tasks that entail lower cognitive requirements but may benefit from improved gross motor function associated with reduced RPE (e.g., long-distance running, weightlifting etc.) [3,75,77].

5.2. Broader Applications

Although synergism of CAF psychology and pharmacology generally modulated the greatest performance benefits within the current study, when isolated, CAF's psychological impetus appeared to mediate CAF ergogenicity to a greater extent vs. CAF pharmacology. Therefore, expectancies may represent an alternative to CAF dosing prior to late evening sports competitions, ameliorating the quality of exercise recovery, training and preparation which is otherwise impaired due to changes in melatonin production, molecular oscillations and sleep quality [33]. The aforementioned approach may also benefit soccer coaches in planning training sessions after accounting for variances in physical/mental recovery which would be aided by enhanced sleep quality. Moreover, these findings represent important implications for soccer players affected by habituation to CAF's central effects [34–36] and health concerns (e.g., individuals suffering from heart disease, cardiac arrythmia, anxiety and depression) and side effects that are exacerbated/instigated by consumption of CAF and potentially detrimental to exercise performance [10,84–87]. Indeed, CAF expectancies represent minimal health concerns as the consumption of pharmacologically active CAF is not required. Moreover, during instances where CAF is consumed, expectancies may be trained and/or manipulated to enhance overall CAF ergogenicity (as indicated by the treatment 'synergism' during the current study). However, the influence of CAF expectancies has not been compared vs. CAF's pharmacological effect following performance of subsequent games (e.g., soccer tournaments which are common across recreational sport). As such, it is unclear how CAF's psychological effect would compare vs. CAF's central effects here. Further research is required.

The current findings also emphasise the need for future CAF studies to account for any psychological effects which are at present largely overlooked. To achieve this, we recommend implementation of the double-dissociation design which involves manipulating beliefs in accord with the experimental purpose. This decreases the discrepancy of individuals guessing which treatment they have been administered and reduces overlaps between CAF psychology and pharmacology.

5.3. Limitations

Although no participants correctly guessed the deception employed, and treatments were generally referred to as they were administered (i.e., told CAF/PLA) we did not explicitly confirm the success of expectancy manipulation. Future research will benefit from confirming the success (or not) of expectancy manipulation.

We compared the subjective experiences of individuals via template analysis, however, CAF associated changes with respect to an individual's circadian rhythm (i.e., changes in melatonin production and molecular oscillations) could have influenced these comparisons especially as some participants performed sessions in the morning, whilst others in the afternoon [33]. Moreover, subjective references were made to poor sleep quality possibly influencing exercise performance which may have been exacerbated by the timing of CAF consumption. Thus, future studies may benefit from measuring sleep quality prior to trials.

Although the notion of greater T_{LIM} associated with lowered RPE is supported by the psychobiological model of endurance performance [73], we did not measure subjective motivation which is also considered an important psychosomatic determinant of exercise tolerance. Future studies should, therefore, explore changes in motivation across treatments.

Although we explored changes in BLa and BG concentrations, CAF may also influence various other metabolites (e.g., epinephrine, norepinephrine etc.) [88,89] that might contribute to fluctuations in sport and exercise performance. Moreover, genetic assessments related to caffeine metabolism were not checked across participants which may have influenced the efficacy of CAF pharmacology [90,91].

Finally, while expectancies were assessed via the CaffEQ, we did not explore habitual CAF consumption, which has been observed to decrease the pharmacological effect of caffeine due to reduced adenosine receptor sensitivity, for habitual consumers [36]. Consequently, CAF's psychological effect may have been overestimated across the current study. However, the effects of CAF withdrawal are likely minimal as generally participants did not indicate any withdrawal symptoms/sensations via template analysis or BRUMS. Moreover, it is unclear why we observed limited findings with respect of BRUMS, especially as various mentions were made to changes in mood states across all treatments, following template analysis.

6. Conclusions

Through implementation of a double-dissociation design, this study is the first to compare CAF's pharmacological vs. psychological impact on various components of simulated soccer performance. Although all treatments enhanced T_{LIM} vs. placebo, synergism resulted in the greatest improvements. However, when isolated, psychology improved T_{LIM} by 7% (~45 s) vs. pharmacology with all participants displaying improvements for psychology. These findings appeared relative to enhanced expectancies and potentially reduced perceptual exertion but not perceptual states. Interestingly, DRT was impaired for individuals displaying positive CAF perceptions which may be explained by reduced conscious effort associated with CAF over-reliance. This was also observed during the LSPT with the opposite occurring during negative perceptions. Thus, the mechanisms by which expectancies influence exercise performance appear to be dependent on the task performed, with reduced RPE a potential key mediator during endurance capacity. Subsequently, CAF expectancies may better suit tasks that require lesser cognitive/skill specific attributes.

Author Contributions: Conceptualization, M.F.H., A.S. and A.H.; Writing—Original Draft Preparation, A.S.; Writing—Review and Editing, M.F.H., A.H., J.T., B.S.; Data Collection, A.S., O.E., L.S., G.S., M.S.

Funding: This research received no external funding.

Acknowledgments: Thank you to Dylon Spiers and Alex van Enis for their assistance during data collection and to Ceri Heldreich and Kyle Farley for their outstanding technical assistance. Bryan Saunders additional affiliation: Institute of Orthopedics and traumatology, faculty of medicine, FMUSP, University of Sao Paulo, Brazil.

Conflicts of Interest: The authors declare no conflict of interest.

References

1. Bloms, L.P.; Fitzgerald, J.S.; Short, M.W.; Whitehead, J.R. The Effects of Caffeine on Vertical Jump Height and Execution in Collegiate Athletes. *J. Strength Cond. Res.* **2016**, *30*, 1855–1861. [CrossRef] [PubMed]
2. Glaister, M.; Muniz-Pumares, D.; Patterson, S.D.; Foley, P.; McInnes, G. Caffeine supplementation and peak anaerobic power output. *Eur. J. Sport Sci.* **2015**, *15*, 400–406. [CrossRef] [PubMed]
3. Del Coso, J.; Munoz-Fernandez, V.E.; Munoz, G.; Fernandez-Elias, V.E.; Ortega, J.F.; Hamouti, N.; Barbero, J.C.; Munoz-Guerra, J. Effects of a Caffeine-Containing Energy Drink on Simulated Soccer Performance. *PLoS ONE* **2012**, *7*, 1–8. [CrossRef] [PubMed]
4. Lara, B.; Gonzalez-Millan, C.; Salinero, J.J.; Abian-Vicen, J.; Areces, F.; Barbero-Alvarez, J.C.; Munoz, V.; Portillo, L.J.; Gonzalez-Rave, J.M.; Del Coso, J. Caffeine-containing energy drink improves physical performance in female soccer players. *Amino Acids* **2014**, *46*, 1385–1392. [CrossRef] [PubMed]
5. Goldstein, E.R.; Ziegenfuss, T.; Kalman, D.; Kreider, R.; Campbell, B.; Wilborn, C.; Taylor, L.; Willoughby, D.; Stout, J.; Graves, B.S.; et al. International society of sports nutrition position stand: Caffeine and performance. *J. Int. Soc. Sports Nutr.* **2010**, *7*, 1–15. [CrossRef] [PubMed]
6. Russell, M.; Kingsley, M. The efficacy of acute nutritional interventions on soccer skill performance. *Sports Med.* **2014**, *44*, 957–970. [CrossRef] [PubMed]
7. Foskett, A.; Ali, A.; Gant, N. Caffeine enhances cognitive function and skill performance during simulated soccer activity. *Int. J. Sport Nutr. Exerc. Metab.* **2009**, *19*, 410–423. [CrossRef]
8. Jordan, J.B.; Korgaokar, A.; Farley, R.S.; Coons, J.M.; Caputo, J.L. Caffeine supplementation and reactive agility in elite youth soccer players. *Pediatric Exerc. Sci.* **2014**, *26*, 168–176. [CrossRef] [PubMed]
9. Fredholm, B.B.; Battig, K.; Holmen, J.; Nehlig, A.; Zvartau, E.E. Actions of caffeine in the brain with special reference to factors that contribute to its widespread use. *Pharmacol. Rev.* **1990**, *51*, 83–133.
10. Pickering, C.; Kiely, J. Are the Current Guidelines on Caffeine Use in Sport Optimal for Everyone? Inter-individual Variation in Caffeine Ergogenicity, and a Move Towards Personalised Sports Nutrition. *Sports Med.* **2018**, *48*, 7–16. [CrossRef]
11. Reilly, T.; Thomas, V. A motion analysis of work-rate in different positional roles in professional football match-play. *J. Hum. Mov. Stud.* **1976**, *2*, 87–89.
12. Mohr, M.; Krustrup, P.; Bangsbo, J. Match performance of high-standard soccer players with special reference to development of fatigue. *J. Sports Sci.* **2003**, *21*, 519–528. [CrossRef] [PubMed]

13. Stolen, T.; Chamari, K.; Castagna, C.; Wisloff, U. Physiology of soccer: An update. *Sports Med.* **2005**, *35*, 501–536. [CrossRef] [PubMed]
14. Vescovi, J.D.; Favero, T.G. Motion characteristics of women's college soccer matches: Female Athletes in Motion (FAiM) study. *Int. J. Sports Physiol. Perform.* **2014**, *9*, 405–414. [CrossRef] [PubMed]
15. Doherty, M.; Smith, P.M. Effects of caffeine ingestion on exercise testing: A meta-analysis. *Int. J. Sport Nutr. Exerc. Metab.* **2004**, *14*, 626–646. [CrossRef] [PubMed]
16. Pickering, C.; Grgic, J. Caffeine and Exercise: What Next? *Sports Med.* **2019**, *49*, 1007–1030. [CrossRef] [PubMed]
17. Alberti, F.G.; Iaia, M.; Arcelli, E.; Cavaggioni, L.; Rampinini, E. Goal scoring patterns in major European soccer leagues. *Sport Sci. Health* **2013**, *9*, 151–153. [CrossRef]
18. Shabir, A.; Hooton, A.; Tallis, J.; Higgins, M.F. The Influence of Caffeine Expectancies on Sport, Exercise, and Cognitive Performance. *Nutrients* **2018**, *10*, 1528. [CrossRef] [PubMed]
19. Saunders, B.; de Oliveira, L.F.; da Silva, R.P.; de Salles Painelli, V.; Goncalves, L.S.; Yamaguchi, G.; Mutti, T.; Maciel, E.; Roschel, H.; Artioli, G.G.; et al. Placebo in sports nutrition: A proof-of-principle study involving caffeine supplementation. *Scand. J. Med. Sci. Sports* **2017**, *27*, 1240–1247. [CrossRef] [PubMed]
20. Beedie, C.J.; Foad, A.J. The placebo effect in sports performance: A brief review. *Sports Med.* **2009**, *39*, 313–329. [CrossRef]
21. Beedie, C.J.; Stuart, E.M.; Coleman, D.A.; Foad, A.J. Placebo effects of caffeine on cycling performance. *Med. Sci. Sports Exerc.* **2006**, *38*, 2159–2164. [CrossRef] [PubMed]
22. Duncan, M.J.; Lyons, M.; Hankey, J. Placebo effects of caffeine on short-term resistance exercise to failure. *Int. J. Sport Physiol.* **2009**, *4*, 244–253. [CrossRef]
23. Harrell, P.T.; Juliano, L.M. Caffeine expectancies influence the subjective and behavioral effects of caffeine. *Psychopharmacology* **2009**, *207*, 335–342. [CrossRef] [PubMed]
24. Denson, T.F.; Jacobsen, M.; von Hippel, W.; Kemp, R.I.; Mak, T. CAF expectancies but not CAF reduce depletion-induced aggression. *Psychol. Addict. Behav.* **2012**, *26*, 140–144. [CrossRef] [PubMed]
25. Pollo, A.; Carlino, E.; Benedetti, F. The top-down influence of ergogenic placebos on muscle work and fatigue. *Eur. J. Neurosci.* **2008**, *28*, 379–388. [CrossRef] [PubMed]
26. Tallis, J.; Muhammad, B.; Islam, M.; Duncan, M.J. Placebo effects of caffeine on maximal voluntary concentric force of the knee flexors and extensors. *Muscle Nerve* **2016**, *54*, 479–486. [CrossRef] [PubMed]
27. Foad, A.J.; Beedie, C.J.; Coleman, D.A. Pharmacological and psychological effects of caffeine ingestion in 40-km cycling performance. *Med. Sci. Sports Exerc.* **2008**, *40*, 158–165. [CrossRef] [PubMed]
28. Brietzke, C.; Asano, R.Y.; Russi de Lima, F.D.; Pinheiro, F.A.; Alvarenga, F.; Ugrinowitsch, C.; Pires, F.O. Caffeine effects on VO2max test outcomes investigated by a placebo perceived-as-caffeine design. *Nutr. Health* **2017**, *23*, 231–238. [CrossRef]
29. Pires, F.O.; dos Anjos, C.A.S.; Covolan, R.J.M.; Fontes, E.B.; Noakes, T.D.; Gibson, A.S.C.; Magalhaes, F.H.; Ugrinowitsch, C. Caffeine and placebo Improved Maximal Exercise Performance Despite Unchanged Motor Cortex Activation and Greater Prefontal Cortex Deoxygenation. *Front. Physiol.* **2018**. [CrossRef]
30. Dawkins, L.; Shahzad, F.Z.; Ahmed, S.S.; Edmonds, C.J. Expectation of having consumed caffeine can improve performance and mood. *Appetite* **2011**, *57*, 597–600. [CrossRef]
31. Oei, A.; Hartley, L.R. The effects of caffeine and expectancy on attention and memory. *Hum. Psychopharmacol.* **2005**, *20*, 193–202. [CrossRef] [PubMed]
32. Fillmore, M.; Vogel-Sprott, M. Expected effect of caffeine on motor performance predicts the type of response to placebo. *Psychopharmacology* **1992**, *106*, 209–214. [CrossRef] [PubMed]
33. Burke, T.M.; Markwald, R.R.; McHill, A.W.; Chinoy, E.D.; Snider, J.A.; Bessman, S.C.; Jung, C.M.; O'Neill, J.S.; Wright, K.P., Jr. Effects of caffeine on the human circadian clock in vivo and in vitro. *Sci. Transl. Med.* **2015**, *16*, 305. [CrossRef] [PubMed]
34. Schicatano, E.J.; Blumenthal, T.D. The effects of different doses of caffeine on habituation of the human acoustic startle reflex. *Pharmacol. Biochem. Behav.* **1995**, *52*, 231–236. [CrossRef]
35. Svenningsson, P.; Nomikos, G.G.; Fredholm, B.B. The stimulatory action and the development of tolerance to caffeine is associated with alterations in gene expression in specific brain regions. *J. Neurosci.* **1999**, *19*, 4011–4022. [CrossRef] [PubMed]
36. Pickering, G.; Kiely, J. What Should We Do About Habitual Caffeine Use in Athletes? *Sports Med.* **2019**, *49*, 833–842. [CrossRef] [PubMed]

37. Nicholas, C.W.; Nuttall, F.E.; Williams, C. The Loughborough Intermittent Shuttle Test: A field test that simulates the activity pattern of soccer. *J. Sports Sci.* **2000**, *18*, 97–104. [CrossRef]
38. Elliman, N.A.; Ash, J.; Green, M.W. Pre-existent expectancy effects in the relationship between caffeine and performance. *Appetite* **2010**, *55*, 355–358. [CrossRef]
39. Van Soeren, M.H.; Graham, T.E. Effect of caffeine on metabolism, exercise endurance, and catecholamine responses after withdrawal. *J. Appl. Physiol.* **1998**, *85*, 1493–1501. [CrossRef]
40. Irwin, C.; Desbrow, B.; Ellis, A.; O'Keeffe, B.; Grant, G.; Leveritt, M. Caffeine withdrawal and high-intensity endurance cycling performance. *J. Sports Sci.* **2011**, *29*, 509–515. [CrossRef]
41. Fernandes, A.L.; Lopes-Silva, J.P.; Bertuzzi, R.; Casarini, D.E.; Arita, D.Y.; Bishop, D.J.; Lima-Silva, A.E. Effect of Time of Day on Performance, Hormonal and Metabolic Response during a 1000-m Cycling Time Trial. *PLoS ONE* **2014**, *9*, e109954. [CrossRef]
42. Strasbourg. *Testing Physical Fitness, Eurofit Experimental Battery Provisional Handbook, Sports Section of the Council of Europe*; Bitworks Design and Consultancy: Cheltenham, UK, 1983.
43. Borg, G.A.V. Psychophysical bases of perceived exertion. *Med. Sci. Sports Exerc.* **1982**, *14*, 377–381. [CrossRef]
44. McGregor, S.J.; Nicholas, C.W.; Lakomy, H.K.A.; Williams, C. The influence of intermittent high intensity shuttle running and fluid ingestion on the performance of a soccer skill. *J. Sports Sci.* **1990**, *17*, 895–903. [CrossRef]
45. Online Tone Generator. Available online: http://www.szynalski.com/tone-generator/ (accessed on 1 July 2017).
46. Lane, A.M.; Lane, H.J. Predictive effectiveness of mood measures. *Percept. Mot. Ski.* **2002**, *94*, 785–791. [CrossRef]
47. Graham, T.E.; Spriet, L.L. Metabolic, catecholamine, and exercise performance responses to various doses of caffeine. *J. Appl. Physiol.* **1995**, *78*, 867–874. [CrossRef]
48. The Science of Caffeine: The Worlds Most Popular Drug. Available online: https://www.youtube.com/watch?v=YuJOhpNS0IY (accessed on 1 July 2017).
49. Fat Albert "JATO" Take-Off 2009. Available online: https://www.youtube.com/watch?v=VHOvoO-6nWQ (accessed on 1 July 2017).
50. Huntley, E.D.; Juliano, L.M. Caffeine Expectancy Questionnaire (CaffEQ): Construction, psychometric properties, and associations with caffeine use, caffeine dependence, and other related variables. *Psychol. Assess* **2011**, *24*, 592–607. [CrossRef]
51. Ando, S.; Kida, N.; Oda, S. Central and peripheral visual reaction time of soccer players and nonathletes. *Percept. Mot. Ski.* **2001**, *92*, 786–794. [CrossRef]
52. Ricotti, L.; Rigosa, J.; Niosi, A.; Menciassi, A. Analysis of balance, rapidity, force and reaction times of soccer players at different levels of competition. *PLoS ONE* **2013**, *8*, e77264. [CrossRef]
53. Ellison, P.H.; Sparks, S.A.; Murphy, P.N.; Carnegie, E.; Marchant, D.C. Determining eye-hand coordination using the sport vision trainer: An evaluation of test-retest reliability. *Res. Sports Med.* **2014**, *22*, 36–48. [CrossRef]
54. Terry, P.C.; Lane, A.M.; Fogarty, G.J. Construct Validity of the POMS-A for use with adults. *J. Sport Exerc. Psychol.* **2003**, *4*, 125–139. [CrossRef]
55. Brooks, J.; McCluskey, S.; Turley, E.; King, N. The Utility of Template Analysis in Qualitative Psychology Research. *Qual. Res. Psychol.* **2015**, *12*, 202–222. [CrossRef]
56. Weber, R.P. *Basic Content Analysis*; Sage: Beverly Hills, CA, USA, 1990.
57. Glaser, B.G.; Strauss, A.L. *The Discovery of Grounded Theory: Strategies for Qualitative Research*; Aldine Publishing Company: Chicago, IL, USA, 1967.
58. Braun, V.; Clarke, V. Using thematic analysis in psychology. *Qual. Res. Psychol.* **2006**, *3*, 77–101. [CrossRef]
59. Jackson, S.A. Factors influencing the occurrence of flow state in elite athletes. *J. Appl. Sport Psychol.* **1995**, *4*, 161–180. [CrossRef]
60. Lincoln, Y.S.; Guba, E.G. *Naturalistic Inquiry*; Sage Publication: Newbury Park, CA, USA, 1985.
61. Patton, M. *Qualitative Evaluation and Research Methods*; Sage: Beverly Hills, CA, USA, 1990.
62. van Manen, M. *Researching Lived Experience: Human Science for and Action Sensitive Pedagogy*; SUNY Press: Albany, NY, USA, 1990.
63. Field, A. (Ed.) *Reliability Analysis*, 2nd ed.; Discovering Statistics Using SPSS; Sage Publication: London, UK, 2005.
64. Armstrong, R.A. When to use the Bonferroni correction. *Ophalmic Physiol. Opt.* **2014**, *34*, 502–508. [CrossRef]

65. Nakagawa, S.; Cuthill, I.C. Effect size, confidence interval and statistical significance: A practical guide for biologists. *Biol. Rev. Camb. Philos. Soc.* **2007**, *82*, 591–605. [CrossRef]
66. Ivarsson, A.; Johnson, U.; Podlog, L. Psychological predictors of injury occurrence: A prospective investigation of professional Swedish soccer players. *J. Sport Rehabil.* **2013**, *22*, 19–26. [CrossRef]
67. Higgins, M.F.; Wilson, S.; Hill, C.; Price, M.J.; Duncan, M.; Tallis, J. Evaluating the effects of caffeine and sodium bicarbonate, ingested individually or in combination, and a taste-matched placebo on high-intensity cycling capacity in healthy males. *Appl. Physiol. Nutr. Metab.* **2016**, *41*, 354–361. [CrossRef]
68. Higgins, M.F.; James, R.S.; Price, M.J. Familiarisation to and reproducibility of cycling at 110% peak power output. *J. Sports Med. Phys. Fit.* **2014**, *54*, 139–146.
69. Benedetti, F.; Mayberg, H.S.; Wager, T.D.; Stohler, C.S.; Zubieta, J.K. Neurobiological mechanisms of the placeo effect. *J. Neurosci.* **2005**, *25*, 10390–10402. [CrossRef]
70. Pageaux, B.; Lepers, R.; Dietz, K.C.; Marcora, S.M. Response inhibition impairs subsequent self-paced endurance performance. *Eur. J. Appl. Physiol.* **2014**, *114*, 1095–1105. [CrossRef]
71. Pageaux, B.; Lepers, R. Fatigue Induced by Physical and Mental Exertion Increases Perception of Effort and Impairs Subsequent Endurance Performance. *Front. Physiol.* **2016**, *7*, 587. [CrossRef] [PubMed]
72. Broelz, E.K.; Enck, P.; Niess, A.M.; Schneeweiss, P.; Wolf, S.; Weimer, K. The neurobiology of placebo effects in sports: EEG frontal alpha asymmetry increases in response to a placebo ergogenic aid. *Sci. Rep.* **2019**, *9*, 2381. [CrossRef] [PubMed]
73. Smirmaul, B.P.C.; Dantas, J.L.; Nakamura, F.Y.; Pereira, G. The psychobiological model: A new explanation to intensity regulation and (in)tolerance in endurance exercise. *Rev. Bras. Educ. Fís.* **2013**, *27*, 333–340. [CrossRef]
74. Meeusen, R.; Roelands, B.; Spriet, L.L. Caffeine, exercise and the brain. *Nestle Nutr. Inst. Workshop Ser.* **2013**, *76*, 1–12. [PubMed]
75. Duvnjak-Zaknich, D.M.; Dawson, B.T.; Wallman, K.E.; Henry, G. Effect of caffeine on reactive agility time when fresh and fatigued. *Med. Sci. Sports Exerc.* **2011**, *43*, 1523–1530. [CrossRef]
76. McLellan, T.M.; Caldwell, J.A.; Lieberman, H.R. A review of caffeine's effects on cognitive, physical and occupational performance. *Neurosci. Biobehav. Rev.* **2016**, *71*, 294–312. [CrossRef]
77. Plaskett, C.J.; Cafarelli, E. Caffeine increases endurance and attenuates force sensation during submaximal isometric contractions. *J. Appl. Physiol.* **2001**, *91*, 1535–1544. [CrossRef]
78. Benowitz, N.L. Clinical pharmacology of caffeine. *Annu. Rev. Med.* **1990**, *41*, 277–288. [CrossRef]
79. Gant, N.; Ali, A.; Foskett, A. The influence of caffeine and carbohydrate coingestion on simulated soccer performance. *Int. J. Sport Nutr. Exerc. Metab.* **2010**, *20*, 191–197. [CrossRef]
80. Coyle, E.F. Physiological determinants of endurance exercise performance. *J. Sci. Med. Sport* **1999**, *2*, 181–189. [CrossRef]
81. Sahlin, K. Muscle glucose metabolism during exercise. *Ann. Med.* **1990**, *22*, 85–89. [PubMed]
82. Burton, D.A.; Stokes, K.; Hall, G.M. Physiological effects of exercise. *BJA Educ.* **2004**, *4*, 185–188. [CrossRef]
83. Yerkes, R.M.; Dodson, J.D. The relation of strength of stimulus to rapidity of habit-formation. *J. Comp. Neurol.* **1908**, *18*, 459–482. [CrossRef]
84. Bchir, F.; Dogui, M.; Ben Fradj, R.; Arnaud, M.J.; Saguem, S. Differences in pharmacokinetic and electroencephalographic responses to caffeine in sleep-sensitive and non-sensitive subjects. *Comptes Rendus Biol.* **2006**, *329*, 512–519. [CrossRef] [PubMed]
85. Hartley, T.R.; Sung, B.H.; Pincomb, G.A.; Whitsett, T.L.; Wilson, M.F.; Lovallo, W.R. Hypertension risk status and effect of caffeine on blood pressure. *Hypertension* **2000**, *36*, 137–141. [CrossRef] [PubMed]
86. Green, P.J.; Kirby, R.; Suls, J. The effects of caffeine on blood pressure and heart rate: A review. *Ann. Behav. Med.* **1996**, *18*, 201–216. [CrossRef]
87. Abraham, J.; Mudd, J.O.; Kapur, N.K.; Klein, K.; Champion, H.C.; Wittstein, I.S. Stress cardiomyopathy after intravenous administration of catecholamines and beta-receptor agonists. *J. Am. Coll. Cardiol.* **2009**, *53*, 1320–1325. [CrossRef]
88. Lane, J.D.; Pieper, C.F.; Phillips-Bute, B.G.; Bryant, J.E.; Kuhn, C.M. Caffeine affects cardiovascular and neuroendocrine activation at work and home. *Psychosom. Med.* **2002**, *64*, 595–603.
89. Van Soeren, M.; Mohr, T.; Kjaer, M.; Graham, T.E. Acute effects of caffeine ingestion at rest in humans with impaired epinephrine responses. *J. Appl. Physiol.* **1996**, *80*, 999–1005. [CrossRef]

90. Southward, K.; Rutherfurd-Markwick, K.; Badenhorst, C.; Ali, A. The Role of Genetics in Moderating the Inter-Individual Differences in the Ergogenicity of Caffeine. *Nutrients* **2018**, *10*, 1352. [CrossRef] [PubMed]
91. Yang, A.; Palmer, A.A.; de Wit, H. Genetics of caffeine consumption and responses to caffeine. *Psychopharmacology* **2010**, *211*, 245–257. [CrossRef] [PubMed]

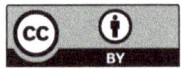

© 2019 by the authors. Licensee MDPI, Basel, Switzerland. This article is an open access article distributed under the terms and conditions of the Creative Commons Attribution (CC BY) license (http://creativecommons.org/licenses/by/4.0/).

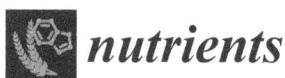

Review

Effect of Caffeine Supplementation on Sports Performance Based on Differences Between Sexes: A Systematic Review

Juan Mielgo-Ayuso [1,*], Diego Marques-Jiménez [2], Ignacio Refoyo [3], Juan Del Coso [4], Patxi León-Guereño [5] and Julio Calleja-González [6]

1. Department of Biochemistry, Molecular Biology and Physiology, Faculty of Health Sciences, University of Valladolid, 42004 Soria, Spain
2. Academy Department, Deportivo Alavés SAD, 01007 Vitoria-Gasteiz, Spain; dmarques001@ikasle.ehu.eus
3. Department of Sports, Faculty of Physical Activity and Sports Sciences (INEF), Universidad Politécnica de Madrid, 28040 Madrid, Spain; ignacio.refoyo@upm.es
4. Centre for Sport Studies. Rey Juan Carlos University, 28943 Fuenlabrada, Spain; juandelcosogarrigos@gmail.com
5. Faculty of Psychology and Education, University of Deusto, Campus of Donostia-San Sebastián, 20012 San Sebastián, Guipúzcoa, Spain; patxi.leon@deusto.es
6. Laboratory of Human Performance, Department of Physical Education and Sport, Faculty of Education, Sports Section, University of the Basque Country, 01007 Vitoria, Spain; julio.calleja.gonzalez@gmail.com
* Correspondence: juanfrancisco.mielgo@uva.es; Tel.: +34-975-129187

Received: 22 August 2019; Accepted: 27 September 2019; Published: 30 September 2019

Abstract: Most studies that have shown the positive effects of caffeine supplementation on sports performance have been carried out on men. However, the differences between sexes are evident in terms of body size, body composition, and hormonal functioning, which might cause different outcomes on performance for the same dosage of caffeine intake in men vs. women. The main aim of this systematic review was to analyze and compare the effects of caffeine intake between men and women on sports performance to provide a source of knowledge to sports practitioners and coaches, especially for those working with women athletes, on the use of caffeine as an ergogenic aid. A structured search was carried out following the Preferred Reporting Items for Systematic Review and Meta-Analyses (PRISMA) guidelines in the Web of Science, Cochrane Library, and Scopus databases until 28 July 2019. The search included studies in which the effects of caffeine supplementation on athletic performance were compared between sexes and to an identical placebo situation (dose, duration and timing). No filters were applied for participants' physical fitness level or age. A total of 254 articles were obtained in the initial search. When applying the inclusion and exclusion criteria, the final sample was 10 articles. The systematic review concluded that four investigations (100% of the number of investigations on this topic) had not found differences between sexes in terms of caffeine supplementation on aerobic performance and 3/3 (100%) on the fatigue index. However, four out of seven articles (57.1%) showed that the ergogenicity of caffeine for anaerobic performance was higher in men than women. In particular, it seems that men are able to produce more power, greater total weight lifted and more speed with the same dose of caffeine than women. In summary, caffeine supplementation produced a similar ergogenic benefit for aerobic performance and the fatigue index in men and women athletes. Nevertheless, the effects of caffeine to produce more power, total weight lifted and to improve sprint performance with respect to a placebo was higher in men than women athletes despite the same dose of caffeine being administered. Thus, the ergogenic effect of acute caffeine intake on anaerobic performance might be higher in men than in women.

Keywords: recovery; strength; power; sprint performance; menstrual cycle

1. Introduction

Numerous studies have shown the effectiveness of caffeine supplementation on sports performance in which aerobic [1], anaerobic [2–4] or mixed [5–7] metabolism is prioritized. Current guidelines recommend the ingestion of low-to-moderate doses of caffeine, ranging from 3 to 6 mg/kg, approximately 60 min prior to exercise to get these improvements [8,9]. Higher doses of caffeine (9–13 mg/kg) do not result in an additional improvement in physical performance [10], while these higher doses might increase the incidence and magnitude of main caffeine-related side effects. In addition, high doses of caffeine might end in urine caffeine concentrations greater than 15 µg/ml, which is prohibited in the National Collegiate Athletic Association (NCAA) [11].

In general, several mechanisms have been proposed to explain the effects of caffeine supplementation on sports performance [3,12]. However, the most well-recognized mechanism at present is that caffeine acts in the central nervous system (CNS) as a competitor for adenosine in its receptors, inhibiting the negative effects that adenosine induces on neurotransmission, excitation and pain perception [13]. In addition, the hypoalgesic effect of caffeine decreases the perception of pain and effort during exercise and therefore might also be considered as a supplementary mechanism of action, at least for exercise situations that induce pain [3,12]. As a result, lower pain perception could maintain or increase the firing rates of the motor units and possibly produce a more sustainable and forceful muscle contraction, and consequently, allow greater strength production [3,14].

Caffeine can affect the use of energy substrates during exercise. In particular, it has been suggested that caffeine supplementation acts as a glycogen saver as it increases the mobilization of free fatty acids by adrenaline (epinephrine) induction [15]. Although this mechanism could favor aerobic and anaerobic sports that depend on muscle glycogen, it is currently known that there are other mechanisms by which athletic performance would be favored such as increased calcium mobilization and phosphodiesterase inhibition [3,9]. In addition, it has been proposed that caffeine supplementation causes a greater activity of the Na^+/K^+ pump to enhance excitation contraction coupling [16].

Given that sex has been identified as an important determinant of athletic performance through the impact of body composition, aerobic capacity or anaerobic thresholds due to hormonal differences [17], specific recommendations for each sex should be in agreement with these sex differences to achieve better results in sports performance. In this respect, while there is a position and recommendations about the use of caffeine supplements in athletes [18,19], there is not enough comparative information on the effects of caffeine on athletic performance between men and women athletes [20]. For that reason, caution would be needed in extrapolating the recommendations made for men to women, since the vast majority of the studies included only male participants [1,2,5,21]. In fact, only ~13% of participants in investigations aimed to determine the ergogenic effect of caffeine are women, while the effect of caffeine in women at high (>9 mg/kg) or very low doses (<1 mg/kg) is unexplored [22]. In addition, due to the menstrual cycle, women are subject to hormonal changes that could affect sports performance [23,24]. For instance, it has been shown that the phase of the menstrual cycle influences the development of strength [25]. Also, the consumption of oral contraceptives has effects on the metabolism of caffeine, extending its half-life and prolonging the responses in the human body [26], although very few studies take these aspects into account [27].

In this respect, studies conducted with the general population have already shown that the stimulating effects (less drowsiness and greater activation) of caffeine are greater in men than in women [28]. Still, few studies have shown the differences in the effect of caffeine supplementation on sports performance between men and women, and their results are controversial [29–37]. While some studies have shown a comparable ergogenic effect of caffeine between sexes on sports performance, others have presented a greater effectiveness of caffeine to increase sprint power [29], isolated forehand stroke peak and average speed [37], total weight lifted [38] and a shorter time to perform a repeated modified agility test (RMAT) [30] in men compared to women. Unifying the data from these different studies could provide knowledge regarding the effect that caffeine supplementation has on sports performance based on the athlete's sex. This analysis might help to enhance the recommendations for caffeine supplementation based on sex and the type of exercise performed. Therefore, it was proposed to carry out a systematic review of the relevant articles published in the scientific literature. The main objective of which was to discern the possible effects of caffeine supplementation on sports performance based on the participant's sex. Specifically, this systematic review focuses on determining the different responses between the sexes to the same caffeine supplementation protocol depending on whether the exercise will be classified as aerobic, anaerobic or when the protocol induced some type of fatigue that could be evaluated (i.e., index of fatigue).

2. Methodology

2.1. Search Strategy

This article is a systematic review focused on the performance effects of caffeine in men athletes vs. women athletes. It was carried out following the Preferred Reporting Items for Systematic Review and Meta-Analyses (PRISMA) guidelines [39]. A structured search was carried out in the Web of Science (WOS), which includes other databases such as BCI, BIOSIS, CCC, DIIDW, INSPEC, KJD, MEDLINE, RSCI, SCIELO, and the Cochrane Library and Scopus, sources of high-quality information in the field of health sciences, thus guaranteeing complete bibliographic support. The search strategy ended on 28 July 2019. The search terms included a mix of medical subject headings (MeSH) and free-text words for key concepts related to caffeine, the sex of the athletes under investigation and different forms of exercise and sports performance. The following search equation was used to find the relevant articles: ("caffeine"[MeSH Terms] OR "caffeine"[All Fields]) AND ((("female"[MeSH Terms] OR "female"[All Fields]) OR ("women"[MeSH Terms] OR "women"[All Fields])) (("male"[MeSH Terms] OR "male"[All Fields]) OR ("men"[MeSH Terms] OR "men"[All Fields] OR "woman"[All Fields])) AND ((("exercise"[MeSH Terms] OR "exercise"[All Fields]) OR ("sports"[MeSH Terms] OR "sports"[All Fields] OR "sport"[All Fields])) AND performance [All Fields]. No filters were applied to the athlete's physical fitness level, race, or age to increase the power of the analysis. The search for published studies was independently performed by 2 different authors (JMA and JCG).

2.2. Inclusion and Exclusion Criteria

The PICOS model was used to determine the inclusion criteria [40]: P (Population): "men and women athletes", I (Intervention): "caffeine supplementation", C (Comparators): "identical conditions for caffeine and placebo experimental trials", O (Outcome): "physical and/or sports performance measurements", and S (study design): "single- or double-blind and randomized design".

As a result, the studies included in this systematic bibliographic review had to meet all the following criteria: (i) populations were elite or amateur athletes or active people, men and women of any age; (ii) participants performed any form of physical exercise or sport using caffeine as an ergogenic aid, which could be administered in the form of capsules/pills, energy or sports drinks, commercial drinks with caffeine content, chewing gum or coffee; (iii) the effects of caffeine were compared on both sexes to an identical placebo condition and the protocols used were similar for male and female participants; (iv) articles examined the effects of caffeine supplementation on physical performance measurements, physiological responses, perceptual measures; (v) study designs were randomized, single- or double-blind, and placebo-controlled. The following exclusion criteria were applied to the experimental protocols of the investigation: (i) studies that were conducted only in men or in women athletes; (ii) studies that were performed for clinical purposes or therapeutic use; (iii) the absence of a true placebo condition or different experimental protocols used for male and female participants; (iv) studies carried out using participants with a previous cardiovascular, metabolic, or musculoskeletal disorder.

2.3. Study Selection

Two authors identified papers through a database search (JMA and JCG). The titles and abstracts of publications identified by the search strategy were screened for a subsequent full-text review and were cross-referenced to identify duplicates. All trials assessed for eligibility and classified as relevant were retrieved and the full text was peer-reviewed (JMA and JCG). Moreover, the reference sections of all relevant articles were also examined applying the snowball strategy. Based on the information within the full reports, inclusion and exclusion criteria were used to select the studies eligible for inclusion in the systematic review. Disagreements were resolved through discussions between the different authors (JMA and JCG).

2.4. Data Extraction

Once the inclusion/exclusion criteria were applied to each study, the following data were extracted: study source (author/s and year of publication); population of the sample indicating the level of activity or sports discipline, age, sex and number of participants; habitual caffeine intake (mg/day); dose of caffeine intake, source from which it is obtained and its administration protocol; and performance outcomes in men and women.

2.5. Quality Assessment and Risk of Bias

In order to carefully consider the potential limitations of the included studies to obtain reliable conclusions, and following Cochrane Collaboration Guidelines [41], two authors independently assessed the methodological quality and risk of bias (JMA and DMJ) of each investigation, and disagreements were resolved by third-party evaluation (JCG). In the Cochrane Risk of Bias tool, the following items are included and divided into different domains: (1) selection bias (items: random sequence generation, allocation concealment), (2) performance bias (blinding of participants and personnel), (3) detection bias (blinding of outcome assessment), (4) attrition bias (incomplete outcome data), (5) reporting bias (selective reporting), and (6) other bias (other sources of bias). The assessment of the risk of bias was characterized as low risk (plausible bias unlikely to seriously alter the results), unclear risk (plausible bias that raises some doubt about the results), or high risk (plausible bias that seriously weakens confidence in the results).

3. Results

3.1. Search Strategy

After applying the search equation, a total of 202 records were identified through database searches and six studies through reference list searches. From these 208 articles, 45 of them were removed because they were duplicates. In addition, 33 studies were excluded after screening the abstract. As a result, 129 studies were assessed for eligibility. From the 129 full-text articles assessed, another 119 papers were removed because they were unrelated to the topic of this systematic review. The topics and number of studies that were excluded were as follows: those excluded because the subjects were inappropriate for the inclusion criteria ($n = 51$; in animals $n = 10$; and in the general population $n = 41$), those that used an unsuitable methodology ($n = 33$; outcomes in men and women separately, or did not compare the responses for both sexes), and those with unsuitable outcomes ($n = 29$; cognitive function and sleep $n = 23$; and toxicological and genetic studies $n = 5$; and bibliographic reviews $n = 7$). Consequently, 10 studies met the previously defined inclusion criteria and were included in this final systematic review (Figure 1).

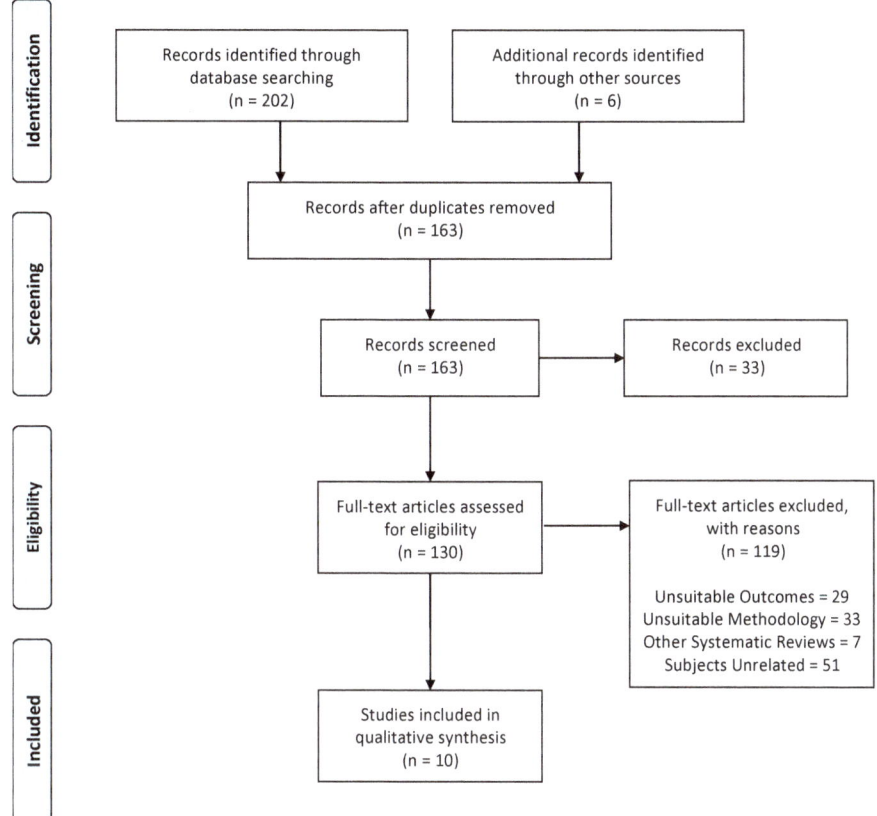

Figure 1. Selection of studies (Preferred Reporting Items for Systematic Review and Meta-Analyses (PRISMA), 2009 Flow Diagram).

3.2. Caffeine Supplementation

The total sample consisted of 221 participants ($n = 113$ males; $n = 108$ females) [29–38]. All studies were performed using adult populations. Healthy active students were selected in three studies [30,31,37] while the remaining studies included participants catalogued as athletes because they train for a specific sport. Athletes from endurance sports such as cycling, triathlon [29,32,36], and from resistance training modalities were used in the investigations [35,38]. Moreover, two trials were performed with elite collegiate athletes from several disciplines such as tennis, basketball and soccer [33,34].

The sources of caffeine supplementation were varied, including commercial drinks used by Jacobson et al. (2018) [37], Tinsley et al. (2017) [35], high chlorogenic coffee (Turkish coffee) used by Nieman et al. (2017) [32], dry anhydrous caffeine mixed with 300 mL water and a sugar-free peach squash solution proposed by Sabblah et al. (2015) [38], and caffeine gum used by Paton et al. (2015) [29]. The other authors of this systematic review used capsules to administer the scheduled doses of caffeine in their studies [31,33,34,36].

In the included studies, caffeine was administered in different doses, based on an individual's body mass, or with an absolute dose. The doses based on the participant's body mass used between 3 and 6 mg/kg of body mass. Skinner et al. (2019) used 3 mg/kg [36], Paton et al. (2015) used 3–4 mg/kg [29], and Tinsley et al. (2017) provided 4 mg/kg of caffeine for men and 3.6 mg/kg of caffeine for women using a caffeinated supplement [35]. Besides, Jebabli et al. (2016) [30] and Sabblah et al. (2015) [38] used 5 mg/kg in the caffeine administration protocol, while Chen et al. (2015) [33], Chen et al., (2019) [34], and Suvi et al. (2016) [31] used a dose of 6 mg/kg. In relation to studies that provided an absolute dose, participants in the study by Jacobson et al. (2018) [37] consumed a commercially available energy drink with 240 mg (≈3.1 mg/kg) of caffeine, and Nieman et al. (2017) [32] used 474 mg (men: ≈6.7 mg/kg and women: ≈7.5 mg/kg) of caffeine from a cup of coffee in their study.

In general, the time of the ingestion of caffeine was between 30 and 60 min before testing. Thus, Chen et al. (2015) [33], Chen et al. (2019) [34] and Sabblah et al. (2015) [38] agreed on administering this type of supplementation 60 min before testing, and Tinsley et al. (2017) [35] and Jacobson et al. (2018) [37] prescribed caffeine supplementation 30 min before testing. However, 45 min before [30] and 90 min before [36] testing were also selected as time-points of caffeine supplementation. Likewise, Suvi et al. (2016) [31] fractionated the dose into two portions: 60 min before (4 mg/kg) and immediately prior to testing (2 mg/kg). A different strategy for supplementation was chosen by Nieman et al. (2017) [32], who proposed a protocol of chronic intake of Turkish coffee every morning for two weeks. In contrast, only one study [29] administered caffeine supplementation during exercise (after completing one third of a 30 km test), and another one after exercise [34], where participants ingested caffeine at 24 and 48 h post-exercise.

3.3. Outcome Variables

Studies included in this systematic review measured a large range of variables. Consequently, studies were clustered by the character of the measurements, such as aerobic performance (Table 1), anaerobic performance (Table 2) and the fatigue index (Table 3). As a result, the effects of caffeine supplementation on aerobic performance were analyzed in four studies [29,31,32,36], on anaerobic performance in seven studies [29–38] and on the fatigue index in three studies [30,33,34].

3.4. Quality Assessment and Risk of Bias

In relation to selection bias, random sequence generation was characterized as low risk only in three studies [35–37], while in the remaining studies, the bias was unclear [29–34,38]. Allocation concealment was categorized as low risk in all experiments [29–38]. Regarding performance bias, the blinding of participants was categorized as low risk in nine studies [29,31–38] and high risk in one trial [30], whereas the blinding of personnel was categorized as low risk in four studies [33–36], unclear in five trials [29–32,37], and high risk in one trial [38]. The domain attrition bias, measured by incomplete outcome data, shows that six studies can be characterized as low risk [29–32,37,38], and four studies can be considered as unclear risk [33–36]. In relation to reporting bias, evaluated through selective reporting, five trials were considered to be of low risk [31,33,34,36,37], three to be of unclear risk [29,35,38] and two to be of high risk [30,32]. Finally, six studies were characterized as low risk of other bias [29,31,33,34,36,38], two trials as unclear risk [32,35] and two studies as high risk [30,37]. Full details for all these risks are given in Figures 2 and 3.

Table 1. Summary of studies included in the systematic review that investigated the effect of caffeine ingestion between sexes on aerobic performance.

Author/s	Population	Intervention	Main Outcome Analyzed	Effect on Men vs. Women
Paton et al. (2015) [29]	Trained cyclists 10 Men (36 ± 10 years) 10 Women (25 ± 7 years)	3–4 mg/kg in caffeinated gum During exercise (10-km point at 1st sprint)	• Time trial performance	• ↔ • ↔ • ↔
Suvi et al. (2016) [31]	Healthy active students 13 Men (24.9 ± 4.1) 10 Women (22.5 ± 2.0 years)	6 mg/kg of gelatin in capsule in two doses 4 mg/kg 60 min before 2 mg/kg pre-test	• Time to exhaustion (minute)	• ↔
Nieman et al. (2017) [32]	Cyclists 10 Men (56.1 ± 3.3) Five Women (43.0 ± 4.5 years)	474 mg of Turkish coffee (men: ≈6.7 mg/kg and women: ≈7.5 mg/kg) Each morning for two weeks	• Time trial performance	• ↔
Skinner et al. (2019) [36]	Endurance-trained cyclists and triathletes 16 Men (32.6 ± 8.3) 11 Women (29.7 ± 5.3 years)	3 mg/kg in opaque capsules 90 min before	• Time trial performance	• ↔

↔ The effect of caffeine supplementation was not statistically different between sexes.

Table 2. Summary of studies included in the systematic review that investigated the effect of caffeine ingestion between sexes on anaerobic performance.

Author/s	Population	Intervention	Main Outcome Analyzed	Effect on Men vs. Women
Chen et al. (2015) [33]	Elite collegiate athletes (tennis, basketball, soccer) 10 Men (20.10 ± 2.18 years) 10 Women (19.9 ± 0.99 years)	6 mg/kg in capsules taken with 500 mL water 60 min before	• MVIC (Nm/kg) • SVIFP (s) • MVIC (Nm/kg)	• ↔ • ↔ • ↔
Paton et al. (2015) [29]	Trained cyclists 10 Men (36 ± 10 years) 10 Women (25 ± 7 years)	3–4 mg/kg in caffeinated gum During exercise (10-km point at 1st sprint)	• 0.2-km sprints each 10-km of a 30-km cycling time trial	• ↑ in men
Sabblah et al. (2015) [38]	Moderately active resistance-trained individuals 10 Men (24.4 ± 3.2 years) Eight Women (27.9 ± 6.13)	5 mg/kg of dry anhydrous caffeine mixed with 300 mL water and a sugar-free peach squash solution 60 min before	• Bench press 1RM • Squat 1RM • Number of bench press reps to failure at 40% 1RM (total weight lifted)	• ↔ • ↔ • ↑ in men
Jebabli et al. (2016) [30]	Healthy active students of Sports Sciences 10 Men (22.9 ± 1.46 years) Eight Women (21.8 ± 0.45 years)	5 mg/kg (Undefined) 45 min before	• RMAT total time (s) • RMAT peak time (s)	• ↓ in men • ↔
Tinsley et al. (2017) [35]	Resistance-trained adults Nine Men (20.7 ± 2.8 years) 12 Women (21.5 ± 2.0 years)	Commercially available multi-ingredient pre-workout supplements 4.0 mg/kg for men 3.6 mg/kg for women 30 min before	• Maximal concentric force (N) • Maximal eccentric force (N)	• ↔ • ↔
Jacobson et al. (2018) [37]	Healthy active students 17 Men and 19 Women (19–26 years)	240 mg of Energy drink shot (57 mL) 30 min before	• IFS peak velocity (m/s) • IFS average velocity (m/s) • CMJ power (W) • CMJ peak velocity (m/s)	• ↓ in men • ↓ in men • ↔ • ↔
Chen et al. (2019) [34]	Elite collegiate athletes (tennis, basketball, soccer) 10 Men (21.1 ± 2.1 years) 10 Women (20.4 ± 1.2 years)	6 mg/kg in capsule taken with 500 mL water 24/48 h post-exercise	• MVIC (Nm/kg) • SVIFP (Tlim) (s) • MVIC post Tlim (Nm/kg)	• ↔ • ↔ • ↔

↔ The effect of caffeine supplementation was not statistically different between sexes; ↓ ↑ in men: the effect of caffeine supplementation was statistically different (higher and lower, respectively) in men than in women. 1RM: One maximal repetition; CMJ: countermovement jump; IFS: Isolated forehand stroke; MVIC: Maximal voluntary isometric contractions; RMAT: Repeated Modified Agility Test; SVIFP: Submaximal voluntary isometric fatigue protocol.

Table 3. Summary of studies included in the systematic review that investigated the effect of caffeine ingestion between sexes on the fatigue index.

Author/s	Population	Intervention	Main Outcome Analyzed	Effect on Men vs. Women
Chen et al. (2015) [33]	Elite collegiate athletes (tennis, basketball, soccer) 10 Men (20.10 ± 2.18 years) 10 Women (19.9 ± 0.99 years)	6 mg/kg in capsules taken with 500 mL water 60 min before	• Fatigue index (%)	• ↔
Jebabli et al. (2016) [30]	Healthy active students of Sports Sciences 10 Men (22.9 ± 1.46 years) Eight Women (21.8 ± 0.45 years)	5 mg/kg (Undefined) 45 min before	• RMAT fatigue index (%)	• ↔
Chen et al. (2019) [34]	Elite collegiate athletes (tennis, basketball, soccer) 10 Men (21.1 ± 2.1 years) 10 Women (20.4 ± 1.2 years)	6 mg/kg in capsule taken with 500 mL water 24/48 h post-exercise	• Fatigue index (%)	• ↔

↔ The effect of caffeine supplementation was not statistically different between sexes. RMAT: Repeated Modified Agility Test.

Study	Sequence generation (selection bias)	Allocation concealment (selection bias)	Blinding of participants (performance bias)	Blinding of personnel (performance bias)	Incomplete outcome data (attrition bias)	Selective outcome reporting (reporting bias)	Other sources of bias
Chen et al. (2015) [33]	?	+	+	+	?	+	+
Paton et al. (2015) [29]	?	+	+	?	+	?	+
Sabblah et al. (2015) [38]	?	+	+	−	+	?	+
Jebabli et al. (2016) [30]	?	+	−	?	+	−	−
Suvi et al. (2016) [31]	?	+	+	?	+	+	+
Nieman et al. (2017) [32]	?	+	+	?	+	−	?
Tinsley et al. (2017) [35]	+	+	+	+	?	?	?
Jacobson et al. (2018) [37]	+	+	+	?	+	+	−
Chen et al. (2019) [34]	?	+	+	+	?	+	+
Skinner et al. (2019) [36]	+	+	+	+	?	+	+

+ indicates low risk of bias, ? indicates unclear risk of bias, and − indicates high risk of bias.

Figure 2. Risk of bias summary: review of authors' judgements about each risk of bias item presented as percentages across all included studies.

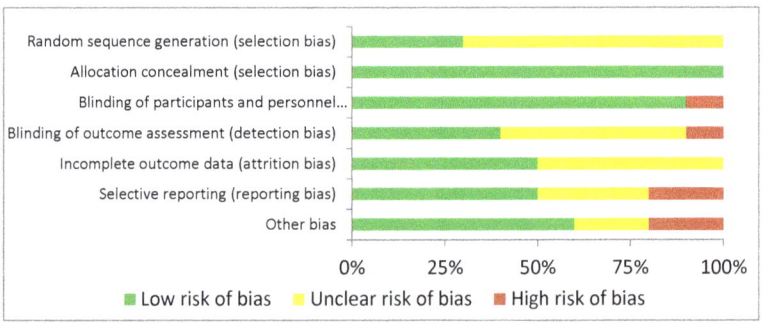

Figure 3. Risk of bias graph: review authors' judgements about each risk of bias item for each included study.

4. Discussion

The main aim of this systematic review was to summarize the differences, if any, in the ergogenic effect of caffeine supplementation between men and women. This systematic review focuses on different responses between sexes to the same caffeine supplementation protocol when the exercise was categorized as aerobic, anaerobic or when the protocol induced some kind of fatigue that could be assessed (i.e., fatigue index). Knowing that caffeine is one of the most popular ergogenic aids with demonstrated effects on physical performance [6,18,19], it was considered that this systematic review might show a global vision of the ergogenic effect of caffeine in men and women, gathering all studies published in this field. Generally, the investigations analyzed reflect that there are no differences between men and women. However, some investigations showed some subtle differences between sexes, indicating that males might experience an increased ergogenic effect of caffeine, especially to produce more power, greater total weight lifted and higher speed with the same dose of caffeine. These results suggest that, in general, both men and women athletes benefit from caffeine supplementation to the same extent. Nevertheless, it seems that ergogenicity might be greater in men for exercise activities with an anaerobic component. Interestingly, none of the investigations depicted a negative effect of acute caffeine intake on physical performance. All this information indicates that the current guidelines for caffeine supplementation can be equally valid for men and women athletes.

4.1. Effects of Caffeine on Aerobic Performance

Caffeine has been popularly used in long-lasting sports given that some improvements are observed over time to exhaustion [8,9], mainly due to a hypothetical glycogen-sparing effect of caffeine [15] and the stimulation in the CNS of this substance, capable of attenuating pain [42]. In fact, numerous studies have used the duration of a test and the time to complete it as an indicator of aerobic endurance performance, in which the effect of a supplement such as caffeine can be measured [29–32,36].

Regarding the differences between men and women, there are more studies in which there are no significant differences between sexes in time trials. For example, Paton et al., (2015) [29] showed improvements of a similar magnitude in the aerobic performance of both sexes, but without differences between them. However, these authors found that men showed significant improvements in anaerobic performance with respect to women, probably due to the increase in activity of the CNS. One of the main reasons why they did not find significant differences between sexes could be the great interindividual variability, which could be associated with individual differences in the metabolism of caffeine or the absorption rate [43].

Suvi et al. (2016) [31] did not show significant differences between sexes in endurance capacity in hot environments (42 °C, 20% relative humidity) after taking 6 mg/kg of caffeine in two doses (4 mg/kg 60 min before the test and 2 mg/kg immediately before it). Similarly, Nieman et al. (2017) [32] did not find sex differences after chronic intake of 474 mg of caffeine for 2 weeks either. Moreover, Skinner et al. (2019) [36] showed significant and comparable improvements in endurance performance in both sexes. The performance improvements observed in women were similar to those in men, even though women showed higher plasma caffeine concentrations. Thus, Skinner et al. (2019) [36] suggested that current recommendations for caffeine supplementation, which are derived from studies conducted in men, could also be applied to women, in particular in aerobic endurance events. The results of these studies suggest that caffeine supplementation is equally effective in terms of improving the aerobic capacity in both men and women athletes.

4.2. Effects of Caffeine on Anaerobic Performance

Regarding anaerobic actions, it has been demonstrated that caffeine produces positive effects on performance among others due to the activation of the CNS [3,44]. Caffeine might antagonistically bind adenosine receptors and decrease adenosine-mediated fatigue [45]. Moreover, a recent study has also suggested that caffeine in physiological concentrations (~40 μmol/L) may improve calcium release from the sarcoplasmic reticulum during muscle contraction [46]. To the best of the authors' knowledge, only one study conducted by Jababli et al. (2016) [30] compared the caffeine supplementation effect on the glycolytic pathway in both sexes. The authors observed that the effect of caffeine to reduce the total time employed to complete several repetitions of an agility test was higher in men than women. The authors indicated that one explanation could be the increase in alertness, leading to more concentration during the execution of this type of test, especially during the changes of direction [30]. However, the effect of caffeine was similar when only the best time in the agility test was taken into account. The controversies between these results may be due to either the sex selection or the selected study population. Due to the scarcity of data comparing the effect of caffeine on agility in men and women, more studies are necessary to confirm these results.

Anaerobic capacity manifests the rapid use of the phosphagen system (adenosine triphosphate (ATP) and creatine phosphate) in the muscles, with type II fibers providing the greatest contribution. Anaerobic capacity can be estimated by numerous laboratory and field tests such as anaerobic speed test, mean power output and peak power output [47]. In addition, there is evidence about the ergogenic effect of caffeine on anaerobic capacity [3,30,44], but the causes remain unclear [48]. It is now accepted that caffeine induces higher levels of Ca^{2+} and K^+. The influx of Ca^{2+} from the sarcoplasmic reticulum favors the formation of cross bridges and therefore increases muscle power, whereas the serum increase in K^+ causes increases in the Na^+ / K^+ ATPase activity, so that it can attenuate muscle fatigue [33,49].

Regarding the potential sex differences of caffeine supplementation on muscle power, Paton et al. (2015) [29] presented similar increases in mean power in the last 10 km between men and women after 3–4 mg/kg caffeine chewing gum supplementation during a 30 km continuous cycling exercise with varying intensity. However, the men showed greater sprint power induced by caffeine than the women, due to the inclusion of aerobic phases of exercise prior to the sprints performed in the test, as well as the inter-individual variability in the response to caffeine [8]; thus, posing a possible sex -based difference that affects high intensity anaerobic measurements [50].

Jacobson et al. (2018) [37] found that only women improved forehand stroke velocity after the intake of 240 mg of caffeine, while the caffeine-induced changes on vertical jump was similar between sexes. Opposite results were shown in the Warren et al. (2010) meta-analysis [48], where it is stated that caffeine has more impact on exercise that involves large muscles than small muscles, such as in the arms. These differences could be, (a) related to the dose of caffeine supplementation because it could be adequate to improve the performance of small muscle groups, but insufficient to improve the performance of muscle groups in the legs and (b) the caffeine amount was the same for all participants, so that the differences in body mass and body composition between sexes could cause the women to receive more caffeine than the men [37].

Therefore, based on the results included in the studies of this systematic review, there are differences between the manifestation of variables associated with muscle power and speed between men and women. However, given the small number of studies, it is difficult to attribute the causes. Jebabli et al. (2016) [30] indicated that a dose of 5 mg/kg of caffeine 45 min before a repeated agility test decreased the total time more in men than in women [30]. The authors attributed these results to the increase in neuromuscular activity that facilitates the neural transmission observed in the men, of which there is no evidence in the women [51].

Another physical capacity included in anaerobic performance may be strength. In this respect, strength is based on a combination of morphological and neural factors that include the cross-sectional area of the muscle and architecture, musculotendinous stiffness, motor unit recruitment, frequency coding, motor unit synchronization and neuromuscular inhibition [52]. However, the effects of caffeine supplementation on strength are not so clear. Some studies found an acute effect of caffeine on increasing strength, while others did not present a response to supplementation with caffeine [48,53]. In any case, few studies have analyzed the potential differences between sexes evaluating the variables associated with strength.

Chen et al. (2015) [33] and Chen et al. (2019) [34] showed that 6 mg/kg of caffeine supplementation improved the maximum voluntary isometric strength (measured by isometric contractions) of the knee extensors after 60 min of caffeine ingestion, and 24/48 h post-exercise, respectively, but without significant differences between sexes. According to the authors, one of the main factors that may have influenced the absence of sex differences was that the women's sample was homogenized in relation to the menstrual cycle (all were in the early follicular phase) [33,34]. In this respect, although some investigators have reported an inotropic effect of estrogens on muscle because of a switching of muscle cross-bridges from low- to high-force generation [54,55], in general muscle strength does not appear to fluctuate significantly during an ovulatory menstrual cycle [47].

In the same line of research, Tinsley et al. (2017) [35] did not show significant differences between sexes in the production of strength after caffeine supplementation (men: 4.0 mg/kg and women: 3.6 mg/kg of caffeine). However, the effect size showed that the caffeine supplement contributed to small increases (not significant) in the men's concentric strength (5–20%, d = 0.2–0.4 relative to placebo), but not in the women's. In this study, the women's menstrual cycle phase was not taken into account. However, women participants were given 75% of the supplement given to men participants to match the differences in body composition between both sexes [35], which could have impacted the slightly lower response to caffeine in the women.

Sabblah et al. (2015) [38] found that 5 mg/kg of caffeine had positive effects on 1RM for both sexes trained in resistance. However, it showed that the women's reaction was smaller than men's, as evidenced by a tendency to improve total weight lifted for men with no such effect in this variable for women. Besides, the authors showed that the perception of pain in both sexes revealed no differences after caffeine supplementation. The greater activation that caffeine has shown in men compared to women could be the potential cause of these differences in the total weight lifted [28].

Therefore, although there are equivocal results, there are more than reasonable doubts to consider that the effect of caffeine supplementation influences men and women differently as regards strength.

4.3. Effects of Caffeine on the Fatigue Index

The consumption of pre-workout supplements makes it possible to experience physiological effects, as well as the psychological effects on performance [35]. In this case, caffeine may delay the onset of fatigue or block the perception of pain or fatigue, using the same mechanisms involved in perception variables [33]. However, regarding rated perceived exertion there is scarcely any scientific evidence that could show significant differences between sexes. Three of the studies included in this systematic review do not show significant differences between men and women in the fatigue index [30,33–35]. Only the study published by Suvi et al. (2016) [31] showed that caffeine supplementation reduced the perception of fatigue in men, but not in women, when exercising in hot environments. The authors attributed this result to the greater sensitivity of men to acute caffeine ingestion compared to women, as shown by previous research [28,56–58].

5. Conclusions

In summary, 10 studies met the previously defined inclusion/exclusion criteria and were included in this systematic review, aimed to analyze the between-sex differences in the effect of caffeine supplementation on physical/sports performance. The total sample consisted of 221 participants (n = 113 males; n = 108 females), while caffeine supplementation was given by using different sources of caffeine between 30 and 60 min before testing. Studies included in this systematic review measured a large range of variables such as aerobic and anaerobic performance and the fatigue index. Overall, the caffeine supplementation produced a similar ergogenic benefit for aerobic performance and the fatigue index in men and women athletes. However, the effects of caffeine to produce more power, total weight lifted and to improve sprint performance with respect to a placebo was greater in men than women athletes despite the same dose of caffeine being administered. Specifically, the men experienced greater mean power than the women during the final 10-km cycling test after ~3–4 mg/kg caffeine supplementation. Likewise, the ergogenic effect of 5 mg/kg of caffeine to increase the total weight lifted was higher in men than in women, in particular the ergogenic effect of acute caffeine intake on anaerobic performance.

Strengths, Limitations and Future Lines of Research

The main strength of the present study is its novelty, given that no previous systematic review has analyzed the effect of caffeine supplementation on performance between sexes. The main limitations were the scarcity of information and the low sample sizes used in most investigations. Besides, differences in physical tests and caffeine supplementation protocols make it difficult to generalize the recommendations. Finally, it is of great importance to continue the work in future research on supplementation with caffeine in female populations. Specifically, it is necessary to determine whether women athletes benefit from acute caffeine intake in other forms of exercise or in sports where several physical fitness variables affect overall performance. In addition, the between-sex difference in the response to other dietary supplements should also be investigated to ascertain whether the findings of previous investigations with males are also applicable to women athletes. Lastly, it is necessary to take into account women's menstrual cycle when investigating caffeine ergogenicity to determine whether this substance exerts positive performance effects in all phases of the menstrual cycle.

Author Contributions: J.M.-A. and J.C.-G.: conceived and designed the investigation, analyzed and interpreted the data, drafted the paper, and approved the final version submitted for publication. D.M.-J. and J.D.C.: analyzed and interpreted the data, critically reviewed the paper and approved the final version submitted for publication. I.R. and P.L.-G.: critically reviewed the paper and approved the final version submitted for publication.

Funding: The authors declare no funding sources.

Conflicts of Interest: The authors declare no conflict of interest.

References

1. Ganio, M.S.; Klau, J.F.; Casa, D.J.; Armstrong, L.E.; Maresh, C.M. Effect of caffeine on sport-specific endurance performance: A systematic review. *J. Strength Cond. Res.* **2009**, *23*, 315–324. [CrossRef] [PubMed]
2. Lopez-Gonzalez, L.M.; Sanchez-Oliver, A.J.; Mata, F.; Jodra, P.; Antonio, J.; Dominguez, R. Acute caffeine supplementation in combat sports: A systematic review. *J. Int. Soc. Sports Nutr.* **2018**, *15*, 60. [CrossRef] [PubMed]
3. Davis, J.K.; Green, J.M. Caffeine and anaerobic performance: ergogenic value and mechanisms of action. *Sports Med.* **2009**, *39*, 813–832. [CrossRef] [PubMed]
4. San Juan, A.F.; Lopez-Samanes, A.; Jodra, P.; Valenzuela, P.L.; Rueda, J.; Veiga-Herreros, P.; Perez-Lopez, A.; Dominguez, R. Caffeine supplementation improves anaerobic performance and neuromuscular efficiency and fatigue in Olympic-level boxers. *Nutrients* **2019**, *11*, 2120. [CrossRef] [PubMed]
5. Salinero, J.J.; Lara, B.; del Coso, J. Effects of acute ingestion of caffeine on team sports performance: A systematic review and meta-analysis. *Res. Sports Med.* **2019**, *27*, 238–256. [CrossRef] [PubMed]
6. Mielgo-Ayuso, J.; Calleja-Gonzalez, J.; del Coso, J.; Urdampilleta, A.; León-Guereño, P.; Fernández-Lázaro, D. Caffeine supplementation and physical performance, muscle damage and perception of fatigue in soccer players: A systematic review. *Nutrients* **2019**, *11*, 440. [CrossRef]
7. Durkalec-Michalski, K.; Nowaczyk, P.M.; Glowka, N.; Grygiel, A. Dose-dependent effect of caffeine supplementation on judo-specific performance and training activity: A randomized placebo-controlled crossover trial. *J. Int. Soc. Sports Nutr.* **2019**, *16*, 1–14. [CrossRef] [PubMed]
8. Pickering, C.; Kiely, J. Are the current guidelines on caffeine use in sport optimal for everyone? Inter-individual variation in caffeine ergogenicity, and a move towards personalised sports nutrition. *Sports Med.* **2018**, *48*, 7–16. [CrossRef]
9. Goldstein, E.R.; Ziegenfuss, T.; Kalman, D.; Kreider, R.; Campbell, B.; Wilborn, C.; Taylor, L.; Willoughby, D.; Stout, J.; Graves, B.S.; et al. International society of sports nutrition position stand: caffeine and performance. *J. Int. Soc. Sports Nutr.* **2010**, *7*, 5. [CrossRef]
10. Pasman, W.J.; van Baak, M.A.; Jeukendrup, A.E.; de Haan, A. The effect of different dosages of caffeine on endurance performance time. *Int. J. Sports Med.* **1995**, *16*, 225–230. [CrossRef]

11. The National Collegiate Athletic Association. *2019–2020 NCAA Banned Substances*; The National Collegiate Athletic Association: Indianapolis, IN, USA, 2019.
12. Tallis, J.; Duncan, M.J.; James, R.S. What can isolated skeletal muscle experiments tell us about the effects of caffeine on exercise performance? *Br. J. Pharmacol.* **2015**, *172*, 3703–3713. [CrossRef] [PubMed]
13. Tarnopolsky, M.A. Effect of caffeine on the neuromuscular system—Potential as an ergogenic aid. *Appl. Physiol. Nutr. Metab.* **2008**, *33*, 1284–1289. [CrossRef] [PubMed]
14. Stojanovic, E.; Stojiljkovic, N.; Scanlan, A.T.; Dalbo, V.J.; Stankovic, R.; Antic, V.; Milanovic, Z. Acute caffeine supplementation promotes small to moderate improvements in performance tests indicative of in-game success in professional female basketball players. *Appl. Physiol. Nutr. Metab.* **2019**, *44*, 849–856. [CrossRef] [PubMed]
15. Laurent, D.; Schneider, K.E.; Prusaczyk, W.K.; Franklin, C.; Vogel, S.M.; Krssak, M.; Petersen, K.F.; Goforth, H.W.; Shulman, G.I. Effects of caffeine on muscle glycogen utilization and the neuroendocrine axis during exercise. *J. Clin. Endocrinol. Metab.* **2000**, *85*, 2170–2175. [CrossRef] [PubMed]
16. Lindinger, M.I.; Willmets, R.G.; Hawke, T.J. Stimulation of Na^+, K^+-pump activity in skeletal muscle by methylxanthines: Evidence and proposed mechanisms. *Acta Physiol. Scand.* **1996**, *156*, 347–353. [CrossRef]
17. Thibault, V.; Guillaume, M.; Berthelot, G.; El Helou, N.; Schaal, K.; Quinquis, L.; Nassif, H.; Tafflet, M.; Escolano, S.; Hermine, O. Women and men in sport performance: The gender gap has not evolved since 1983. *J. Sports Sci. Med.* **2010**, *9*, 214–223.
18. Burke, L.M. Caffeine and Sports Performance. *Appl. Physiol. Nutr. Metab.* **2008**, *33*, 1319–1334. [CrossRef]
19. Thomas, D.T.; Erdman, K.A.; Burke, L.M. American college of sports medicine joint position statement. Nutrition and athletic performance. *Med. Sci. Sports Exerc.* **2016**, *48*, 543–568.
20. Grgic, J.; Grgic, I.; Pickering, C.; Schoenfeld, B.J.; Bishop, D.J.; Pedisic, Z. Wake up and smell the coffee: Caffeine supplementation and exercise performance—An umbrella review of 21 published meta-analyses. *Br. J. Sports Med.* **2019**. [CrossRef]
21. Grgic, J.; Mikulic, P.; Schoenfeld, B.J.; Bishop, D.J.; Pedisic, Z. The influence of caffeine supplementation on resistance exercise: A review. *Sports Med.* **2019**, *49*, 17–30. [CrossRef]
22. Salinero, J.J.; Lara, B.; Jimenez-Ormeno, E.; Romero-Moraleda, B.; Giraldez-Costas, V.; Baltazar-Martins, G.; del Coso, J. More research is necessary to establish the ergogenic effect of caffeine in female athletes. *Nutrients* **2019**, *11*, 1600. [CrossRef] [PubMed]
23. Julian, R.; Hecksteden, A.; Fullagar, H.H.; Meyer, T. The effects of menstrual cycle phase on physical performance in female soccer players. *PLoS ONE* **2017**, *12*, e0173951. [CrossRef] [PubMed]
24. Tounsi, M.; Jaafar, H.; Aloui, A.; Souissi, N. Soccer-related performance in eumenorrheic Tunisian high-level soccer players: Effects of menstrual cycle phase and moment of day. *J. Sports Med. Phys. Fit.* **2018**, *58*, 497–502.
25. Dos, M.S.A.; Mascarin, N.C.; Foster, R.; de Jarmy di Bella, Z.I.; Vancini, R.L.; de Lira, C.A.B. Is muscular strength balance influenced by menstrual cycle in female soccer players? *J. Sports Med. Phys. Fit.* **2017**, *57*, 859–864.
26. Ribeiro-Alves, M.A.; Trugo, L.C.; Donangelo, C.M. Use of oral contraceptives blunts the calciuric effect of caffeine in young adult women. *J. Nutr.* **2003**, *133*, 393–398. [CrossRef] [PubMed]
27. Ali, A.; O'Donnell, J.; Foskett, A.; Rutherfurd-Markwick, K. The influence of caffeine ingestion on strength and power performance in female team-sport players. *J. Int. Soc. Sports Nutr.* **2016**, *13*, 46. [CrossRef]
28. Adan, A.; Prat, G.; Fabbri, M.; Sanchez-Turet, M. Early effects of caffeinated and decaffeinated coffee on subjective state and gender differences. *Prog. Neuropsychopharmacol. Biol. Psychiatry* **2008**, *32*, 1698–1703. [CrossRef]
29. Paton, C.; Costa, V.; Guglielmo, L. Effects of caffeine chewing gum on race performance and physiology in male and female cyclists. *J. Sports Sci.* **2015**, *33*, 1076–1083. [CrossRef] [PubMed]
30. Jebabli, N.; Ouerghi, N.; Bouabid, J.; Bettaib, R. Effect of caffeine on the repeated modified agility test from some cardiovascular factors, blood glucose and rating of perceived exertion in young people. *Iran. J. Public. Health* **2017**, *46*, 755–761.
31. Suvi, S.; Timpmann, S.; Tamm, M.; Aedma, M.; Kreegipuu, K.; Ööpik, V. Effects of caffeine on endurance capacity and psychological state in young females and males exercising in the heat. *Appl. Physiol. Nutr. Metab.* **2016**, *42*, 68–76. [CrossRef]

32. Nieman, D.C.; Goodman, C.L.; Capps, C.R.; Shue, Z.L.; Arnot, R. Influence of 2-weeks ingestion of high chlorogenic acid coffee on mood state, performance, and postexercise inflammation and oxidative stress: A randomized, placebo-controlled trial. *Int. J. Sport Nutr. Exerc. Metab.* **2018**, *28*, 55–65. [CrossRef] [PubMed]
33. Chen, H.Y.; Wang, H.S.; Tung, K.; Chao, H.H. Effects of gender difference and caffeine supplementation on anaerobic muscle performance. *Int. J. Sports Med.* **2015**, *36*, 974–978. [CrossRef] [PubMed]
34. Chen, H.Y.; Chen, Y.C.; Tung, K.; Chao, H.H.; Wang, H.S. Effects of caffeine and sex on muscle performance and delayed onset muscle soreness after exercise-induced muscle damage: A double-blind randomized trial. *J. Appl. Physiol.* **2019**. [CrossRef] [PubMed]
35. Tinsley, G.M.; Hamm, M.A.; Hurtado, A.K.; Cross, A.G.; Pineda, J.G.; Martin, A.Y.; Uribe, V.A.; Palmer, T.B. Effects of two pre-workout supplements on concentric and eccentric force production during lower body resistance exercise in males and females: A counterbalanced, double-blind, placebo-controlled trial. *J. Int. Soc. Sports Nutr.* **2017**, *14*, 46. [CrossRef] [PubMed]
36. Skinner, T.L.; Desbrow, B.; Arapova, J.; Schaumberg, M.A.; Osborne, J.; Grant, G.D.; Anoopkumar-Dukie, S.; Leveritt, M.D. Women experience the same ergogenic response to caffeine as men. *Med. Sci. Sports Exerc.* **2019**, *51*, 1195–1202. [CrossRef] [PubMed]
37. Jacobson, B.H.; Hester, G.M.; Palmer, T.B.; Williams, K.; Pope, Z.K.; Sellers, J.H.; Conchola, E.C.; Woolsey, C.; Estrada, C. Effect of energy drink consumption on power and velocity of selected sport performance activities. *J. Strength Cond. Res.* **2018**, *32*, 1613–1618. [CrossRef] [PubMed]
38. Sabblah, S.; Dixon, D.; Bottoms, L. Sex differences on the acute effects of caffeine on maximal strength and muscular endurance. *Comp. Exerc. Physiol.* **2015**, *11*, 89–94. [CrossRef]
39. Liberati, A.; Altman, D.G.; Tetzlaff, J.; Mulrow, C.; Gotzsche, P.C.; Ioannidis, J.P.; Clarke, M.; Devereaux, P.J.; Kleijnen, J.; Moher, D. The PRISMA statement for reporting systematic reviews and meta-analyses of studies that evaluate healthcare interventions: Explanation and elaboration. *BMJ* **2009**, *339*. [CrossRef]
40. O'Connor, D.; Green, S.; Higgins, J.P. Defining the review question and developing criteria for including studies. In *Cochrane Handbook for Systematic Reviews of Interventions: Cochrane Book Series*; John Wiley & Sons: Hoboken, NJ, USA, 2008; pp. 81–94.
41. Green, S.; Higgins, J.P. *Cochrane Handbook for Systematic Reviews of Interventions, Version 5.0.2*; The Cochrane Library; Wiley Online Library: Chichester, West Sussex, UK, 2009.
42. Cappelletti, S.; Daria, P.; Sani, G.; Aromatario, M. Caffeine: Cognitive and physical performance enhancer or psychoactive drug? *Curr. Neuropharmacol.* **2015**, *13*, 71–88. [CrossRef]
43. Nehlig, A. Interindividual differences in caffeine metabolism and factors driving caffeine consumption. *Pharmacol. Rev.* **2018**, *70*, 384–411. [CrossRef]
44. Pickering, C.; Grgic, J. Caffeine and exercise: What next? *Sports Med.* **2019**, *49*, 1007–1030. [CrossRef] [PubMed]
45. Mansour, T.E. Phosphofructokinase activity in skeletal muscle extracts following administration of epinephrine. *J. Biol. Chem.* **1972**, *247*, 6059–6066. [PubMed]
46. Tallis, J.; James, R.S.; Cox, V.M.; Duncan, M.J. The effect of a physiological concentration of caffeine on the endurance of maximally and submaximally stimulated mouse soleus muscle. *J. Physiol. Sci.* **2013**, *63*, 125–132. [CrossRef] [PubMed]
47. Constantini, N.W.; Dubnov, G.; Lebrun, C.M. The menstrual cycle and sport performance. *Clin. Sports Med.* **2005**, *24*, e51–e82. [CrossRef]
48. Warren, G.L.; Park, N.D.; Maresca, R.D.; McKibans, K.I.; Millard-Stafford, M.L. Effect of caffeine ingestion on muscular strength and endurance: A meta-analysis. *Med. Sci. Sports Exerc.* **2010**, *42*, 1375–1387. [CrossRef]
49. Sokmen, B.; Armstrong, L.E.; Kraemer, W.J.; Casa, D.J.; Dias, J.C.; Judelson, D.A.; Maresh, C.M. Caffeine use in sports: Considerations for the athlete. *J. Strength Cond. Res.* **2008**, *22*, 978–986. [CrossRef] [PubMed]
50. Yanovich, R.; Evans, R.; Israeli, E.; Constantini, N.; Sharvit, N.; Merkel, D.; Epstein, Y.; Moran, D.S. Differences in physical fitness of male and female recruits in gender-integrated army basic training. *Med. Sci. Sports Exerc.* **2008**, *40*, S654–S659. [CrossRef]
51. McLellan, T.M.; Caldwell, J.A.; Lieberman, H.R. A review of caffeine's effects on cognitive, physical and occupational performance. *Neurosci. Biobehav. Rev.* **2016**, *71*, 294–312. [CrossRef]
52. Suchomel, T.J.; Nimphius, S.; Bellon, C.R.; Stone, M.H. The importance of muscular strength: Training considerations. *Sports Med.* **2018**, *48*, 765–785. [CrossRef]

53. Astorino, T.A.; Rohmann, R.L.; Firth, K. Effect of caffeine ingestion on one-repetition maximum muscular strength. *Eur. J. Appl. Physiol.* **2008**, *102*, 127–132. [CrossRef]
54. Phillips, S.K.; Sanderson, A.G.; Birch, K.; Bruce, S.A.; Woledge, R.C. Changes in maximal voluntary force of human adductor pollicis muscle during the menstrual cycle. *J. Physiol.* **1996**, *496*, 551–557. [CrossRef] [PubMed]
55. Sarwar, R.; Niclos, B.B.; Rutherford, O.M. Changes in muscle strength, relaxation rate and fatiguability during the human menstrual cycle. *J. Physiol.* **1996**, *493*, 267–272. [CrossRef] [PubMed]
56. Botella, P.; Parra, A. Coffee increases state anxiety in males but not in females. *Hum. Psychopharmacol. Clin. Exp.* **2003**, *18*, 141–143. [CrossRef] [PubMed]
57. Temple, J.L.; Bulkley, A.M.; Briatico, L.; Dewey, A.M. Sex differences in reinforcing value of caffeinated beverages in adolescents. *Behav. Pharmacol.* **2009**, *20*, 731–741. [CrossRef] [PubMed]
58. Temple, J.L.; Dewey, A.M.; Briatico, L.N. Effects of acute caffeine administration on adolescents. *Exp. Clin. Psychopharmacol.* **2010**, *18*, 510–520. [CrossRef] [PubMed]

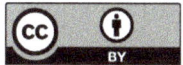

© 2019 by the authors. Licensee MDPI, Basel, Switzerland. This article is an open access article distributed under the terms and conditions of the Creative Commons Attribution (CC BY) license (http://creativecommons.org/licenses/by/4.0/).

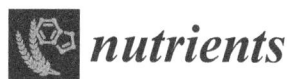

Review

Caffeine Supplementation and Physical Performance, Muscle Damage and Perception of Fatigue in Soccer Players: A Systematic Review

Juan Mielgo-Ayuso [1,*], Julio Calleja-Gonzalez [2], Juan Del Coso [3], Aritz Urdampilleta [4], Patxi León-Guereño [5] and Diego Fernández-Lázaro [6]

1. Department of Biochemistry and Physiology, School of Physical Therapy, University of Valladolid, 42004 Soria, Spain
2. Laboratory of Human Performance, Department of Physical Education and Sport, Faculty of Physical Activity and Sport, University of the Basque Country, 01007 Vitoria, Spain; julio.calleja.gonzalez@gmail.com
3. Exercise Physiology Laboratory, Camilo José Cela University, 28692 Madrid, Spain; jdelcoso@ucjc.edu
4. Elikasport, Nutrition, Innovation & Sport, 08290 Barcelona, Spain; a.urdampilleta@drurdampilleta.com
5. Faculty of Psychology and Education, University of Deusto, Campus of Donostia-San Sebastián, 20012 San Sebastián, Guipúzcoa, Spain; patxi.leon@deusto.es
6. Department of Cellular Biology, Histology and Pharmacology. Faculty of Physical Therapy, University of Valladolid. Campus de Soria, 42004 Soria, Spain; diego.fernandez.lazaro@uva.es
* Correspondence: juanfrancisco.mielgo@uva.es; Tel.: +34-975-129-187

Received: 21 January 2019; Accepted: 15 February 2019; Published: 20 February 2019

Abstract: Soccer is a complex team sport and success in this discipline depends on different factors such as physical fitness, player technique and team tactics, among others. In the last few years, several studies have described the impact of caffeine intake on soccer physical performance, but the results of these investigations have not been properly reviewed and summarized. The main objective of this review was to evaluate critically the effectiveness of a moderate dose of caffeine on soccer physical performance. A structured search was carried out following the Preferred Reporting Items for Systematic Review and Meta-Analyses (PRISMA) guidelines in the Medline/PubMed and Web of Science databases from January 2007 to November 2018. The search included studies with a cross-over and randomized experimental design in which the intake of caffeine (either from caffeinated drinks or pills) was compared to an identical placebo situation. There were no filters applied to the soccer players' level, gender or age. This review included 17 articles that investigated the effects of caffeine on soccer-specific abilities ($n = 12$) or on muscle damage ($n = 5$). The review concluded that 5 investigations (100% of the number of investigations on this topic) had found ergogenic effects of caffeine on jump performance, 4 (100%) on repeated sprint ability and 2 (100%) on running distance during a simulated soccer game. However, only 1 investigation (25%) found as an effect of caffeine to increase serum markers of muscle damage, while no investigation reported an effect of caffeine to reduce perceived fatigue after soccer practice. In conclusion, a single and moderate dose of caffeine, ingested 5–60 min before a soccer practice, might produce valuable improvements in certain abilities related to enhanced soccer physical performance. However, caffeine does not seem to cause increased markers of muscle damage or changes in perceived exertion during soccer practice.

Keywords: football; RPE; DOMS; sport performance; supplementation; ergogenic aids

1. Introduction

Soccer is considered one of the most popular sports worldwide. According to the Fédération Internationale de Football Association (FIFA) Big Count survey, there are 265 million active soccer players and the number is progressively increasing, especially in women's football [1]. In addition, soccer attracts millions of television spectators while the socio-economic impact of elite soccer affects almost every culture worldwide [2]. Thus, the study of soccer and the variables that affect performance in this complex team sport can have a great impact on sport sciences. Briefly, modern soccer is characterized by the continuous combination of short sprints, rapid accelerations/decelerations and changes of direction interspersed with jumping, kicking, tackling and informal times for recovery [3]. In addition to these physical fitness variables, players' techniques and cognitive capacity, team tactics, and psychological factors might also have an impact on overall soccer performance [4,5]. Unlike other team sports, such as basketball or handball, soccer is a low-scoring game and, thus, the margins of victory are close/reduced, particularly at the elite level. In consequence, the study of the effects of ergogenic aids on performance have become an important subject for players, coaches and sport scientists associated with soccer because it has the potential to increase success in the game [6].

Caffeine (1, 3, 7-trimethylxanthine) is one of the most popular supplements among athletes for its potent stimulant effects and due to its easy availability in the market in different commercial forms (energy drinks, caffeinated beverages, pills, pre-workout and thermogenic supplements, etc.). In addition, the ergogenic effects of the acute ingestion of caffeine have been widely reported on different forms of exercise, although most of the classic studies focused on endurance performance [7,8]. In the last few years, several investigations have found that caffeine can also increase anaerobic and sprint performance, although the direct application of these research outcomes to the complexity of soccer is complicated [9–11]. According to the Australian Institute of Sport (AIS), the potential ergogenicity of caffeine reflects level 1 evidence, which allocates it as a safe supplement to use in sport [12]. In addition, the International Olympic Committee indicates, in its recent consensus statement for dietary supplements, that caffeine intake results in performance gains when ingested before exercise in doses ranging from 3 to 6 mg/kg. Finally, two recent systematic reviews have concluded that caffeine might be ergogenic in team sport athletes [6,13]. With this background, one might suppose that caffeine is also ergogenic in soccer although the information regarding this sport has not been summarized. In the last few years, several studies have investigated the effects of caffeine intake on soccer physical performance [14–21] and in the opinion of the authors, the results of these investigations need to be objectively reviewed and summarized. Therefore, the objective of this systematic review was to critically evaluate the effectiveness of a moderate dose of caffeine on soccer physical performance, muscle damage and perception of fatigue in order to provide more objective and comprehensive information about the positive and negative impact of caffeine on soccer players.

2. Methods

2.1. Search Strategies

The present article is a systematic review focusing on the impact of caffeine intake on soccer physical performance and it was conducted following the Preferred Reporting Items for Systematic Review and Meta-Analyses (PRISMA) guidelines and the PICOS model for the definition of the inclusion criteria: P (Population): "soccer players", I (Intervention): "impact of caffeine on soccer physical performance, muscle damage and perception of fatigue", C (Comparators): "same conditions with placebo", O (Outcome): "soccer-specific abilities, serum markers of muscle damage and perceived fatigue (RPE) and heart rate", and S (study design): "double-blind and randomized cross-over design" [22].

A structured search was carried out in the Medline (PubMed) database and in the Web of Science (WOS) which includes other databases such as BCI, BIOSIS, CCC, DIIDW, INSPEC, KJD, MEDLINE, RSCI, SCIELO, both high quality databases which guarantee good bibliographic support. The search covered from July 2006, when Hespel et al., [23] suggested the use of caffeine as an effective supplement for soccer athletic performance, to November 2018. Search terms included a mix of Medical Subject Headings (MeSH) and free-text words for key concepts related to caffeine and soccer physical performance, muscle damage or perceived fatigue as follows: ("football"(All Fields) OR "soccer"(All Fields)) AND ("caffeine"(All Fields) OR "energy drink"(All Fields)) AND (("physical performance"(All Fields) OR performance(All Fields))) OR (("muscles"(MeSH Terms) OR "muscles" (All Fields) OR "muscle" (All Fields))) OR damage(All Fields) OR (RPE(All Fields) OR "perceived fatigue "(All Fields)). Through this search, relevant articles in the field were obtained applying the snowball strategy. All titles and abstracts from the search were cross-referenced to identify duplicates and any potential missing studies. Titles and abstracts were then screened for a subsequent full-text review. The search for published studies was independently performed by two authors (JMA and JCG) and disagreements about physical parameters were resolved through discussion.

2.2. Inclusion and Exclusion Criteria

For the articles obtained in the search, the following inclusion criteria were applied to select studies: articles (1) depicting a well-designed experiment that included the ingestion of an acute dose of caffeine—or a caffeine-containing product—before and/or during exercise in humans; (2) with an identical experimental situation related to the ingestion of a placebo performed on a different day; (3) testing the effects of caffeine on soccer-specific tests and/or real or simulated matches; (4) with a double-blind, and randomized cross-over design; (5) with clear information regarding the administration of caffeine (relative dose of caffeine per kg of body mass and/or absolute dose of caffeine with information about body mass; timing of caffeine intake before the onset of performance measurements, etc.); (6) where caffeine was administered in the form of a beverage, coffee gum or pills; (7) on soccer players with previous training backgrounds in soccer; (8) the languages were restricted to English, German, French, Italian, Spanish and Portuguese. The following exclusion criteria were applied to the experimental protocols of the investigation: (1) the use of caffeine doses below 1 mg/kg or above 9 mg/kg; (2) the absence of a true placebo condition; (3) the absence of pre-experimental standardizations such as elimination of dietary sources of caffeine 24 h before testing; (4) carried out in participants with a previous condition or injury. There were no filters applied to the soccer players' level, sex or age to increase the power of the analysis. Moreover, the Physiotherapy Evidence Database scale (PEDro), the key factors of which assess eligibility criteria, random allocation, baseline values, success of the blinding procedures, power of the key outcomes, correct statistical analysis and measurement of participants' distribution of studies, was used to evaluate whether the selected randomized controlled trials were scientifically sound: 9–10 = excellent, 6–8 = good, 4–5 = fair, and <4 = poor) [24]. Papers with a poor PEDro score were excluded (i.e., <4 points).

Once the inclusion/exclusion criteria were applied to each study, data on study source (including authors and year of publication), study design, caffeine administration (dose and timing), sample size, characteristics of the participants (level and sex), and final outcomes of the interventions were extracted independently by two authors (JMA and JCG) using a spreadsheet (Microsoft Inc, Seattle, WA, USA). Subsequently, disagreements were resolved through discussion until a consensus was reached. Experiments were clustered by the type of test used to assess the effects of caffeine on soccer physical performance and groups of experiments were created on the effects of caffeine physical performance, muscle damage and perception of fatigue because of its importance to overall soccer performance [4].

3. Results

3.1. Main Search

The literature search provided a total of 135 articles related to the selected descriptors, but only 17 articles met all the inclusion/exclusion criteria (see Figure 1). The number of articles and their exclusion criteria were: 32 papers were removed because they were duplicated; 4 papers were removed because they were performed on a non-human population; another 4 papers were removed because they were narrative or systematic reviews; 13 studies were not carried out during the range of dates included in the inclusion criteria. From the remaining 40 articles, another 23 papers were removed because they were unrelated to the effects of caffeine on soccer physical performance. The topics and number of studies that were excluded were: 1 because of lack of information on body mass, 1 because the caffeine content was found in nutritional supplements with other drugs, 1 because it was a suggestion for future research, 1 because the sport investigated was not specified, 4 because they dealt with recovery or sleep processes, 4 because they investigated other team sports (1 rugby, 1 volleyball, 1 tennis, 1 Gaelic football), and the remaining 11 articles because they studied other subjects unrelated to the focus of this systematic review. Thus, the current systematic review includes 17 studies.

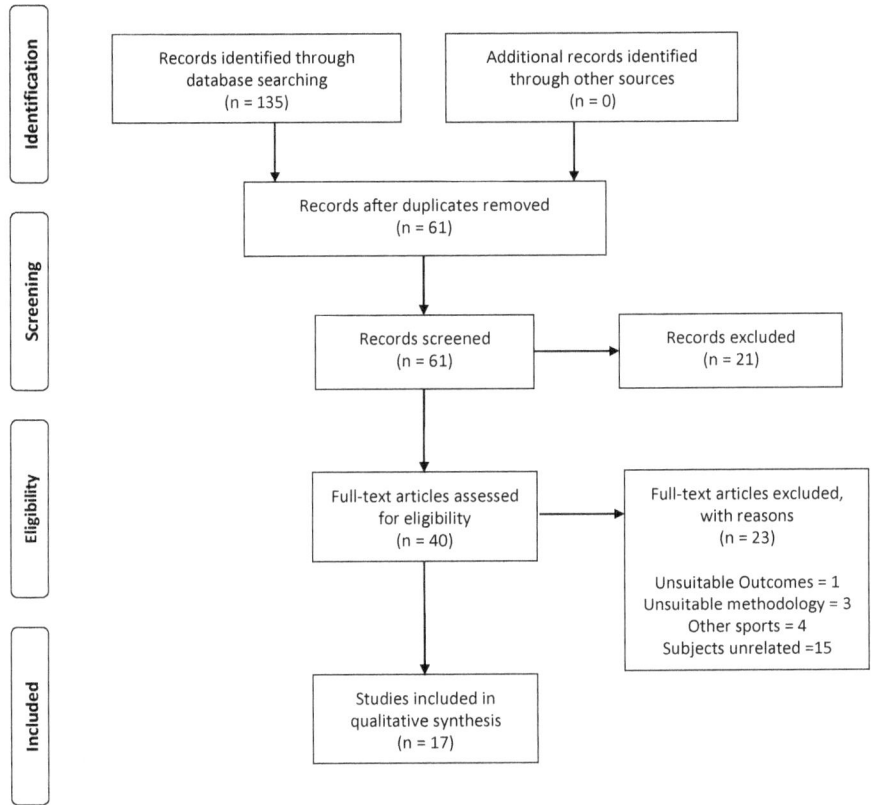

Figure 1. Selection of studies.

3.2. Caffeine Supplementation

The participants' samples included players of both genders (241 males and 33 females), who competed in professional or elite ($n = 108$), semi-professional ($n = 19$) and amateur teams ($n = 147$). In addition, 70 players were adolescents. Out of the 17 investigations, only 2 studies included female soccer players. In 12 out of 17 studies, caffeine was administered based on the soccer player's body mass, while an absolute dose was provided for all participants in 5 studies. In 2 studies the caffeine dose employed was less than 3 mg/kg, 3 studies used a caffeine dose of around 3 mg/kg, in 2 studies it was 4.5 mg/kg, in 3 studies it was around 5 mg/kg, in 4 studies the dose was 6 mg/kg and 2 studies included a dose above 6 mg/kg (i.e., 7.2 mg/kg). In 1 study, soccer players took different doses (1, 2 and 3 mg/kg). Regarding the form of administration, 9 investigations used capsules filled with caffeine, 3 investigations used caffeinated energy drinks, 3 investigations used a caffeinated sport drink, 1 investigation employed a 20% carbohydrate solution and 1 investigation employed caffeinated chewing gum.

Most investigations administered caffeine 30–60 min prior to testing, with the exception of the studies conducted by Andrade-Souza et al. (2015) where the consumption of caffeine was carried out 3 h after a practice session, 4 h after its effects were evaluated in a simulated match [25]. Also, Guttierres et al. (2013) used a protocol that included the ingestion of caffeine 1 h before the test and every 15 min during the protocol [26]. Finally, Ranchordas et al. (2018) employed caffeine 5 min before the tests because they used caffeinated gums [17]. In summary, different studies examined the effect of caffeine on soccer physical performance by using a variety of times of ingestion prior to the testing (5 min–60 min).

3.3. Outcome Measures

Tables 1–3 include information about author/s and year of publication; the sample investigated, with details of sport level, sex and the number of participants; the study design cites the control group if the study included one; the supplementation protocol that specifies the type of caffeine used, the dose and the time that it was administered; the parameters analyzed or main effects either on sport performance ($n = 12$; Table 1) and muscle damage ($n = 5$; Table 2) and finally results or main conclusions. Additionally, some studies also presented data on the effects of caffeine on perceived exertion and heart rate ($n = 6$; Table 3).

Table 1. Summary of studies included in the systematic review that investigated the effect of caffeine ingestion as compared to a placebo on soccer-specific abilities.

Author/s	Population	Intervention	Outcomes Analyzed	Main Conclusion
Ellis M. et al. 2018 [21]	15 male elite youth players (16 ± 1 years)	1, 2 or 3 mg/kg of caffeine capsules 60 min before the start	20-m sprint Arrowhead agility CMJ Yo-Yo IR1	↑ 20-m sprint ↑ Arrowhead agility † CMJ † Yo-Yo IR1
Apostolidis A. et al. 2018 [19]	20 well-trained male players High ($n=11$) and low ($n=9$) responders (21.5 ± 4 years)	6 mg/kg of caffeine capsules 60 min before the start	CMJ Reaction time Time to fatigue	† CMJ ↑ Reaction time ↑ Time to fatigue
Guerra MA Jr. et al. 2018 [18]	12 male professional players (23 ± 6 years)	5 mg/kg of caffeine + 20% carbohydrate solution 60 min before the start	CMJ at 1, 3 and 5 min after the conditioning stimulus	↑ CMJ
Ranchordas et al. 2018 [17]	10 male university-standard players (19 ± 1 years)	200 mg (≈2.7 g/kg) of caffeinated gum 5 min before the start	20-m sprint CMJ Yo-Yo IR1	↑ 20-m sprint † CMJ ↑ Yo-Yo IR1
Andrade Souza, V. et al. 2015 [25]	11 male amateur players (25.4 ± 2.3 years)	6 mg/kg of caffeine capsules 3 h after the LIST	30-m Repeated-Sprint test CMJ LSPT	↑ 30-m Repeated-sprint test † CMJ † LSPT
Jordan, J et al. 2014 [16]	17 male elite young players (14.1 ± 3.5 years)	6 mg/kg of caffeine capsules 60 min before the start	Sprint time Reaction time	† Sprint time ↑ Reaction time on non-dominant leg
Lara, B. et al. 2014 [27]	18 female semi-professional players (21 ± 2 years)	3 mg/kg of caffeinated energy drinks 60 min before the start	Height and power of jump Average speed of running Total distance covered Number of sprints	↑ Height and power of jump ↑ Average speed of running ↑ Total distance covered ↑ Number of sprints
Astorino, T. et al. 2012 [20]	15 female collegiate players (19.5 ± 1.1 years)	255 mL (≈1.3 mg/kg) of caffeinated energy drinks (Redbull) 60 min before the start	Sprint time	† Sprint time
Del Coso, J. et al. 2012 [6]	19 male semi-professional players (2. ± 2 years)	3 mg/kg of caffeine in energy drink 60 min before the start	Maximum height jump Maximum running speed Distance covered Caffeine concentration in urine	↑ Maximum height jump ↑ Maximum running speed ↑ Distance covered ↑ Caffeine concentrations in urine
Gant, N. et al. 2010 [28]	15 male first team level players (21.3 ± 3 years)	160 mg/L (≈3.7 mg/kg) of caffeinated sport drinks 60 min before the start and every 15 min during the test	Sprint times Jump power Test of passes Blood lactate Post-exercise caffeine in urine	↑ Sprint times ↑ Jump power ↑ Test of passes ↑ Blood lactate ↑ Post-exercise caffeine in urine
Foskett et al. 2009 [15]	12 male professional players (23.8 ± 4.5 years)	6 mg/kg of caffeine capsules 60 min before the start	LSPT CMJ	↑ LSPT † CMJ
Guttierres, A. P. et al. 2009 [29]	18 male junior players (16.1 ± 0.7 years)	250 mg/L (≈7.2 mg/kg) of caffeinated sport drinks 20 min before and every 15 min during the test	Jump height Illinois agility test	↑ Jump height † Illinois agility test

↑: statistically significant increase; †: change with no statistical significance; ↓: statistically significant decrease. CMJ: countermovement jump; LIST: Loughborough Intermittent Shuttle Test; LSPT: Loughborough Soccer Passing Test; Yo-Yo IR1: Yo-Yo intermittent recovery test level-1

Table 2. Summary of studies included in the systematic review that investigated the effect of caffeine ingestion as compared to a placebo on serum markers of muscle damage.

Author/s	Population	Intervention	Outcomes Analyzed	Main Conclusion
Guttierres, A. P. et al. 2013 [26]	20 male young players (16.1 ± 0.7 years)	7.2 mg/kg of caffeinated sport drinks 20 min before and every 15 min during the test	Blood glucose Blood lactate Plasma caffeine Free fatty acids Urine caffeine	↑ Blood glucose ↑ Blood lactate ↑ Plasma caffeine † Free fatty acids † Urine caffeine
Machado, M. et al. 2010 [30]	15 male players (18.4 ± 0.8 years)	4.5 mg/kg of caffeine capsules Immediately before the test	CK LDH ALT AST basophils, eosinophils, neutrophils, monocyte lymphocytes	† CK † LDH † ALT † AST † basophils, eosinophils, neutrophils, monocyte lymphocytes
Machado, M. et al. 2009 [31]	20 male players (18.8 ± 1 years)	4.5 mg/kg of caffeine capsules Immediately before the test	Basic hemogram CK LDH ALT AST AP γ-GT	† Basic hemogram † CK † LDH † ALT † AST † AP † γ-GT
Machado, M. et al. 2009 [32]	15 male professional players (19 ± 1 years)	5.5 mg/kg of caffeine capsules Immediately before the test	CK LDH ALT AST	† CK † LDH † ALT † AST
Bassini-Cameron, A. et al. 2007 [33]	22 male professional players (26.0 ± 1.6 years)	5 mg/kg of caffeine capsules 60 min before the start	CK LDH ALT AST	↑ CK † LDH ↑ALT † AST

↑: statistically significant increase; †: change with no statistical significance; ↓: statistically significant decrease. CK: creatine kinase; LDH: lactate dehydrogenase; ALT: alanine aminotransferase; AST: aspartate aminotransferase; AP: alkaline phosphorylase; γ-GT: γ-glutamyl transferase.

Table 3. Summary of studies included in the systematic review that investigated the effect of caffeine ingestion as compared to a placebo on perceived fatigue and heart rate.

Author/s	Population	Intervention	Outcomes Analyzed	Main Conclusion
Andrade Souza, V. et al. 2015 [25]	11 male amateur players (25.4 ± 2.3 years)	6 mg/kg of caffeine capsules 3 h after the LIST	Perceived effort	↑ Perceived effort
Jordan, J. et al. 2014 [16]	17 male elite young players (14.1 ± 0.5 years)	6 mg/kg of caffeine capsules 60 min before the start	Heart rate	⁺ Heart rate
Lara, B. et al. 2014 [27]	18 female semi-professional players (21 ± 2 years)	3 mg/kg of caffeinated energy drinks 60 min before the start	Heart rate	⁺ Heart rate
Guttierres, A. P. et al. 2013 [26]	20 male young players (16.1 ± 0.7 years)	7.2 mg/kg of caffeinated sport drinks 20 min before and every 15 min during the test	Perceived effort	⁺ Perceived effort
Astorino, T. et al. 2012 [20]	15 female collegiate players (19.5 ± 1.1 years)	255 mL (≈1.3 mg/kg) of caffeinated energy drinks (Redbull) 60 min before the start	Perceived effort Heart rate	⁺ Perceived effort ⁺ Heart rate
Foskett et al. 2009 [15]	12 male professional players (23.8 ± 4.5 years)	6 mg/kg of caffeine capsules 60 min before the start	Heart rate	⁺ Heart rate

↑: statistically significant increase; ⁺ change with no statistical significance; ↓: statistically significant decrease.

4. Discussion

The purpose of this systematic review was to summarize all scientific evidence for the effect of acute caffeine ingestion on variables related to soccer physical performance. Due to the differences of the effects studied among the investigations included in the analysis, the following variables have been clustered for a more comprehensive scrutiny.

4.1. Impact on Sports Performance

A total of 12 investigations carried out research protocols that studied the effects of caffeine on one or more variables related to soccer-specific abilities. Overall, these investigations showed an improvement in soccer-related skills with the pre-exercise ingestion of caffeine (Table 1). Specifically, Foskett et al., [15], with 12 first division football players (age: 23.8 ± 4.5 years), observed that the consumption of 6 mg/kg of caffeine before exercise increased passing accuracy and accrued significantly less penalty time during two validated tests to assess soccer skill performance (intermittent shuttle-running protocol and Loughborough Soccer Passing Test; LSPT). In addition, this investigation also found that caffeine improved the functional power of the leg measured by a vertical jump. In the study conducted by Jordan et al., 17 soccer players from the elite youth category (age: 14.1 ± 0.5 years) performed an agility test (reactive agility test) validated for football [34]. These authors indicated, based on the results of their investigation, the intake of 6 mg/kg of caffeine 60 min before the test significantly improved the reaction time of the players in their non-dominant leg [16]. In another study conducted with 15 elite young players (age: 16 ± 1 years) that were administered low doses of caffeine (1, 2 and 3 mg/kg), Ellis et al., [21] observed that improvements in physical performance depended on the dose and the type of task. Specifically, they concluded that 3 mg/kg of caffeine seems to be the optimal dose to obtain positive effects on soccer-specific tests (20 m sprint, arrowhead agility and CMJ). However, the authors also suggested that even higher doses of caffeine might be required to improve endurance performance, as measured by the Yo-Yo intermittent recovery test level 1 (Yo-Yo IR1).

In this line, Apostolidis et al., [19] showed that 6 mg/kg of caffeine ingested 60 min previous to a battery of tests improved aerobic endurance (time to fatigue) and neuromuscular performance (CMJ) in 20 well-trained soccer players (age: 21.5 ± 4 years). Since these authors did not find any change in substrate oxidation with caffeine, measured by indirect calorimetry during the testing, they commented that performance improvements could only be attributed to positive effects on the central nervous system and/or neuromuscular function, although the precise mechanism of caffeine ergogenicity was not indicated in this investigation. Finally, Guerra et al., [18] investigated the addition of caffeine (5 mg/kg) to a post-activation potentiation protocol that included plyometrics and sled towing. These authors found that, in a group of 12 male professional soccer players (age: 23 ± 5 years), caffeine augmented the effects of the post-activation potentiation, as measured by CMJ. These investigations, taken together, suggest that caffeine might be effective to improve performance in players' abilities and soccer-specific skills (jumps, sprint, agility, aerobic endurance, accuracy of passes and ball control).

Caffeinated energy drinks are considered as one of the most common ways to provide caffeine before exercise [14], and the effect of this type of beverages have been also investigated in soccer players. Del Coso et al., [16] chose 19 semi-professional players (age: 21 ± 2 years) in order to determine if the caffeine, provided via a commercially-available energy drink (3 mg/kg), improved performance during several soccer-specific tests (single and repeated jump tests and repeated sprint ability test) and during a simulated soccer match. For this investigation, players ingested either an energy drink without sugar but with caffeine (i.e., sugar-free Redbull), or a sugar-free soda (Pepsi diet without caffeine) 60 min prior to testing. The results showed that the consumption of the caffeinated energy drink increased the ability to jump, to repeat sprints, and it affected positively total running distance and the running distance at >13 km/h covered during the simulated game. In another similar study carried out with 18 semi-professional women soccer players (age: 21 ± 2 years), Lara et al., [34] demonstrated that the consumption of an energy drink containing 3 mg/kg of caffeine improved jump height, the ability to perform sprints, the total running distance and the distance covered at high running intensity (i.e., >18 km/h). These two investigations together suggest that caffeine in the form of an energy drink, can improve the physical demands associated with high performance in soccer, such as sprints, rapid accelerations/decelerations and constant changes of direction [35,36].

Thanks to the collaboration of 18 junior soccer players (age: 16.1 ± 0.7 years), Guttierres et al., [29] evaluated whether the physical performance of these players increased with the consumption of a caffeinated sports drink (250 mg/L ≈ 7.2 mg/kg) compared to a commercial carbonated drink. They concluded that the caffeine-based sport drink significantly increased jump height and improved the power in the lower limbs, another determinant factor in soccer physical performance [37]. However, positive effects were not demonstrated in the "Illinois Agility Test", a validated routine to assess agility in team sports players [38]. This lack of positive effects was possibly due to the fact that players' agility is a complex process that depends on the coordination of factors such as decision making and speed in the changes of direction, both aspects of which are trained and constantly improved in training [39]. Gant et al., [28] used a caffeine-containing carbonated drink in 15 professional soccer players (age: 21.3 ± 3 years) and were able to evidence that the addition of caffeine to a carbonated drink, in a dose of 3.7 mg/kg (60 min before starting and every 15 min during the test), improved sprint performance and the vertical jump in soccer players. Andrade-Souza et al., [25] proposed a very interesting study where the aim was to investigate the effect of a carbohydrate-based drink, with (6 mg/kg) and without caffeine, and they compared these trials to the isolated ingestion of caffeine. The study was carried out with 11 college football players (age: 25.4 ± 2.3 years) with the ingestion of the drinks after the morning training session to see the effects of the 20% carbohydrate solutions on the afternoon training session of the same day. The main finding of Andrade-Souza's study was that none of the drinks was able to increase performance. This fact could be related to reduction of the glycogen levels from the morning to the afternoon training sessions, a factor that was either not considered or measured in the study. According to Jacobs [40], a reduction in the content of muscle glycogen below a critical threshold can affect anaerobic strength and performance. In the Andrade-Souza's study, the recovery time between the two practice sessions was very short (4 h) and the nutritional strategies chosen were not optimal to replenish muscle glycogen [25]. Thus, it is likely that the reduction of glycogen stores might have precluded the ergogenic effect of caffeine in this experimental design.

Chewing gum provides an alternative mode of caffeine administration that is more rapidly absorbed (via the buccal mucosa) than capsules and drinks (i.e., 5 min vs. 45 min, respectively) and less likely to cause gastrointestinal distress [41]. Along these lines, Ranchordas et al., reported that caffeinated chewing gum, containing 200 mg of caffeine, can enhance aerobic capacity (Yo-Yo IR1) by 2% and increase CMJ performance by 2.2% in 10 male university soccer players (age: 19 ± 1 years) [17]. Therefore, chewing gum could be beneficial for soccer players where the time between ingestion and performance is short, (e.g., for substitutes that would come on when called upon by the coach and for players who cannot tolerate caffeinated beverages or capsules because of gastrointestinal distress before kick-off [17]).

4.2. Impact on Muscle Damage

A total of 5 investigations studied the effect of caffeine on the levels of muscle damage after a soccer practice (Table 2). In soccer, muscle damage is a very important physiological variable because all the high-intensity exercises produced in this sport (sprints, accelerations/decelerations, changes of directions and even tackles) may be associated with myofibril damage [42]. In this way, Machado et al. carried out three studies on this specific topic: one with 20 healthy soccer players (age: 18.8 ± 1 years) [31]; another one with 15 male soccer players (age: 19 ± 1 years) [32] and the last one with 15 male soccer athletes (age: 18.4 ± 0.8 years) [30]. The main goal of these three investigations was to determine whether consumption of caffeine in single and acute doses (4.5–5.5 mg/kg) negatively affected blood markers typically used to assess the level of muscle damage. The authors concluded that these markers (creatine kinase, lactate dehydrogenase, aspartate aminotransferase and alanine aminotransferase) increased with exercise, but they did not find that this increase was exacerbated with the consumption of caffeine. On the other hand, a study conducted by Bassini-Cameron et al., [33] which measured hematological variables, muscle proteins and liver enzymes in 22 professional soccer players (age: 26.0 ± 1.6 years), concluded that 5 mg/kg of caffeine ingested 60 min before the start of a game increased the risk of muscle damage in players because there was an increase in the white blood cell count. However, the serum concentration of white blood cells is not a definitive marker of muscle damage level during exercise, as other factors can increase the count of leukocytes during exercise. In summary, although most of studies found an absence of effect of caffeine on exercise-induced muscle damage in soccer players, further research is necessary to confirm this notion [43].

Guttierres et al., [26], in an experiment with 20 youth soccer players (age: 16.1 ± 0.7 years), observed the effect of caffeine (contained in a sport drinks) on free fatty acids mobilization. Participants consumed the beverage 20 min before a soccer match and every 15 min during the game with a total caffeine consumption of 7.2 mg/kg. The authors certified that the caffeine did not increase the mobilization of free fatty acids. Anyway, the caffeinated beverage was also rich in carbohydrates, increasing blood glucose concentration, promoting more insulin and therefore inhibiting the mobilization of fatty acids. Graham, et al., [44] showed that caffeine with glucose increased insulin secretion versus glucose consumption alone. In the Guttierres study, blood glucose concentrations were higher possibly due to an increase in sympathetic nervous system activity [26], increasing adrenaline and noradrenaline and glycogenolysis [45,46]. Moreover, blood lactate concentrations increased with the ingestion of caffeine, likely indicating, in an indirect manner, that players achieved a greater intensity in the trial with caffeine. These outcomes could suggest that soccer players exercised at a higher percentage of their maximum heart rate (caffeine: 80.6 % versus control: 74.7% of maximum heart rate) with the ingestion of caffeine.

4.3. Impact on the Perception of Fatigue

Astorino et al., [20] concluded that the consumption of a serving portion of an energy drink (Redbull), with 1.3 mg/kg of caffeine, did not alter the perception of fatigue or heart rate in 15 semi-professional soccer players (age: 19.5 ± 1.1 years; Table 3). An important limitation of this study was that the amount of caffeine consumed was very low (80 mg) and thus, the effects of caffeine would have been limited due to dosage. On the contrary, Guttierres et al., [26] and Lara et al., [28] found that caffeine tended to cause an increase in exercise heart rate with a concomitant reduction in the perception of fatigue. While caffeine has been proven to reduce perception of fatigue in exercise protocols that used a fixed exercise intensity [47], these investigations [20,26,28] used exercise protocols more applicable to soccer, where exercise intensity can be freely chosen, as happens during soccer play. Under these specific conditions, caffeine served to increase exercise intensity (as indicated by higher running distances and higher average heart rate) while perception of fatigue was unaffected or tended to be reduced. Thus, it might be speculated that caffeine might have the capacity to enhance soccer physical performance without producing higher values of fatigue, which can be understood as a positive property of this stimulant.

4.4. Caffeine Dose and Inter-Individual Responses to Caffeine Administration

The dose of caffeine administered in the experiments ranged from 1.3 to ~7.2 mg/kg and thus, the ergogenic effects of caffeine on soccer players must be attributed to this range of dosage. However, it is still possible that dose-response effects exist or even that a caffeine dose threshold is necessary to obtain benefits from caffeine in soccer, as recently suggested by Chia et al., for ball sports [6]. Based on previous investigations with other different forms of exercise [48–50], or soccer [20,21], it can be suggested that doses below 2 mg of caffeine per kg of body mass might not be effective to increase soccer physical performance. All the experiments included in this systematic review reported their findings as a group mean comparing caffeine vs. placebo trials. Nevertheless, recent investigations have shown that not all individuals experience enhanced physical performance after the ingestion of moderate doses of caffeine [51–54]. These studies have identified the presence of athletes who obtain minimal ergogenic effects or only slight ergolytic effects after acute administration of caffeine, and such participants have been catalogued as "non-responders to caffeine" [55]. To date, there is still no clear explanation for the lack of ergogenic effects after the acute administration of caffeine in some individuals, although factors such as training status, habitual daily caffeine intake, tolerance to caffeine, and genotype variation have been proposed as possible modifying factors for the ergogenicity of caffeine [55]. Whilst this systematic review suggests that the ingestion of 3–6 mg/kg of caffeine is ergogenic for soccer players, it might not be optimal for everyone. The inter-individual variability in the ergogenic response to acute caffeine ingestion suggests that caffeine should be recommended in a customized manner. The development of more precise and individualized guidelines would seem necessary for soccer players.

4.5. Strengths, Limitations and Future Lines of Research

The current systematic review presents some limitations related to the different research protocols and performance tests used in the investigations included. Although we selected investigations in which caffeine was compared to an identical situation without caffeine administration, in some investigations, caffeine was co-ingested with other ingredients (e.g., carbohydrates). It is still possible that some of these ingredients produced a synergistic or antagonistic effect on performance. In addition, the dose of caffeine and posology were not uniform among investigations, which could influence some of the outcomes of the research included in the review. In addition, in the investigations included in the analysis there were different competitive levels and age categories while the low number of articles impeded us from knowing if the effect of caffeine on soccer physical performance depends on level or players' age. Despite these limitations, this review suggests a positive effect of caffeine in increasing soccer players' physical performance with no or little effect on the levels of muscle damage, perceived effort, or exercising heart rate. Because soccer is a complex sport in which the variables investigated in this systematic review represent only a small proportion of the factors necessary for succeeding, further investigations are necessary to determine the effects of caffeine on more complex and ecological soccer-specific tests, especially involving decision-making situations. In the same way, studies should be undertaken into whether the effect of caffeine is different according to the competitive level or soccer player's age.

5. Conclusions

In summary, acute caffeine intake of a moderate dose of caffeine before exercise has the capacity to improve several soccer-related abilities and skills such as vertical jump height, repeated sprint ability, running distances during a game and passing accuracy. Likewise, so far, it has been shown that a single and acute dose of caffeine does not have a negative impact on the increase of variables related to muscle damage during official matches. However, more studies are needed to assess whether chronic caffeine consumption could alter muscle damage markers. Moreover, caffeine supplementation does not cause changes in either the perception of effort or heart rate during regular high-intensity intermittent soccer exercises.

Despite this investigation suggesting several benefits of caffeine in soccer, the use of this stimulant should only be recommended after a careful evaluation of the drawbacks typically associated with the use of caffeine [56]. With this aim, the minimal dose with a positive impact would be recommended (i.e., 3 mg/kg), while it can be consumed in either powder (capsules) or liquid (energy drink or sport drink) forms. Caffeine should only be recommended to athletes who are willing to use ergogenic aids to increase performance and it should be recommended only on an individual basis under careful supervision, in order to avoid the use of this substance in non-responders or athletes who report negative side-effects. Experimenting with caffeine while training, before use in any competition, and avoiding caffeine tolerance may also be further recommendations when using this substance to increase soccer physical performance.

Author Contributions: J.M.-A.: conceived and designed the investigation, analysed and interpreted the data, drafted the paper, and approved the final version submitted for publication. J.C.-G.: and J.D.C.: analysed and interpreted the data, critically reviewed the paper and approved the final version submitted for publication. A.U., P.L.-G. and D.F.-L. critically reviewed the paper and approved the final version submitted for publication.

Funding: The authors declare no funding sources.

Conflicts of Interest: The authors declare no conflict of interest.

References

1. FIFA Communications Division. The FIFA Big Count 2006: 230 Million Active in Football. 2007. Available online: https://www.fifa.com/mm/document/fifafacts/bcoffsurv/bigcount.statspackage_7024.pdf (accessed on 18 July 2018).
2. Cornelissen, S.; Maennig, W. On the Political Economy of 'feel-good' effects at Sport Mega-Events: Experiences from FIFA Germany 2006 and Prospects for South Africa 2010. *Alternation* **2010**, *17*, 96–120.
3. Haycraft, J.A.; Kovalchik, S.; Pyne, D.B.; Robertson, S. Physical characteristics of players within the Australian football league participation pathways: A systematic review. *Sports Med. Open* **2017**, *3*, 46. [CrossRef] [PubMed]
4. Sporis, G.; Jukic, I.; Ostojic, S.M.; Milanovic, D. Fitness profiling in soccer: Physical and physiologic characteristics of elite players. *J. Strength Cond. Res.* **2009**, *23*, 1947–1953. [CrossRef] [PubMed]
5. Krustrup, P.; Mohr, M.; Steensberg, A.; Bencke, J.; Kjaer, M.; Bangsbo, J. Muscle and blood metabolites during a soccer game: Implications for sprint performance. *Med. Sci. Sports Exerc.* **2006**, *38*, 1165–1174. [CrossRef] [PubMed]
6. Chia, J.S.; Barrett, L.A.; Chow, J.Y.; Burns, S.F. Effects of caffeine supplementation on performance in ball games. *Sports Med.* **2017**, *47*, 2453–2471. [CrossRef] [PubMed]
7. Holway, F.E.; Spriet, L.L. Sport-specific nutrition: Practical strategies for team sports. *J. Sports Sci.* **2011**, *29*, S115–S125. [CrossRef] [PubMed]
8. Bishop, D. Dietary supplements and team-sport performance. *Sports Med.* **2010**, *40*, 995–1017. [CrossRef]
9. Davis, J.K.; Green, J.M. Caffeine and anaerobic performance: Ergogenic value and mechanisms of action. *Sports Med.* **2009**, *39*, 813–832. [CrossRef]
10. Trexler, E.T.; Smith-Ryan, A.E.; Roelofs, E.J.; Hirsch, K.R.; Mock, M.G. Effects of coffee and caffeine anhydrous on strength and sprint performance. *Eur. J. Sport Sci.* **2015**. [CrossRef]
11. Glaister, M.; Muniz-Pumares, D.; Patterson, S.D.; Foley, P.; McInnes, G. caffeine supplementation and peak anaerobic power output. *Eur. J. Sport. Sci.* **2015**, *15*, 400–406. [CrossRef]
12. Australian Institute of Sport. Australian Institute of Sport. 2014. Available online: https://www.sportaus.gov.au/ais (accessed on 25 October 2017).
13. Salinero, J.J.; Lara, B.; Del Coso, J. Effects of acute ingestion of caffeine on team sports performance: A systematic review and meta-analysis. *Res. Sports Med.* **2018**. [CrossRef] [PubMed]
14. Del Coso, J.; Munoz-Fernandez, V.E.; Munoz, G.; Fernandez-Elias, V.E.; Ortega, J.F.; Hamouti, N.; Barbero, J.C.; Munoz-Guerra, J. Effects of a caffeine-containing energy drink on simulated soccer performance. *PLoS ONE* **2012**, *7*, e31380. [CrossRef] [PubMed]
15. Foskett, A.; Ali, A.; Gant, N. Caffeine enhances cognitive function and skill performance during simulated soccer activity. *Int. J. Sport Nutr. Exerc. Metab.* **2009**, *19*, 410–423. [CrossRef] [PubMed]
16. Jordan, J.B.; Korgaokar, A.; Farley, R.S.; Coons, J.M.; Caputo, J.L. Caffeine supplementation and reactive agility in elite youth soccer players. *Pediatr. Exerc. Sci.* **2014**, *26*, 168–176. [CrossRef]
17. Ranchordas, M.K.; King, G.; Russell, M.; Lynn, A.; Russell, M. Effects of caffeinated gum on a battery of soccer-specific tests in trained university-standard male soccer players. *Int. J. Sport Nutr. Exerc. Metab.* **2018**. [CrossRef] [PubMed]
18. Guerra, M.A., Jr.; Caldas, L.C.; De Souza, H.L.; Vitzel, K.F.; Cholewa, J.M.; Duncan, M.J.; Guimaraes-Ferreira, L. The acute effects of plyometric and sled towing stimuli with and without caffeine ingestion on vertical jump performance in professional soccer players. *J. Int. Soc. Sports Nutr.* **2018**. [CrossRef] [PubMed]
19. Apostolidis, A.; Mougios, V.; Smilios, I.; Rodosthenous, J.; Hadjicharalambous, M. Caffeine supplementation: Ergogenic in both high and low caffeine responders. *Int. J. Sports Physiol. Perform.* **2018**, *14*, 1–25. [CrossRef]

20. Astorino, T.A.; Matera, A.J.; Basinger, J.; Evans, M.; Schurman, T.; Marquez, R. Effects of red bull energy drink on repeated sprint performance in women athletes. *Amino Acids* **2012**, *42*, 1803–1808. [CrossRef]
21. Ellis, M.; Noon, M.; Myers, T.; Clarke, N. Low doses of caffeine: Enhancement of physical performance in elite adolescent male soccer players. *Int. J. Sports Physiol. Perform.* **2018**, *9*, 1–21. [CrossRef]
22. Liberati, A.; Altman, D.G.; Tetzlaff, J.; Mulrow, C.; Gotzsche, P.C.; Ioannidis, J.P.; Clarke, M.; Devereaux, P.J.; Kleijnen, J.; Moher, D. The PRISMA statement for reporting systematic reviews and meta-analyses of studies that evaluate healthcare interventions: Explanation and elaboration. *BMJ* **2009**, *339*, b2700. [CrossRef]
23. Hespel, P.; Maughan, R.J.; Greenhaff, P.L. Dietary supplements for football. *J. Sports Sci.* **2006**, *24*, 749–761. [CrossRef] [PubMed]
24. Maher, C.G.; Sherrington, C.; Herbert, R.D.; Moseley, A.M.; Elkins, M. Reliability of the PEDro scale for rating quality of randomized controlled trials. *Phys. Ther.* **2003**, *83*, 713–721. [PubMed]
25. Andrade-Souza, V.A.; Bertuzzi, R.; de Araujo, G.G.; Bishop, D.; Lima-Silva, A.E. Effects of isolated or combined carbohydrate and caffeine supplementation between 2 daily training sessions on soccer performance. *Appl. Physiol. Nutr. Metab.* **2015**, *40*, 457–463. [CrossRef] [PubMed]
26. Guttierres, A.P.M.; Alfenas, R.d.C.; Gatti, K.; Lima, J.R.P.; Silva, Â.A.; Natali, A.J.; Marins, J.C.B. Metabolic effects of a caffeinated sports drink consumed during a soccer match. *Motriz: Revista de Educação Física* **2013**, *19*, 688–695.
27. Lara, B.; Gonzalez-Millan, C.; Salinero, J.J.; Abian-Vicen, J.; Areces, F.; Barbero-Alvarez, J.C.; Munoz, V.; Portillo, L.J.; Gonzalez-Rave, J.M.; Del Coso, J. Caffeine-containing energy drink improves physical performance in female soccer players. *Amino Acids* **2014**, *46*, 1385–1392. [CrossRef] [PubMed]
28. Gant, N.; Ali, A.; Foskett, A. The influence of caffeine and carbohydrate coingestion on simulated soccer performance. *Int. J. Sport Nutr. Exerc. Metab.* **2010**, *20*, 191–197. [CrossRef] [PubMed]
29. Guttierres, A.P.M.; Natali, A.J.; Alfenas, R.D.C.G.; Marins, J.C.B. Ergogenic Effect of a caffeinated sports drink on performance in soccer specific abilities tests. *Revista Brasileira de Medicina do Esporte* **2009**, *15*, 450–454. [CrossRef]
30. Machado, M.; Koch, A.J.; Willardson, J.M.; dos Santos, F.C.; Curty, V.M.; Pereira, L.N. Caffeine does not augment markers of muscle damage or leukocytosis following resistance exercise. *Int. J. Sports Physiol. Perform.* **2010**, *5*, 18–26.
31. Machado, M.; Antunes, W.D.; Tamy, A.L.M.; Azevedo, P.G.; Barreto, J.G.; Hackney, A.C. Effect of a single dose of caffeine supplementation and intermittent-interval exercise on muscle damage markers in soccer players. *J. Exerc. Sci. Fit.* **2009**, *7*, 91–97. [CrossRef]
32. Machado, M.; Breder, A.C.; Ximenes, M.C.; Simões, J.R.; Vigo, J.F.F. Caffeine supplementation and muscle damage in soccer players. *Braz. J. Pharm.* **2009**, *45*, 257–261. [CrossRef]
33. Bassini-Cameron, A.; Sweet, E.; Bottino, A.; Bittar, C.; Veiga, C.; Cameron, L.C. Effect of caffeine supplementation on haematological and biochemical variables in elite soccer players under physical stress conditions. *Br. J. Sports Med.* **2007**, *41*, 523–530. [CrossRef] [PubMed]
34. Sheppard, J.M.; Young, W.B.; Doyle, T.L.; Sheppard, T.A.; Newton, R.U. An evaluation of a new test of reactive agility and its relationship to sprint speed and change of direction speed. *J. Sci. Med. Sport* **2006**, *9*, 342–349. [CrossRef] [PubMed]
35. Reilly, T.; Williams, A.M.; Nevill, A.; Franks, A. A Multidisciplinary approach to talent identification in soccer. *J. Sports Sci.* **2000**, *18*, 695–702. [CrossRef] [PubMed]
36. Little, T.; Williams, A.G. Specificity of acceleration, maximum speed, and agility in professional soccer players. *J. Strength Cond Res.* **2005**, *19*, 76–78.
37. Bangsbo, J. The Physiology of soccer—With special reference to intense intermittent exercise. *Acta Physiol. Scand. Suppl.* **1994**, *619*, 1–155. [PubMed]
38. Roozen, M. Illinois Agility Test. *NSCA's Perform. Train. J.* **2004**, *3*, 5–6.
39. Serrano, J.; Shahidian, S.; Sampaio, J.; Leite, N. The importance of sports performance factors and training contents from the perspective of futsal coaches. *J. Hum. Kinet.* **2013**, *38*, 151–160. [CrossRef] [PubMed]
40. Jacobs, I. Lactate, muscle glycogen and exercise performance in man. *Acta Physiol. Scand.* **1981**, *495*, 1–35.
41. Kamimori, G.H.; Karyekar, C.S.; Otterstetter, R.; Cox, D.S.; Balkin, T.J.; Belenky, G.L.; Eddington, N.D. The rate of absorption and relative bioavailability of caffeine administered in chewing gum versus capsules to normal healthy volunteers. *Int. J. Pharm.* **2002**, *234*, 159–167. [CrossRef]

42. Thorpe, R.; Sunderland, C. Muscle damage, endocrine, and immune marker response to a soccer match. *J. Strength Cond. Res.* **2012**, *26*, 2783–2790. [CrossRef]
43. Clarkson, P.M.; Hubal, M.J. Exercise-induced muscle damage in humans. *Am. J. Phys. Med. Rehabil.* **2002**, *81*, S52–S69. [CrossRef] [PubMed]
44. Graham, T.E.; Sathasivam, P.; Rowland, M.; Marko, N.; Greer, F.; Battram, D. Caffeine ingestion elevates plasma insulin response in humans during an oral glucose tolerance test. *Can. J. Physiol. Pharmacol.* **2001**, *79*, 559–565. [CrossRef] [PubMed]
45. Davis, J.M.; Zhao, Z.; Stock, H.S.; Mehl, K.A.; Buggy, J.; Hand, G.A. Central nervous system effects of caffeine and adenosine on fatigue. *Am. J. Physiol. Regul. Integr. Comp. Physiol.* **2003**, *284*, R399–R404. [CrossRef] [PubMed]
46. Yeo, S.E.; Jentjens, R.L.; Wallis, G.A.; Jeukendrup, A.E. Caffeine increases exogenous carbohydrate oxidation during exercise. *J. Appl. Physiol.* **2005**, *99*, 844–850. [CrossRef] [PubMed]
47. Doherty, M.; Smith, P. Effects of caffeine ingestion on rating of perceived exertion during and after exercise: A Meta-analysis. *Scand. J. Med. Sci. Sports* **2005**, *15*, 69–78. [CrossRef] [PubMed]
48. Del Coso, J.; Ramirez, J.A.; Munoz, G.; Portillo, J.; Gonzalez-Millan, C.; Munoz, V.; Barbero-Alvarez, J.C.; Munoz-Guerra, J. Caffeine-containing energy drink improves physical performance of elite rugby players during a simulated match. *Appl. Physiol. Nutr. Metab.* **2013**, *38*, 368–374. [CrossRef]
49. Astorino, T.A.; Cottrell, T.; Lozano, A.T.; Aburto-Pratt, K.; Duhon, J. Effect of caffeine on RPE and perceptions of pain, arousal, and pleasure/displeasure during a cycling time trial in endurance trained and active men. *Physiol. Behav.* **2012**, *106*, 211–217. [CrossRef]
50. Turley, K.; Eusse, P.A.; Thomas, M.M.; Townsend, J.R.; Morton, A.B. Effects of different doses of caffeine on anaerobic exercise in boys. *Pediatr. Exerc. Sci.* **2015**, *27*, 50–56. [CrossRef]
51. Doherty, M.; Smith, P.M.; Davison, R.C.; Hughes, M.G. Caffeine is ergogenic after supplementation of oral creatine monohydrate. *Med. Sci. Sports Exerc.* **2002**, *34*, 1785–1792. [CrossRef]
52. Grgic, J.; Mikulic, P. Caffeine ingestion acutely enhances muscular strength and power but not muscular endurance in resistance-trained men. *Eur. J. Sport Sci.* **2017**, *17*, 1029–1036. [CrossRef]
53. Lara, B.; Ruiz-Vicente, D.; Areces, F.; Abian-Vicen, J.; Salinero, J.J.; Gonzalez-Millan, C.; Gallo-Salazar, C.; Del Coso, J. Acute consumption of a caffeinated energy drink enhances aspects of performance in sprint swimmers. *Br. J. Nutr.* **2015**, *114*, 908–914. [CrossRef] [PubMed]
54. Skinner, T.L.; Jenkins, D.G.; Coombes, J.S.; Taaffe, D.R.; Leveritt, M.D. Dose response of caffeine on 2000-m rowing performance. *Med. Sci. Sports Exerc.* **2010**, *42*, 571–576. [CrossRef] [PubMed]
55. Pickering, C.; Kiely, J. Are the current guidelines on caffeine use in sport optimal for everyone? Inter-individual variation in caffeine ergogenicity, and a move towards personalised sports nutrition. *Sports Med.* **2018**, *48*, 7–16. [CrossRef] [PubMed]
56. Salinero, J.J.; Lara, B.; Abian-Vicen, J.; Gonzalez-Millán, C.; Areces, F.; Gallo-Salazar, C.; Ruiz-Vicente, D.; Del Coso, J. The use of energy drinks in sport: Perceived ergogenicity and side effects in male and female athletes. *Br. J. Nutr.* **2014**, *112*, 1494–1502. [CrossRef] [PubMed]

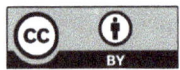

© 2019 by the authors. Licensee MDPI, Basel, Switzerland. This article is an open access article distributed under the terms and conditions of the Creative Commons Attribution (CC BY) license (http://creativecommons.org/licenses/by/4.0/).

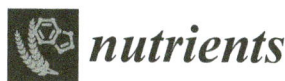

Article

The Effects of Caffeine on Metabolomic Responses to Muscle Contraction in Rat Skeletal Muscle

Satoshi Tsuda [1], Tatsuya Hayashi [1] and Tatsuro Egawa [1,2,*]

[1] Laboratory of Sports and Exercise Medicine, Graduate School of Human and Environmental Studies, Kyoto University, Kyoto 606-8501, Japan
[2] Laboratory of Health and Exercise Sciences, Graduate School of Human and Environmental Studies, Kyoto University, Kyoto 606-8501, Japan
* Correspondence: egawa.tatsuro.4u@kyoto-u.ac.jp; Tel.: +81-75-753-6613; Fax: +81-75-753-6885

Received: 4 July 2019; Accepted: 5 August 2019; Published: 7 August 2019

Abstract: Exercise has beneficial effects on our health by stimulating metabolic activation of skeletal muscle contraction. Caffeine is a powerful metabolic stimulant in the skeletal muscle that has ergogenic effects, including enhanced muscle power output and endurance capacity. In the present study, we aim to characterize the metabolic signatures of contracting muscles with or without caffeine stimulation using liquid chromatography-mass spectrometry and capillary electrophoresis coupled to mass spectrometry. Isolated rat epitrochlearis muscle was incubated in the presence or absence or of 3 mM caffeine for 30 min. Electrical stimulation (ES) was used to induce tetanic contractions during the final 10 min of incubation. Principal component analysis and hierarchical clustering analysis detected 184 distinct metabolites across three experimental groups—basal, ES, and ES with caffeine (ES + C). Significance Analysis of Microarray identified a total of 50 metabolites with significant changes in expression, and 23 metabolites significantly changed between the ES and ES + C groups. Changes were observed in metabolite levels of various metabolic pathways, including the pentose phosphate, nucleotide synthesis, β-oxidation, tricarboxylic acid cycle, and amino acid metabolism. In particular, D-ribose 5-phosphate, IMP, O-acetylcarnitine, butyrylcarnitine, L-leucine, L-valine, and L-aspartate levels were higher in the ES + C group than in the ES group. These metabolic alterations induced by caffeine suggest that caffeine accelerates contraction-induced metabolic activations, thereby contributing to muscle endurance performance and exercise benefits to our health.

Keywords: metabolome; skeletal muscle; exercise; muscle contraction; ergogenic effect

1. Introduction

Exercise contributes to health benefits by reducing the risk of several chronic diseases. These effects are partly attributed to metabolic alterations that occur in contracting skeletal muscles. Exercise enhances muscle insulin sensitivity and mitochondrial function by stimulating master metabolic regulators, such as 5′-AMP-activated protein kinase (AMPK), sirtuin 1, and peroxisome proliferator-activated receptor-γ co-activator 1α [1,2]. Recent evidence has suggested that secreted myokines from contracting skeletal muscles have positive effects on metabolic disorders [3]. Therefore, it is accepted that muscle contraction-induced metabolic activation is a key factor for maintaining normal physical function.

Caffeine is a powerful metabolic stimulant in the skeletal muscle. In vitro caffeine treatment of the skeletal muscle promotes insulin-independent glucose transport [4–8], fatty acid oxidation [8,9], Ca^{2+} release from the sarcoplasmic reticulum [10,11], and mitochondrial biogenesis [12]. We have recently demonstrated that caffeine increases the maximal capacity of contraction-stimulated AMPK activation and glucose transport in rat skeletal muscles [6]. Additionally, caffeine is thought to be an important contributor to ergogenic effects in humans. Meta-analyses have shown that caffeine intake has positive effects on muscle power output and endurance performance [13–15]. These findings suggest that caffeine accelerates muscle contraction-induced metabolic activation, thereby contributing to exercise benefits toward health promotion. However, there are no observations investigating the overall effects of caffeine on muscle contraction-induced metabolic activation in the skeletal muscle.

Metabolomic techniques are useful tools for the investigation of complex metabolic responses to muscle contraction [16,17]. In the present study, we aim to characterize the metabolic signatures of contracting muscles with or without caffeine stimulation, using liquid chromatography-mass spectrometry (LC-MS) and capillary electrophoresis coupled to mass spectrometry (CE-MS) analysis.

2. Materials and Methods

2.1. Animals

Male Sprague–Dawley rats (150–160 g) were purchased from Shimizu Breeding Laboratories (Kyoto, Japan). Rats were fed a standard diet (Certified Diet MF; Oriental Koubo, Tokyo, Japan) with *ad libitum* water and were subjected to overnight fasting before the experiments. All animal-related protocols were performed in accordance with the Guide for the Care and Use of Laboratory Animals as adopted and promulgated by the National Institutes of Health (Bethesda, MD, USA) and were approved by the Animal Use Committee at Kyoto University Graduate School of Human and Environmental Studies.

2.2. Muscle Treatment

Muscles were treated as previously described [6]. Rats were killed by cervical dislocation without anesthesia, and the epitrochlearis muscles were removed and mounted on to an incubation apparatus with the tension set to 0.5 g. The epitrochlearis muscle is composed predominantly of fast-twitch glycolytic fibers (60–65% fast-twitch white, 20% fast-twitch red, 15% slow-twitch red) [18], but also has higher oxidative potential than the other fast-twitch muscle [19]. Moreover, it is a small and thin muscle that is suitable for in vitro incubation study. The muscles were pre-incubated in alpha-minimum essential medium (21444-05, nacalai tesque, Kyoto, Japan) containing 1.0 g/L glucose supplemented with 1% penicillin/streptomycin for 40 min and then incubated in fresh medium in the presence or absence of 3 mM caffeine for 30 min. For tetanic contractions, the muscles were stimulated using an electric stimulator (SEN-3401; Nihon Koden, Tokyo, Japan) during the final 10 min of the incubation period (train rate, 1/min; train duration, 10 s; pulse rate, 100 Hz; pulse duration, 0.1 ms; voltage; 10 V). Basal muscles were pre-incubated and incubated without contraction and caffeine treatment. All media were continuously gassed with 95% O_2/5% CO_2 and maintained at 37 °C.

2.3. Metabolomic Analysis

Metabolomic analysis was performed by LSI Medience Corporation (Tokyo, Japan). In brief, the muscle samples (≥50 mg) were homogenized using beads and suspended into 1 mL distilled water. They were then mixed with methanol (2 mL) and chloroform (2 mL) for 10 min at room temperature. After centrifugation at 1000× g for 15 min, the supernatant was evaporated using nitrogen gas and dissolved with 10% acetonitrile aqueous solution (200 μL). After adding internal standards, the samples were subjected to both LC-MS and CE-MS. All peak positions (retention time and *m/z*) and areas were calculated using Markeranalysis (LSI Medience, Tokyo, Japan). All peak areas were aligned into one data sheet, and the errors of peak intensities were corrected using internal standards. Noise peaks were deleted after comparison with the peaks detected in blank samples. The metabolites were identified by comparing the retention times and *m/z* values with a standard dataset provided by LSI Medience Corporation.

2.4. Data Analysis

After applying autoscaling (mean-centered and divided by standard deviation of each variable), principal component analysis (PCA), significance analysis of microarray (SAM), hierarchical clustering analysis (HCA), and one-way ANOVA with Tukey's multiple comparison test were performed using the web-based metabolomic data processing tool MetaboAnalyst 4.0 (http://www.metaboanalyst.ca, Xia Lab, McGill University, Montreal, Canada). In PCA, a score plot of the first and second principal components was generated. HCA was performed to exhibit simultaneous clustering of metabolites and samples by Euclidean distance using Ward's method. Heat maps were generated by coloring the values of all data across their value ranges. False discovery rates (FDR) were calculated to reduce the risk of false positives by adjusted p values. FDR < 0.05 was defined as statistically significant.

3. Results and Discussion

3.1. Pattern Recognition of Metabolites

Metabolomic analysis detected 184 metabolites by LC-MS and CE-MS (Table S1). PCA is a statistical procedure that is used for feature extraction. Using PCA on the detected 184 metabolites, three groups, i.e., basal, electrical stimulation (ES), and ES with caffeine (ES + C), were clearly distinguished on the principal component (PC) 2, although they were overlapped on PC1 (Figure 1). We previously demonstrated that ES in isolated rat skeletal muscles induces metabolic activation [20]. Likewise, the PCA results in this study indicated that ES-induced muscle contraction influences the metabolomic profile of the skeletal muscle. Furthermore, PCA plots in the ES + C group were more distant from basal than in the ES group (Figure 1), suggesting that caffeine accelerates ES-induced metabolic responses.

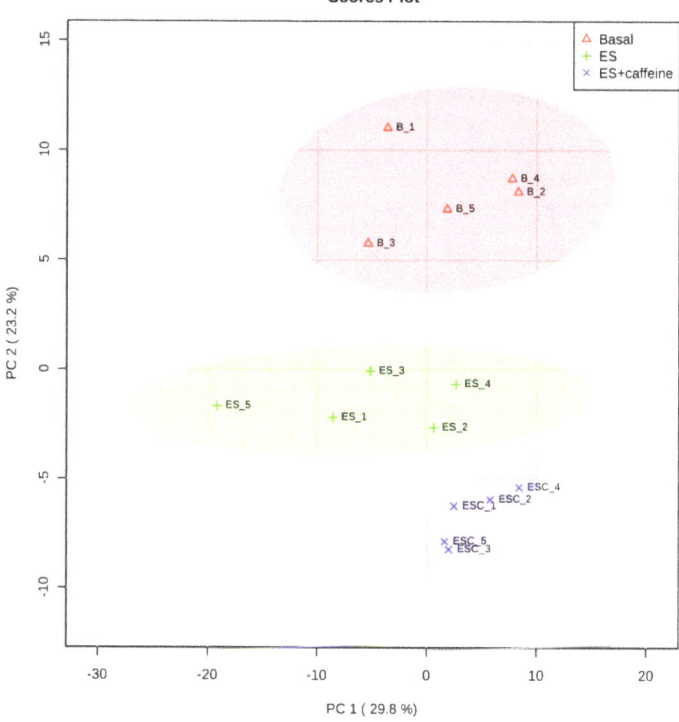

Figure 1. Principal component analysis (PCA) plot of the identified metabolites of the skeletal muscle of three groups, basal (B), electrical stimulation (ES), and electrical stimulation + caffeine (ESC). Principal components (PC1 and PC2) capture 53.0% of the variation in the dataset. The elliptic areas represent the 95% confidence regions.

3.2. Discovery of Differentiating Metabolites

To identify differentially expressed metabolites among the three groups, SAM, a popular method employed in microarray data analysis [21], was used. SAM identified a total of 50 metabolites with FDR = 0.007 (Figure 2). Table 1 lists the identified compounds. HCA of the 50 metabolites showed that each group was tightly clustered and that the caffeine influenced the metabolite profiles of ES toward a high level of contents (Figure 3). Figures 4–7 show the 23 metabolites that significantly changed between the ES and ES + C groups.

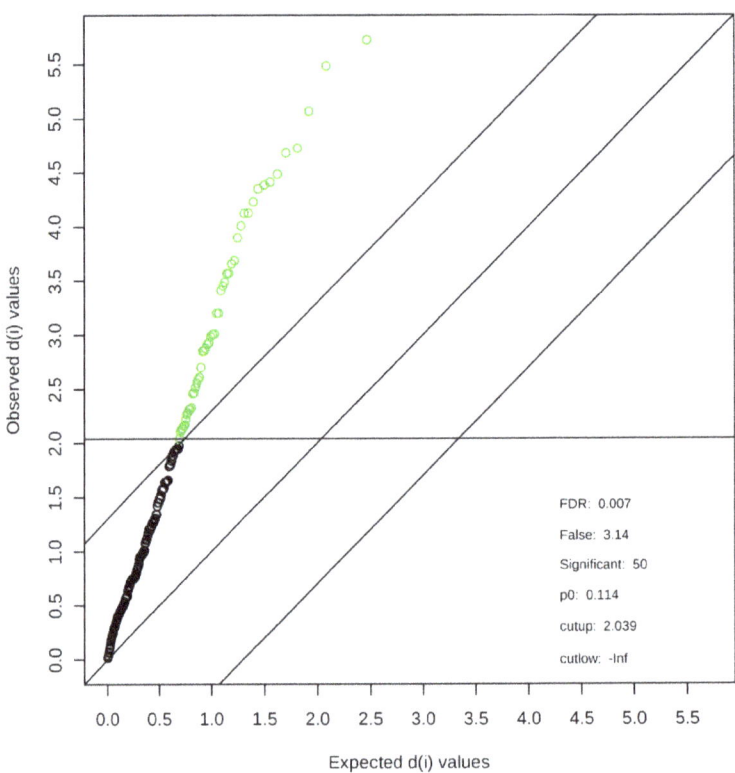

Figure 2. Identification of metabolites with significant changes in expression by significance analysis of microarray (SAM) among the three groups. The SAM plot is a scatter plot of the observed relative difference versus the expected relative difference. The solid diagonal line indicates where these two measures are the same. The dotted lines are drawn at a distance of delta from the solid line. The significant variables are highlighted in green and the details are shown in Table 1.

Table 1. Significant features identified by SAM.

	Name	d Value	SD	p Value	q Value
1	Theobromine	5.7247	0.031023	0.0	0.0
2	Butyrylcarnitine (C4)	5.4855	0.055814	0.0	0.0
3	IMP	5.0676	0.10169	0.0	0.0
4	β-Aminoisobutyric acid	4.7254	0.14193	0.0	0.0
5	L-Lactic acid	4.6827	0.14713	0.0	0.0
6	Cytosine	4.4855	0.1717	5.4348×10^{-5}	1.1445×10^{-4}
7	D-Ribose 5-phosphate	4.4111	0.1812	5.4348×10^{-5}	1.1445×10^{-4}
8	D-Glyceraldehyde	4.3854	0.18452	5.4348×10^{-5}	1.1445×10^{-4}
9	Hypoxanthine	4.3489	0.18926	5.4348×10^{-5}	1.1445×10^{-4}
10	Maltotriose	4.2295	0.205	5.4348×10^{-5}	1.1445×10^{-4}
11	D-Glucosamine 6-phosphate	4.1269	0.21883	1.087×10^{-4}	1.7607×10^{-4}
12	Choline	4.1237	0.21927	1.087×10^{-4}	1.7607×10^{-4}
13	Succinic acid	4.0087	0.2351	1.087×10^{-4}	1.7607×10^{-4}
14	N4-Acetylcytidine	3.8995	0.25048	1.6304×10^{-4}	2.4524×10^{-4}
15	L-Glutamate	3.6907	0.28084	3.2609×10^{-4}	4.2917×10^{-4}
16	Acetylenedicarboxylate	3.6613	0.28523	3.2609×10^{-4}	4.2917×10^{-4}
17	L-Leucine	3.5719	0.29872	4.8913×10^{-4}	5.7223×10^{-4}
18	1-Myristoylglycerophosphocholine	3.5708	0.29889	4.8913×10^{-4}	5.7223×10^{-4}
19	L-Hexanoyl-carnitine (C6)	3.4897	0.31135	5.4348×10^{-4}	6.0234×10^{-4}
20	Serotonin	3.4538	0.31693	5.9783×10^{-4}	6.2945×10^{-4}
21	Threonate	3.4109	0.32367	7.0652×10^{-4}	7.0847×10^{-4}
22	Glycerol-3-phosphate	3.2018	0.35736	0.001413	0.0012937
23	2-Oxobutanoate	3.1997	0.35772	0.001413	0.0012937
24	ATP	3.009	0.38981	0.0021739	0.0018047
25	N-Acetyl-L-alanine	3.0039	0.3907	0.0021739	0.0018047
26	L-Alanine	2.9853	0.39391	0.0022283	0.0018047
27	Xanthine	2.9261	0.40421	0.0023913	0.001865
28	Imidazole lactic acid	2.913	0.40651	0.0025543	0.001921
29	N8-Acetylspermidine	2.8766	0.41292	0.002663	0.0019337
30	NADP	2.8527	0.41718	0.0029348	0.0020305
31	Oxypurinol	2.8504	0.41759	0.0029891	0.0020305
32	Taurine	2.7011	0.44464	0.0040761	0.0026823
33	O-Acetylcarnitine (C2)	2.6096	0.46169	0.0052174	0.0032651
34	Isatin	2.5882	0.46572	0.0052717	0.0032651
35	L-Fucose	2.5586	0.47133	0.0057065	0.0034334
36	Spermidine	2.5126	0.48016	0.0064674	0.0037831
37	1-Palmitoleoylglycerophosphocholine	2.4683	0.48872	0.0071739	0.0040357
38	GDP	2.4586	0.49062	0.0072826	0.0040357
39	Iminodiacetate	2.3301	0.51606	0.0096196	0.0051941
40	L-Methionine	2.3125	0.51962	0.010054	0.0052477
41	γ-Glu-leu	2.3104	0.52004	0.010217	0.0052477
42	Maleamate	2.2816	0.52587	0.010761	0.0052964
43	L-Aspartate	2.2673	0.52879	0.010815	0.0052964
44	Guanidinosuccinic acid	2.2214	0.53822	0.011793	0.0056442
45	L-Valine	2.169	0.54911	0.013478	0.0062447
46	CDP	2.1582	0.55136	0.013641	0.0062447
47	EDTA	2.134	0.55645	0.014511	0.0064614
48	2-Hydroxyisobutyric acid	2.126	0.55815	0.014728	0.0064614
49	Creatinine	2.1072	0.56212	0.015163	0.0065164
50	3-Methyl-2-oxobutyric acid	2.0385	0.57683	0.017065	0.0071872

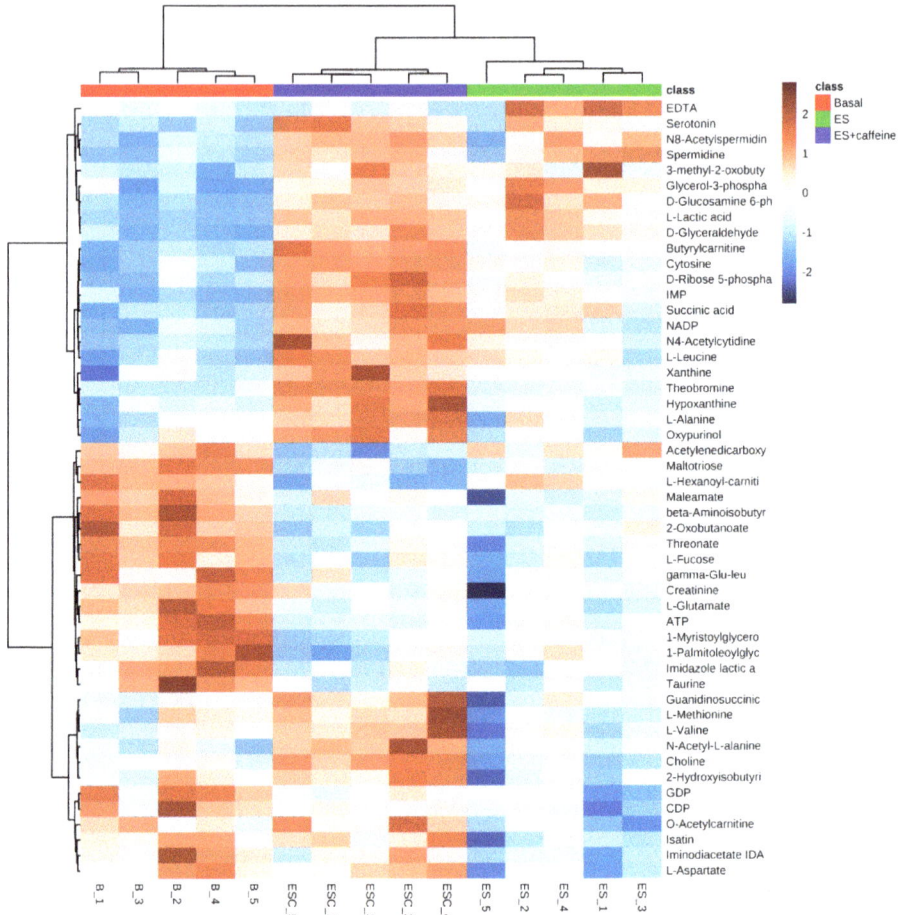

Figure 3. A heat map of hierarchical clustering analysis comparing the 50 different metabolites among groups. The heat map patterns among groups were distinguishable. The color red demonstrates that the relative content of metabolites is high and blue demonstrates that they are low.

3.3. Pentose Phosphate Pathway/Nucleotide Synthesis Pathway

The pentose phosphate pathway is an alternative pathway to glycolysis [22]. It does not lead to ATP formation, but rather, produces ribose 5-phosphate. Intracellular ribose 5-phosphate concentration is an important determinant of rates of de novo purine synthesis [23]. The synthesis of purine nucleotides begins with ribose 5-phosphate and produces the first fully formed nucleotide, IMP. IMP is accumulated in contracted skeletal muscle during exercise and accounted for ATP re-synthesis during recovery phase from exercise [24]. Therefore, pentose phosphate pathway activation and subsequent nucleotide synthesis is suggested to be important for maintaining cellular energy during and following exercise.

In the present study, ES increased D-ribose 5-phophate levels, and caffeine further increased this effect (Figure 4), indicating that caffeine promotes exercise-induced activation of the pentose phosphate pathway in skeletal muscles. It was also found that caffeine in conjunction with ES increased IMP levels, as compared to ES alone (Figure 4). Taken together, the stimulation of the pentose phosphate pathway by caffeine may contribute to recovery from energy depletion following muscle contraction by promoting ATP re-synthesis from IMP. In our previous study, caffeine alleviated muscle fatigue during contraction [6]. Furthermore, it has been suggested that activation of the pentose phosphate pathway stimulates energy production by enhancing mitochondrial function [25]. These metabolic responses may contribute to a positive effect of caffeine on endurance performance.

A small proportion of IMP is converted to inosine and further to hypoxanthine, and hypoxanthine is transformed to xanthine, which is then subsequently converted to uric acid and excreted in the urine [26]. In the present study, hypoxanthine and xanthine levels were increased by caffeine treatment in the contracted muscle (Figure 4), supporting the caffeine-induced accumulation of IMP.

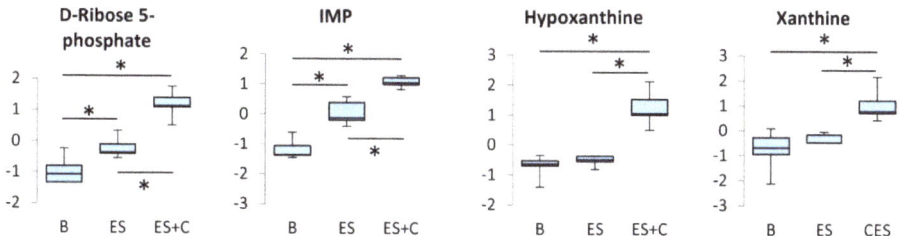

Figure 4. Box plots of the concentration variations of significantly altered metabolites in the pentose phosphate pathway/nucleotide synthesis pathway. Y axes are represented as normalized intensity. The boxes range from the 25% to the 75% percentiles. Medians are indicated by horizontal lines within each box. The ends of the whiskers represent the maximum and minimum of the data. * One-way ANOVA with Tukey's post hoc test indicates a significant difference (false discovery rates (FDR) < 0.05) between groups.

3.4. Acylcarnitine/Tricarboxylic Acid (TCA) Cycle

Acylcarnitines, which are esters of L-carnitine and fatty acyl-coenzyme A (CoA), are important intermediates in the transport of long-chain fatty acyl-CoA into the mitochondria [27]. Intramitochondrial acylcarnitine is converted back to carnitine and long-chain acyl-CoA by carnitine palmitoyltransferase 2, which then undergoes β-oxidation to produce acetyl-CoA. Acetyl-CoA is an essential intermediate metabolite that enters the TCA cycle and is oxidized to yield energy. When the production of short-chain acyl-CoAs exceeds TCA cycle flux, acetyl-CoA is converted to acetylcarnitine by carnitine acetyltransferase [28]. In the present study, caffeine treatment increased O-acetylcarnitine (C2) during skeletal muscle contraction (Figure 5), indicating that substrate catabolism during β-oxidation exceeds the capacity of acetyl-CoA utilization in the TCA cycle.

Muscle contraction-induced AMPK activation inhibits acetyl-CoA carboxylase activity, leading to a decrease in malonyl CoA content [29]. Malonyl CoA is a potent inhibitor of CPT1, an enzyme that combines fatty acyl-CoA with carnitine for transport into the mitochondria for β-oxidation, and the decrease in malonyl CoA during muscle contraction contributes to the increase in absolute lipid oxidation [30]. In addition, it has been demonstrated that the increase in acetylcarinitine level during muscle contraction decreases the availability of free carnitine, a substrate of CPT1, results in low CPT1 activity [31]. Thus, the accumulation of acetylcarnitine within the skeletal muscle leads to a diminished supply of long-chain fatty acyl-CoA to β-oxidation [31]. In fact, an increase in acetylcarnitine was observed concomitantly with a decrease in long-chain fatty acid oxidation during exercise in humans [31]. In the present study, L-hexanoyl-carnitine (C6) was reduced by caffeine treatment (Figure 5), indicating that the increase in muscle acetylcarnitine level by caffeine might inhibit β-oxidation of long-chain fatty acyl-CoA, thereby leading to a decreased supply of short-chain (~C10) fatty acyl-CoA.

However, we found the accumulation of butyrylcarnitine (C4) following caffeine treatment (Figure 5). In accordance with this result, a previous study has demonstrated that the 10 min of treadmill exercise increased C4 acylcarnitine level in rat skeletal muscle [32]. The authors have suggested that the accumulation of C4 acylcarnitine was attributed to a greater utilization of branched chain amino acids (BCAA: leucine, isoleucine, and valine) [32]. We also found that caffeine treatment increased L-leucine and L-valine levels in contracted muscle (Figure 6). Therefore, it is suggested that the increase in butyrylcarnitine (C4) level originates from the amino acids metabolism.

Succinic acid is a key TCA cycle metabolite, the levels of which can be increased by both long-term exercise training as well as an individual bout of exercise [17,33]. In the present study, caffeine increased succinic acid levels in the contracted muscle (Figure 5). This result suggests that the TCA cycle is activated by caffeine treatment during muscle contraction. However, succinic acid level is reflected by the activity of succinate dehydrogenase, which catalyze succinic acid into fumarate in the TCA cycle. Therefore, to determine the effect of caffeine on the activity level of the TCA cycle during muscle contraction, succinate dehydrogenase level and/or another enzyme activity and metabolite levels need to be investigated.

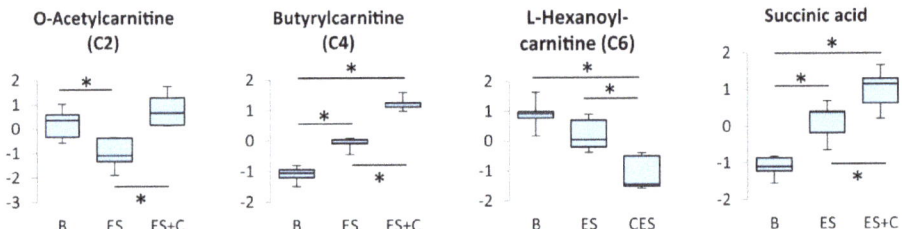

Figure 5. Box plots of the concentration variations of significantly altered metabolites in the Acylcarnitine/ TCA cycle. * One-way ANOVA with Tukey's post hoc test indicates a significant difference (FDR < 0.05) between groups.

In the present study, glycolysis was not affected by caffeine (Figure 8), suggesting that an increase in acetylcarnitine following caffeine treatment can be attributed to the acceleration of acetyl-CoA production from β-oxidation. Maintaining the acetylcarnitine recycling system is critical for muscle contractile performance and fatigue resistance [34]. Therefore, caffeine may stimulate the acetylcarnitine recycling system, thereby contributing to enhanced muscle endurance capacity. To assess this possibility, further study is required to measure the effects of caffeine on carnitine.

3.5. Amino Acid/Amino Acid Metabolism

Protein degradation and subsequent amino acid oxidation contribute slightly to energy supply during exercise as well as to glucose and fatty acid oxidation [35]. Six amino acids are metabolized in the skeletal muscle: BCAA (leucine, isoleucine, and valine), asparagine, aspartate, and glutamate [35]. Leucine can be converted to acetyl-CoA and oxidized in the TCA cycle [36]. The catabolic pathway of valine consists of several enzymatic steps and results in the formation of succinyl-CoA, a member of the TCA cycle. Disruption of BCAA metabolism in skeletal muscle impairs endurance capacity [37]. Thus, the supply of BCAA is considered to be an important factor for controlling exercise metabolism and endurance. In the present study, L-leucine and L-valine were higher in the ES + C group than in the ES group (Figure 6), indicating that these amino acids contribute to energy production of caffeine-treated muscle by incorporated into TCA intermediates.

Aspartate has been suggested to have an ergogenic potential [38]. Aspartate is converted to oxaloacetate by aspartate transaminase, which then enters the TCA cycle. A previous study has demonstrated that the administration of potassium-magnesium-aspartate increased the capacity for prolonged exercise in human [39]. This effect has been supported by other studies [38]. In the present study, caffeine suppressed L-aspartate reduction by ES (Figure 6), indicating that the caffeine-induced ergogenic effect may be partly attributed to aspartate preservation during muscle contraction. However, there are a number of negative findings related to aspartate's ergogenic potential [38]. For example, in human volunteers neither the exerted force nor the endurance time increased after oral administration of potassium-magnesium-aspartate [40]. Therefore, further studies are required to clarify the relationship between aspartate and caffeine's ergogenic potential.

Methionine is suggested to be transaminated and is also subjected to transulfuration in the skeletal muscle [41]. Although caffeine increased L-methionine levels (Figure 6) in the contracted muscle, the importance of methionine during exercise is poorly understood.

Alanine is formed from pyruvate and glutamate in the alanine aminotransferase reaction. Increase in skeletal muscle alanine is thought to be due to the enhanced availability of pyruvate and glutamate [42]. Alanine synthesized in the skeletal muscle is released into the blood and taken up by the liver, where it is reconverted into glucose via gluconeogenesis. In the present study, caffeine treatment increased L-alanine during muscle contraction (Figure 6). Considering that pyruvate and glutamate were not changed by caffeine stimulation (Table S1), this caffeine-induced increase in alanine may be attributed to protein degradation. The increase in alanine production may contribute to the increase in N-acetyl-L-alanine levels, which is generated from alanine by phenylalanine N-acetyltransferase, in caffeine and electrically stimulated muscle (Figure 6).

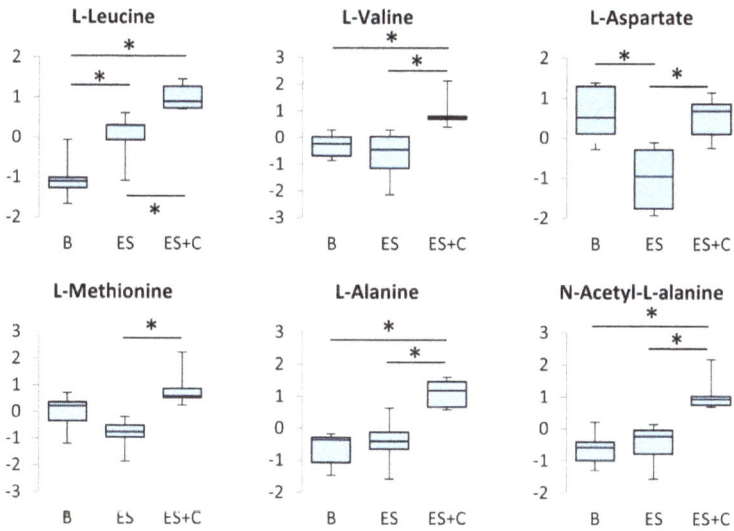

Figure 6. Box plots of the concentration variations of significantly altered metabolites in the amino acid/amino acid metabolism. * One-way ANOVA with Tukey's post hoc test indicates a significant difference (FDR < 0.05) between groups.

3.6. Others

N4-acetylcytidine, choline, cytosine, 2-hydroxyisobutyric acid, isatin, guanidinosuccinic acid, oxypurinol, ethylenediaminetetraacetic acid (EDTA), and acetylenedicarboxylate levels were significantly higher in the ES + C group than in the ES group (Figure 7). However, no previous studies have investigated the association between exercise and these metabolites. The functional significance of increased levels of these metabolites in the caffeine-stimulated group needs to be further investigated.

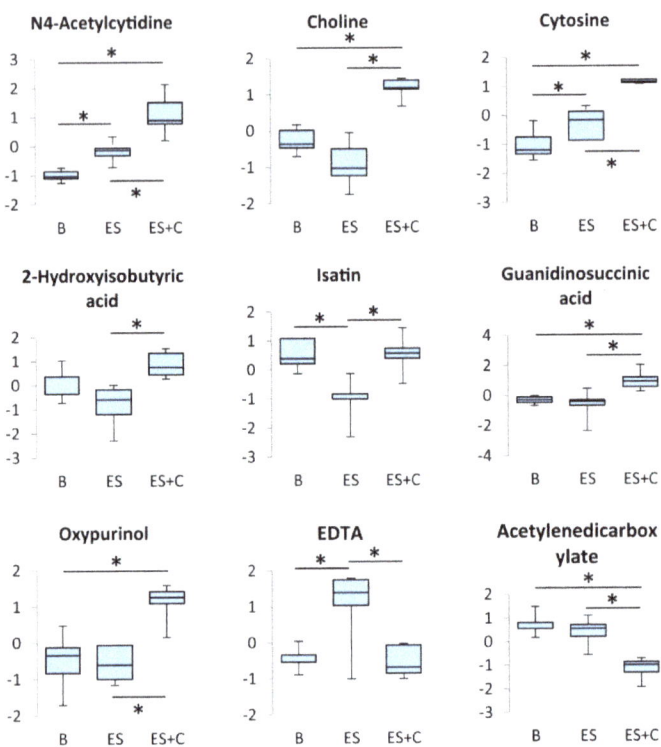

Figure 7. Box plots of the concentration variations of significantly altered metabolites in the other pathways. * One-way ANOVA with Tukey's post hoc test indicates a significant difference (FDR < 0.05) between groups.

3.7. Limitations

Many reactions take place continuously within cells, so concentrations of metabolites are very dynamic. In the present study, we investigated metabolomic responses only 10 min after muscle contraction. Therefore, in a case where increased levels of metabolites are observed, two distinct mechanisms contribute to this observation: either increased production or decreased consumption. For further understanding of caffeine-mediated effects on metabolic changes during muscle contraction, time-course experiments should be conducted.

In this study, we used a concentration of caffeine at 3 mM, which would be toxic to humans [43]. Plasma concentration of caffeine after ingestion of 100 mg (1 cup of coffee) reaches approximately 5 to 10 µM [44], with less than 70 µM being the physiological concentrations [45]. Experiments using isolated skeletal muscle preparation have benefits of eliminating the effects of systemic confounders such as circulatory, humoral and neural factors, and of intestinal absorption of caffeine. Taking advantage of this point, a number of studies have unveiled the direct ergogenic properties of caffeine at the supraphysiological concentrations [10,46–49]. Our previous study have demonstrated that µM concentrations were enough to activate AMPK in vivo, but mM concentrations of caffeine were needed to activate AMPK in isolate rat skeletal muscle [5]. Therefore, we should be careful when comparing the results of in vitro and in vivo studies in terms of caffeine concentrations.

Caffeine is found in foods, beverages, and pharmaceuticals, and the most frequently consumed non-prescription drug. To date, many researchers have discussed the effect of caffeine on energy metabolism and our health [50–52]. However, no study has investigated the caffeine-mediated changes of metabolomic signatures in skeletal muscle and the other organs. Although the present study contributes to unveiling the effect of caffeine on metabolomic responses during muscle contraction condition, the effect of caffeine alone on skeletal muscle metabolism has not been cleared. Further studies are expected to examine the effect of caffeine on muscle's non-contracted condition.

4. Conclusions

The present study reveals for the first time that caffeine influences metabolic responses induced by electrically stimulated muscle contraction in isolated rat skeletal muscles. A schematic representation of the metabolic changes induced by caffeine is shown in Figure 8. Many of these changes are related to energy metabolism. First, caffeine promotes contraction-induced activation of the pentose phosphate pathway and increases IMP production. Second, caffeine stimulates β-oxidation of fatty acyl-CoA, accompanied by increase in acyl-CoA, butylcarnitine and O-acetylcarnitine; however, it does not affect the glycolysis metabolites, glycerol-3-phosphate and L-lactic acid. Third, caffeine increases amino acids levels associated with energy production (L-leucine, L-valine, and L-aspartate). These metabolic alterations induced by caffeine suggest that caffeine accelerates contraction-induced metabolic activations and thereby contributes to muscle endurance performance and exercise benefits to health.

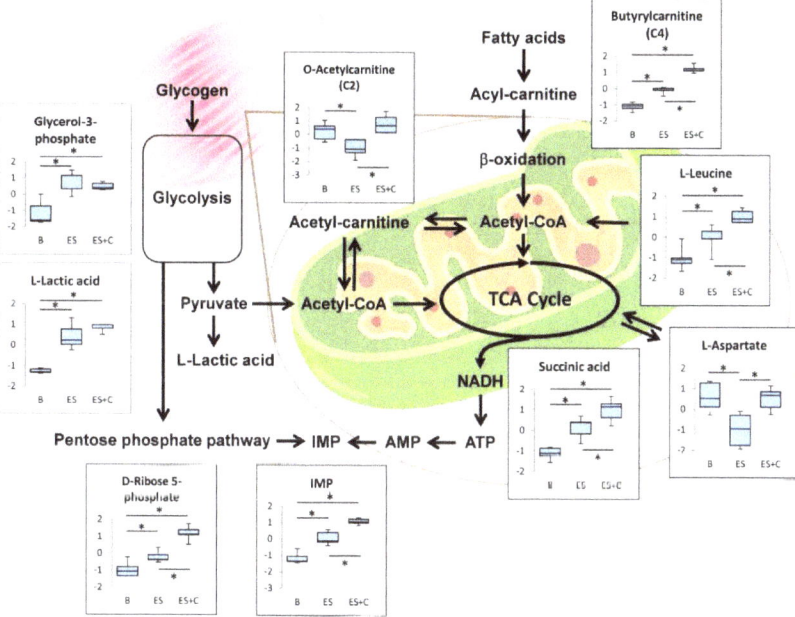

Figure 8. Schematic representation of metabolic pathway changes. * One-way ANOVA with Tukey's post hoc test indicates a significant difference (FDR < 0.05) between groups.

Supplementary Materials: The following are available online at http://www.mdpi.com/2072-6643/11/8/1819/s1, Table S1: List of detected metabolites.

Author Contributions: S.T. performed experiments, analyzed the data and contributed with drafting the manuscript. T.H. conceived and designed the research, and drafted the manuscript. T.E. conceived and designed the research, analyzed the data, and drafted the manuscript. All authors interpreted the results, contributed to the discussion, edited and revised the manuscript and read and approved the final version of the manuscript.

Funding: This study was supported in part by JSPS KAKENHI (Tatsuro Egawa, 18H03148; Tatsuya Hayashi, 19K11520); the Council for Science, Technology and Innovation; SIP (Funding agency: Bio-oriented Technology Research Advancement Institution, NARO) (Tatsuya Hayashi, 14533567). Takeda Research Support (TH, TKDS20170531015).

Conflicts of Interest: The authors declare no conflict of interest.

References

1. Canto, C.; Auwerx, J. PGC-1alpha, SIRT1 and AMPK, an energy sensing network that controls energy expenditure. *Curr. Opin. Lipidol.* **2009**, *20*, 98–105. [CrossRef]
2. Canto, C.; Jiang, L.Q.; Deshmukh, A.S.; Mataki, C.; Coste, A.; Lagouge, M.; Zierath, J.R.; Auwerx, J. Interdependence of AMPK and SIRT1 for metabolic adaptation to fasting and exercise in skeletal muscle. *Cell Metab.* **2010**, *11*, 213–219. [CrossRef] [PubMed]
3. Pedersen, B.K.; Febbraio, M.A. Muscles, exercise and obesity: Skeletal muscle as a secretory organ. *Nat. Rev. Endocrinol.* **2012**, *8*, 457–465. [CrossRef]
4. Egawa, T.; Hamada, T.; Kameda, N.; Karaike, K.; Ma, X.; Masuda, S.; Iwanaka, N.; Hayashi, T. Caffeine acutely activates 5′adenosine monophosphate–activated protein kinase and increases insulin-independent glucose transport in rat skeletal muscles. *Metab. Clin. Exp.* **2009**, *58*, 1609–1617. [CrossRef]
5. Egawa, T.; Hamada, T.; Ma, X.; Karaike, K.; Kameda, N.; Masuda, S.; Iwanaka, N.; Hayashi, T. Caffeine activates preferentially alpha1-isoform of 5′amp-activated protein kinase in rat skeletal muscle. *Acta Physiol.* **2011**, *201*, 227–238. [CrossRef] [PubMed]
6. Tsuda, S.; Egawa, T.; Kitani, K.; Oshima, R.; Ma, X.; Hayashi, T. Caffeine and contraction synergistically stimulate 5′-AMP-activated protein kinase and insulin-independent glucose transport in rat skeletal muscle. *Physiol. Rep.* **2015**, *3*, e12592. [CrossRef] [PubMed]
7. Jensen, T.E.; Rose, A.J.; Hellsten, Y.; Wojtaszewski, J.F.; Richter, E.A. Caffeine-induced ca(2+) release increases ampk-dependent glucose uptake in rodent soleus muscle. *Am. J. Physiol. Endocrinol. Metab.* **2007**, *293*, E286–E292. [CrossRef] [PubMed]
8. Raney, M.A.; Turcotte, L.P. Evidence for the involvement of camkii and ampk in ca2+-dependent signaling pathways regulating fa uptake and oxidation in contracting rodent muscle. *J. Appl. Physiol.* **2008**, *104*, 1366–1373. [CrossRef]
9. Lally, J.S.V.; Jain, S.S.; Han, X.X.; Snook, L.A.; Glatz, J.F.C.; Luiken, J.J.F.P.; McFarlan, J.; Holloway, G.P.; Bonen, A. Caffeine-stimulated fatty acid oxidation is blunted in CD36 null mice. *Acta Physiol.* **2012**, *205*, 71–81. [CrossRef] [PubMed]
10. Allen, D.G.; Westerblad, H. The effects of caffeine on intracellular calcium, force and the rate of relaxation of mouse skeletal muscle. *J. Physiol.* **1995**, *487*, 331–342. [CrossRef]
11. Konishi, M.; Kurihara, S. Effects of caffeine on intracellular calcium concentrations in frog skeletal muscle fibres. *J. Physiol.* **1987**, *383*, 269–283. [CrossRef] [PubMed]
12. Wright, D.C.; Geiger, P.C.; Han, D.H.; Jones, T.E.; Holloszy, J.O. Calcium induces increases in peroxisome proliferator-activated receptor gamma coactivator-1alpha and mitochondrial biogenesis by a pathway leading to p38 mitogen-activated protein kinase activation. *J. Biol. Chem.* **2007**, *282*, 18793–18799. [CrossRef] [PubMed]
13. Shen, J.G.; Brooks, M.B.; Cincotta, J.; Manjourides, J.D. Establishing a relationship between the effect of caffeine and duration of endurance athletic time trial events: A systematic review and meta-analysis. *J. Sci. Med. Sport* **2019**, *22*, 232–238. [CrossRef] [PubMed]
14. Ribeiro, B.G.; Morales, A.P.; Sampaio-Jorge, F.; Tinoco, F.D.S.; De Matos, A.A.; Leite, T.C. Acute effects of caffeine intake on athletic performance: A systematic review and meta-analysis. *Rev. Chil. Nutr.* **2017**, *44*, 283. [CrossRef]
15. Southward, K.; Rutherfurd-Markwick, K.J.; Ali, A. The Effect of Acute Caffeine Ingestion on Endurance Performance: A Systematic Review and Meta-Analysis. *Sports Med.* **2018**, *48*, 1913–1928. [CrossRef] [PubMed]
16. Dotzert, M.S.; Murray, M.R.; McDonald, M.W.; Olver, T.D.; Velenosi, T.J.; Hennop, A.; Noble, E.G.; Urquhart, B.L.; Melling, C.W.J. Metabolomic Response of Skeletal Muscle to Aerobic Exercise Training in Insulin Resistant Type 1 Diabetic Rats. *Sci. Rep.* **2016**, *6*, 26379. [CrossRef] [PubMed]

17. Starnes, J.W.; Parry, T.L.; O'Neal, S.K.; Bain, J.R.; Muehlbauer, M.J.; Honcoop, A.; Ilaiwy, A.; Christopher, P.M.; Patterson, C.; Willis, M.S. Exercise-Induced Alterations in Skeletal Muscle, Heart, Liver, and Serum Metabolome Identified by Non-Targeted Metabolomics Analysis. *Metabolites* **2017**, *7*, 40. [CrossRef] [PubMed]
18. Nesher, R.; Karl, I.E.; Kaiser, K.E.; Kipnis, D.M. Epitrochlearis muscle. I. Mechanical performance, energetics, and fiber composition. *Am. J. Physiol.* **1980**, *239*, E454–E460. [CrossRef]
19. Zetan, N.; Wallberg-Henriksson, H.; Henriksson, J. The rat epitrochlearis muscle: Metabolic characteristics. *Acta Physiol. Scand.* **1988**, *134*, 155–156. [CrossRef]
20. Miyamoto, L.; Egawa, T.; Oshima, R.; Kurogi, E.; Tomida, Y.; Tsuchiya, K.; Hayashi, T. AICAR stimulation metabolome widely mimics electrical contraction in isolated rat epitrochlearis muscle. *Am. J. Physiol. Physiol.* **2013**, *305*, C1214–C1222. [CrossRef]
21. Larsson, O.; Wahlestedt, C.; Timmons, J.A. Considerations when using the significance analysis of microarrays (SAM) algorithm. *BMC Bioinform.* **2005**, *6*, 129. [CrossRef] [PubMed]
22. Stincone, A.; Prigione, A.; Cramer, T.; Wamelink, M.M.; Campbell, K.; Cheung, E.; Olin-Sandoval, V.; Gruning, N.M.; Kruger, A.; Tauqeer Alam, M.; et al. The return of metabolism: Biochemistry and physiology of the pentose phosphate pathway. *Biol. Rev. Camb. Philos. Soc.* **2015**, *90*, 927–963. [CrossRef] [PubMed]
23. Dodd, S.L.; Johnson, C.A.; Fernholz, K.; Cyr, J.A. The role of ribose in human skeletal muscle metabolism. *Med. Hypotheses* **2004**, *62*, 819–824. [CrossRef] [PubMed]
24. Hellsten, Y.; Richter, E.A.; Kiens, B.; Bangsbo, J. AMP deamination and purine exchange in human skeletal muscle during and after intense exercise. *J. Physiol.* **1999**, *520*, 909–920. [CrossRef] [PubMed]
25. Mahoney, D.E.; Hiebert, J.B.; Thimmesch, A.; Pierce, J.T.; Vacek, J.L.; Clancy, R.L.; Sauer, A.J.; Pierce, J.D. Understanding D-Ribose and Mitochondrial Function. *Adv. Biosci. Clin. Med.* **2018**, *6*, 1–5. [CrossRef]
26. Palić, I.R.; Đorđević, A.S.; Ickovski, J.D.; Kostic, D.A.; Dimitrijevic, D.S.; Stojanović, G.S. Xanthine Oxidase: Isolation, Assays of Activity, and Inhibition. *J. Chem.* **2015**, *2015*, 1–8.
27. Schooneman, M.G.; Vaz, F.M.; Houten, S.M.; Soeters, M.R. Acylcarnitines: Reflecting or inflicting insulin resistance? *Diabetes* **2013**, *62*, 1–8. [CrossRef]
28. Furuichi, Y.; Goto-Inoue, N.; Fujii, N.L. Role of carnitine acetylation in skeletal muscle. *J. Phys. Fit. Sports Med.* **2014**, *3*, 163–168. [CrossRef]
29. Hardie, D.G.; Pan, D.A.; Hardie, G. Regulation of fatty acid synthesis and oxidation by the AMP-activated protein kinase. *Biochem. Soc. Trans.* **2002**, *30*, 1064–1070. [CrossRef]
30. Miura, S.; Tadaishi, M.; Kamei, Y.; Ezaki, O. Mechanisms of exercise- and training-induced fatty acid oxidation in skeletal muscle. *J. Phys. Fit. Sports Med.* **2014**, *3*, 43–53. [CrossRef]
31. Kiens, B. Skeletal Muscle Lipid Metabolism in Exercise and Insulin Resistance. *Physiol. Rev.* **2006**, *86*, 205–243. [CrossRef]
32. Overmyer, K.A.; Evans, C.R.; Qi, N.R.; Minogue, C.E.; Carson, J.J.; Chermside-Scabbo, C.J.; Koch, L.G.; Britton, S.L.; Pagliarini, D.J.; Coon, J.J.; et al. Maximal oxidative capacity during exercise is associated with skeletal muscle fuel selection and dynamic changes in mitochondrial protein acetylation. *Cell Metab.* **2015**, *21*, 468–478. [CrossRef]
33. Huffman, K.M.; Koves, T.R.; Hubal, M.J.; Abouassi, H.; Beri, N.; Bateman, L.A.; Stevens, R.D.; Ilkayeva, O.R.; Hoffman, E.P.; Muoio, D.M.; et al. Metabolite signatures of exercise training in human skeletal muscle relate to mitochondrial remodelling and cardiometabolic fitness. *Diabetologia* **2014**, *57*, 2282–2295. [CrossRef]
34. Seiler, S.E.; Koves, T.R.; Gooding, J.R.; Wong, K.E.; Stevens, R.S.; Ilkayeva, O.R.; Wittmann, A.H.; DeBalsi, K.L.; Davies, M.N.; Lindeboom, L.; et al. Carnitine Acetyltransferase Mitigates Metabolic Inertia and Muscle Fatigue During Exercise. *Cell Metab.* **2015**, *22*, 65–76. [CrossRef]
35. Wagenmakers, A.J.M. 11 muscle amino acid metabolism at rest and during exercise: Role in human physiology and metabolism. *Exerc. Sport Sci. Rev.* **1998**, *26*, 287–314. [CrossRef]
36. Zhang, S.; Zeng, X.; Ren, M.; Mao, X.; Qiao, S. Novel metabolic and physiological functions of branched chain amino acids: A review. *J. Anim. Sci. Biotechnol.* **2017**, *8*, 10. [CrossRef]
37. She, P.; Zhou, Y.; Zhang, Z.; Griffin, K.; Gowda, K.; Lynch, C.J. Disruption of bcaa metabolism in mice impairs exercise metabolism and endurance. *J. Appl. Physiol.* **2010**, *108*, 941–949. [CrossRef]
38. Trudeau, F. Aspartate as an Ergogenic Supplement. *Sports Med.* **2008**, *38*, 9–16. [CrossRef]
39. Ahlboro, B.; Ekelund, L.-G.; Nilsson, C.-G. Effect of Potassium-Magnesium-Aspartate on the Capacity for Prolonged Exercise in Man. *Acta Physiol. Scand.* **1968**, *74*, 238–245. [CrossRef]

40. de Haan, A.; van Doorn, J.E.; Westra, H.G. Effects of potassium + magnesium aspartate on muscle metabolism and force development during short intensive static exercise. *Int. J. Sports Med.* **1985**, *6*, 44–49. [CrossRef]
41. Scislowski, P.W.D.; Hokland, B.M.; Thienen, W.I.A.D.-V.; Bremer, J.; Davis, E.J. Methionine metabolism by rat muscle and other tissues. Occurrence of a new carnitine intermediate. *Biochem. J.* **1987**, *247*, 35–40. [CrossRef]
42. Ishikura, K.; Ra, S.-G.; Ohmori, H. Exercise-induced changes in amino acid levels in skeletal muscle and plasma. *J. Phys. Fit. Sports Med.* **2013**, *2*, 301–310. [CrossRef]
43. Fredholm, B.B.; Bättig, K.; Holmén, J.; Nehlig, A.; Zvartau, E.E. Actions of caffeine in the brain with special reference to factors that contribute to its widespread use. *Pharmacol. Rev.* **1999**, *51*, 83–133.
44. Derungs, A.; Donzelli, M.; Berger, B.; Noppen, C.; Krahenbuhl, S.; Haschke, M. Effects of cytochrome p450 inhibition and induction on the phenotyping metrics of the basel cocktail: A randomized crossover study. *Clin. Pharmacokinet.* **2016**, *55*, 79–91. [CrossRef]
45. Graham, T.E. Caffeine and exercise: Metabolism, endurance and performance. *Sports Med.* **2001**, *31*, 785–807. [CrossRef]
46. Rossi, R.; Bottinelli, R.; Sorrentino, V.; Reggiani, C. Response to caffeine and ryanodine receptor isoforms in mouse skeletal muscles. *Am. J. Physiol. Physiol.* **2001**, *281*, C585–C594. [CrossRef]
47. Huddart, H.; Abram, R.G. Modification of excitation-contraction coupling in locust skeletal muscle induced by caffeine. *J. Exp. Zool.* **1969**, *171*, 49–58. [CrossRef]
48. Weber, A.; Herz, R. The Relationship between Caffeine Contracture of Intact Muscle and the Effect of Caffeine on Reticulum. *J. Gen. Physiol.* **1968**, *52*, 750–759. [CrossRef]
49. Luttgau, H.C.; Oetliker, H. The action of caffeine on the activation of the contractile mechanism in striated muscle fibres. *J. Physiol.* **1968**, *194*, 51–74. [CrossRef]
50. Nawrot, P.; Jordan, S.; Eastwood, J.; Rotstein, J.; Hugenholtz, A.; Feeley, M. Effects of caffeine on human health. *Food Addit. Contam.* **2003**, *20*, 1–30. [CrossRef]
51. Grosso, G.; Godos, J.; Galvano, F.; Giovannucci, E.L. Coffee, Caffeine, and Health Outcomes: An Umbrella Review. *Annu. Rev. Nutr.* **2017**, *37*, 131–156. [CrossRef]
52. Harpaz, E.; Tamir, S.; Weinstein, A. The effect of caffeine on energy balance. *J. Basic Clin. Physiol. Pharmacol.* **2017**, *28*, 1–10. [CrossRef]

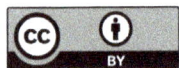

© 2019 by the authors. Licensee MDPI, Basel, Switzerland. This article is an open access article distributed under the terms and conditions of the Creative Commons Attribution (CC BY) license (http://creativecommons.org/licenses/by/4.0/).

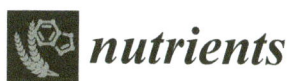

Article

Consumers' Perceptions of Coffee Health Benefits and Motives for Coffee Consumption and Purchasing

Antonella Samoggia * and Bettina Riedel

Department of Agro-Food Sciences and Technologies, Alma Mater Studiorum University of Bologna, Viale Fanin 50, 40127 Bologna, Italy; bettina.riedel@unibo.it
* Correspondence: antonella.samoggia@unibo.it

Received: 15 February 2019; Accepted: 13 March 2019; Published: 18 March 2019

Abstract: Coffee is popular worldwide and consumption is increasing, particularly in non-traditional markets. There is evidence that coffee consumption may have beneficial health effects. Consumers' beliefs in the health benefits of coffee are unclear. The study aimed at analyzing consumers' perceptions of coffee health benefits, consumption and purchasing motives of coffee consumers with positive perceptions of coffee health benefits, and willingness to pay for coffee with associated health claims. Data were collected through a face-to-face survey with consumers, resulting in a convenience sample of 250 questionnaires valid for data elaboration. Results were elaborated with factor analysis and logistic regression analysis. Findings revealed that a relevant minority of consumers believed that coffee could have positive health effects. The consumer with a positive perception of coffee health benefits is mostly male, young, works, is familiar with non-espresso-based coffee, consumes a limited amount of coffee (generally not for breakfast and often in social settings), and buys coffee at retail outlets. Consumers drink coffee for its energetic and therapeutic effects. Coffee consumption is still price-driven, but consumers are interested in purchasing coffee with associated health claims. There is the opportunity to improve the perception of coffee health benefits in consumers' minds.

Keywords: consumer; behavior; perception; coffee; health; consumption motives

---

1. Introduction

Coffee is one of the most consumed beverages worldwide. Global coffee consumption is estimated to increase, particularly in non-traditional coffee drinking countries in Africa, Asia, and Oceania (+4.1%). Demand in traditional markets is estimated to grow by 1% in Europe and by 2.5% in North America [1]. Leading drivers for coffee market growth are innovations in out-of-home consumption, online commerce opportunities, and innovative brewed coffee beverage types [2]. Consumers are interested in coffee product quality and origin, as well as social, environmental, and economic sustainability [3].

Innovative coffee attributes related to the health properties of coffee could be a driver for coffee consumption [4]. Some researchers suggest that coffee might have the potential of a functional food thanks to its biochemical properties and the possible health benefits [5,6]. In particular, there is evidence that coffee consumption may have beneficial effects on non-communicable diseases (NCDs) [7]. This may contribute to the World Health Organization's objective of reducing the relative risk of premature mortality from NCDs by 25% by 2025, by improving the modifiable risk factor of an unhealthy diet [8].

Consumers' beliefs in the health benefits of coffee are unclear. Only 16% of U.S. consumers know about coffee's health benefits, and 66% are prone to limiting their caffeine consumption [9]. Many European consumers are also confused about coffee's impact on health, with 49% believing coffee has negative health effects [10]. On the other hand, consumption of green coffee-based beverages has become popular in recent years due to the belief in its beneficial antioxidant properties (e.g., chlorogenic acids, polyphenols) [5,11,12].

Coffee contributes to the daily intake of dietary antioxidants, more than tea, fruit, and vegetables [13]. A screening of the most consumed beverages for their bioactive non-nutrient contents identified instant coffee as the beverage with the highest total biophenol content [14]. Two other studies observed coffee to be the beverage with the highest total antioxidant capacity as compared to others like green and black tea and herbal infusions [15,16]. The biochemical composition of a cup of coffee depends on the degree of roasting, the type of bean (Arabica versus Robusta), and the coffee brewing method, including grind type [17–19]

There is little scientific knowledge on consumers' attitude towards coffee health benefits. The perception of coffee's health effects in consumers' minds is unclear and has not been thoroughly researched. Past research studied consumer preferences and attitudes towards coffee attributes including sustainability, brands, coffee types, and motives for consumption like taste, energy, pleasure, socialization [20]. The paper aims to fill this gap in the literature and analyze the link between consumers' coffee consumption behavior and their perception of coffee's health benefits and risks. The research adds value to existing literature by analyzing what consumers perceive about coffee's health effects. If coffee has positive effects on human health it would be important to educate consumers about the possible health benefits and the correct consumption of coffee. Therefore, it is important to first study the status of consumers' perceptions about coffee's health effects. Furthermore, this will allow for an exploration into whether there are marketing possibilities for coffee with health benefits considering the increasing consumption trend of healthy food.

In evaluating the healthiness of a cup of coffee it is important to consider that coffee drinking is a complex consumption behavior and that preferences and preparation methods are influenced by culture and tradition. To fully exploit coffee's capability to impact on consumer food dietary lifestyle and health, there is need to better understand consumers' coffee consumption habits, motives, and perception of coffee's health benefits. Therefore, the objective of the research is to analyze consumers' perception of coffee's health benefits, consumption and purchasing motives of coffee consumers with positive perception of coffee health benefits, and willingness to pay for coffee with associated health claims.

Data was collected through a direct face-to-face survey with consumers using questionnaires with closed-ended questions. The structure of the paper is as follows. Section 2 provides a literature review of coffee consumption and purchasing motives and coffee and health, with a detailed review of the relevant literature on coffee's effect on single health conditions. Section 3 describes data gathering and elaboration, and the data sample. Results are presented in Section 4. This section first discusses the results regarding consumers' characteristics and perception of health effects of coffee, followed by insights on consumers' perception of coffee health effects and motives for coffee consumption and purchasing, and concludes with analyzing consumers' willingness to pay a price premium for coffee with associated health claims. Finally, the paper provides a discussion and conclusions on consumers' perceptions of coffee's health effects, profiling consumers according to their attitudes towards health coffee benefits. Section 6 puts the topic into the broader context of consumers' increasing interest in healthy food and eating behavior, and reflects on marketing possibilities for coffee focusing on specific health benefits.

2. Literature Review

2.1. Coffee Consumption Motives

The scientific knowledge on motives and preferences of coffee consumption and purchasing behavior is fragmented. Past research focused strongly on a limited number of specific issues, particularly on aspects of sustainability and fair-trade labelling of coffee. Evidence from a recent systematic review of 54 papers on coffee consumer research [20] identified the leading motives for consumers' coffee consumption and purchasing behaviors. Results suggest that there are several leading motives for coffee consumption: functional, taste and pleasure, habit, tradition and culture, and socialization. The main limiting factors for coffee consumption are a dislike of coffee's taste and a belief in its possible negative health effects. The functional and the pleasure motives are the two leading drivers for coffee consumption and are of similar importance across cultures.

2.2. Coffee Purchasing Motives

Key coffee attributes that impact on consumers' purchasing decisions are sustainability (including organic and fair trade), intrinsic quality attributes (e.g., roast degree, country of origin, variety), extrinsic attributes (packaging, brands), and coffee type (e.g., the espresso type includes black espresso and *macchiato*, that is, with a small amount of milk; other types include American long coffee (i.e., espresso topped with hot water), cappuccino, decaffeinated coffee, filter coffee, iced coffee, and coffee powder) [20]. A recent review on coffee purchasing motives did not identify studies that focused specifically on the relation between coffee price and consumer behavior [20]. There is limited research on consumer preferences for coffee's intrinsic qualities. Preference for different intrinsic qualities depends on expertise and sensory skills of the consumer [21]. The untrained consumer has difficulties in distinguishing quality levels of coffee compared to an expert. The role of familiarity with the product is important in the assessment of its quality [22]. There is not much evidence on the role that extrinsic attributes and marketing play in buying decisions towards coffee; nonetheless, brands and labels are considered essential for the coffee industry. Research on brands, labels and packaging mainly concerns the willingness to pay for sustainability labels and the role of packaging and labels for the communication of sustainability information [23].

2.3. Coffee and Health

Consumers' beliefs in health benefits or risks of coffee are inconclusive. For some the health benefit (e.g., anti-migraine effect) is a driver for consumption [24], others avoid coffee consumption for medical reasons like anxiety and insomnia [25], or because of the belief that coffee is generally bad for health [10]. Coffee drinking is not considered a health-oriented behavior, even if scientific evidence indicates that coffee can be part of a healthy diet [26,27]. The main health concerns arise with regard to the caffeine content of coffee [28]. Consumers see coffee mostly as a stimulant and are not informed about beneficial components and suggested health benefits [10].

Roasted coffee is a mixture of over 1000 bioactive compounds, with potentially therapeutic antioxidant, anti-inflammatory, antifibrotic, and anticancer effects [11,29]. Key active compounds are caffeine, chlorogenic acids, diterpenes, cafestol, and kahweol [7,30]. Coffee is rich in vitamin B3 and magnesium [6], and brewed coffee maintains the potassium concentration of the original seeds [31]. Caffeine is the most studied coffee component.

Scientific research has studied extensively the associations between coffee and all-cause mortality, cancer, cardiovascular diseases, neurological and gastrointestinal as well as liver systems, and all effects on pregnancy, with differing results over the years.

Current research concludes that coffee drinking is safe when consumed by healthy, non-pregnant women and adult persons in moderate quantity, equivalent to three to four cups per day, providing 300 to 400 mg/d of caffeine [7,26,28,32]. The largest reduction in relative risk of all-cause mortality was found with a consumption of three cups per day as compared with no consumption. Results suggest an inverse relationship between coffee drinking and all-cause mortality in men and women [7]. Daily coffee drinkers reduced their risk of dying prematurely compared with non-drinkers by 7–12% [33]. There were beneficial effects of coffee on cancer and cardiovascular diseases, as well as metabolic and neurological conditions [26]. Adverse effects of coffee drinking were mainly limited to pregnancy and to women at increased risk of bone fracture. Negative effects are mainly associated with caffeine rather than any other components in coffee [7,26]. Table 1 provides details on the studies focused on the effects of coffee on single health conditions.

Table 1. Effects of coffee on single health conditions.

Cardiovascular disease	Habitual coffee consumption was consistently associated with a lower risk of cardiovascular diseases mortality [7,31]. Compared to non-coffee drinkers, risk was reduced by 19% and the largest reduction in relative risk was found at three cups per day [7,34,35]. Coffee consumption may have a protective effect on the risk of stroke [36,37], especially in women [38]. Research found a 30% lower risk of mortality from stroke of coffee consumers compared to non-drinkers [7]. The reduced risk for cardiovascular conditions is related to the antioxidant effects of coffee [26,39].
Type-2 Diabetes	Polyphenolic coffee compounds have beneficial effects on insulin and glucose metabolism [26,31]. Coffee consumption was associated with a lower risk of developing type 2 diabetes [7], with a stronger effect for women [40]. An intake of three to four cups of coffee/day seems to lower the risk by 25% compared to no coffee or less than two cups a day [34,41,42]. A meta-analysis concluded that the risk to develop type 2 diabetes decreased by 6% for each cup-per-day increase in consumed coffee [43].
Liver Conditions	Coffee consumption is related to a lower risk of developing several liver conditions [44,45]. There is an inverse association between coffee consumption and liver cancer [46,47]. Phenolic compounds, melanoidins, and caffeine are responsible for antioxidant effects in the liver [26].
Neuro-degenerative disorders	Lifelong, regular and moderate coffee consumption might have a beneficial effect on physiological, age-related cognitive decline/dementia [48,49], Parkinson's disease [50,51], and Alzheimer's disease [52,53]. The potential beneficial effects of coffee on mental health seem to be related to the neuroprotective effect of caffeine [26,50].
Depression and anxiety	Caffeine and other polyphenolic compounds of coffee have been associated with positive effects on mental health, for example behavior, mood, depression, and cognition [7,54]. On the other hand, high caffeine consumption is associated with anxiety and nervousness. Positive effect on mood is influenced by time of consumption, being highest in the late morning [55]. Caffeine seems to be more beneficial for habitual consumers [56]. Coffee consumption had a consistent association with lower risk of depression [26,57] and to relieve depressive symptoms [58].
Cancer	The International Agency for Research on Cancer (IARC) evaluated in 2016 a database of 1000 observational and experimental studies on coffee and cancer and concluded that there are no clear associations between coffee drinking and cancer at any body site. Coffee was classified as an agent "not classifiable as to carcinogenicity to humans". There is evidence for a lower risk of cancer in high versus low coffee consumption [7]. Phytochemical compounds in coffee (diterpenes, melanoidins, polyphenols) may have beneficial effects at the cellular level, for example inhibiting oxidative stress and damage [26]. There is evidence that coffee intake is associated with a reduced risk of certain cancers [30,59].
Lung and gastric cancers	An adverse effect of coffee consumption has been seen in an increased risk of lung and gastric cancers. In this case, it is important to consider the potentially modifying effect of associated smoking habits. A subgroup analysis showed that the association was significant only in studies that did not adjust for smoking behavior [7,26].
Blood pressure	Coffee consumption has been associated with a rise in blood pressure [26]. Coffee intake raises blood pressure in non-coffee-drinkers, but not in habitual coffee drinkers. On the other hand it was observed that the antioxidant compounds of coffee might counteract the effects of caffeine in raising blood pressure [26]. Research results are conflicting and the association between coffee consumption and blood pressure remains unclear [60].
Pregnancy	Negative associations of coffee and caffeine intake were mostly pregnancy-related (low birth weight, pregnancy loss, preterm birth, childhood leukemia) [7,26,61,62]. The European Food Safety Authority (EFSA) [32] recommends that a moderate caffeine intake of 200 mg/day does not increase the risk of any pregnancy-related complication. Still, the association between coffee/caffeine and reproductive health outcomes needs further investigation as available data are insufficient and the role of confounding (e.g., diet, smoking etc.) factors is unclear [61].
Bone fracture	A negative association between coffee consumption and bone fracture was seen in women [7]. A 14% higher risk was found in high versus low coffee consumption [63]. The increased risk in women seems related to caffeine and its potential influence on calcium absorption [64] and bone mineral density [65]. The systematic review by Wikoff et al. [28] concludes that a caffeine intake of 400 mg/day was not associated with negative effects on fracture, bone mineral density, and calcium metabolism.

The main limitation in drawing conclusions on coffee health associations is that existing evidence is observational and of lower quality. More research is needed with data from long-term randomized controlled trials [7,26,28].

3. Materials and Methods

3.1. Data Gathering

Data gathering was based on a direct face-to-face survey. Data was collected using questionnaires with closed-ended questions. The first question aimed at filtering interviewees so as to collect responses only from coffee consumers (i.e., those who generally drink coffee). The questionnaire includes five sections. Section 1 was on coffee consumption habits: types of coffee drunk (e.g., espresso, long coffee, cappuccino, decaffeinated, coffee powder, iced coffee, filter coffee); number of cups of coffee per day; occasions and places of consumption; companionship during consumption; consumption of other caffeinated drinks; type of coffee preparation; and outlets of coffee purchasing. Section 2 focused on motives of coffee consumption and purchasing (Table 2). Section 3 focused on the perception of health benefits of coffee. In particular, the first sub-section included questions aimed at eliciting the view of the consumers as to whether coffee consumption can bring health benefits, can reduce diseases, can be a functional beverage for human wellness, and has nutritional properties that can improve human health. These items are based on coffee health impact literature review, past research studies exploring consumers' perception of food healthiness [4,9,66–71], and the European Food Safety Agency food health and nutrition claims [72]. The second sub-section asked consumers' opinions on the effects of moderate coffee consumption on diminishing the risk of diseases and on influencing a number of physical effects based on scientific-tested studies (Table 1). Then, the third sub-section asked if consumers thought that there was a gender difference in terms of coffee consumption with respect to health, and whether decaffeinated coffee had different health impact compared to caffeinated coffee. These items are based on a coffee health impact literature review. Sections 2 and 3 asked the respondents to rate each question using a 5-point Likert scale of agreement/disagreement (1: "totally disagree" to 5: "totally agree", with scale end values anchored to interpretations), or with other responses options (e.g., "yes"/"no") as reported in the Table notes.

In the fourth section respondents were asked to state their willingness to pay (WTP) for the most common type of coffee product, the coffee brick pack. Only participants that more frequently bought this type of coffee were considered in the analysis. Participants' WTP was assessed by applying the multi price list (MPL) in a hypothetical setting method, widely adopted in experimental economics [73–75]. This mechanism has the great advantage of being transparent and very simple to understand for participants. The minor disadvantage is the interval response with a psychological bias toward the middle of the list [76]. Before eliciting their WTP, participants were provided with a reference price for the product type that was identified based on current retailer prices. The price premiums went from €0.10/brick to €1.50/brick, with 15 price premium options with a €0.10 difference. Section 6 gathered information on the socio-demographic profiles of the respondents.

The questionnaire was tested in trial face-to-face interviews and the items identified as unclear or not important were revised. Interviewers carried out 272 interviews. Data cleaning led to the definition of a convenience sample of 250 questionnaires for data elaboration. The places of interviews were retail outlets, coffee shops, bars, and malls. Interviews were carried out from April to July 2018. At the beginning the interviewer declared the interview was part of a university study, wore a badge with name and university affiliation, and proceeded with the interview if the respondent agreed to participate in the research. The time necessary to carry out each interview was around seven minutes. No reward or token was awarded. Data were collected with the support of the Qualtrics survey program by uploading the answers gathered during the face-to-face interviews.

Table 2. Literature references for studied items in the questionnaire.

Item	Literature References
Functional (awakening and attention, physical energy)	[24,77–79]
Sensory (taste, smell)	[25,77–80]
Pleasure (mood and emotion, comfort, relaxing)	[77–79]
To socialize (with family, friends, coworkers)	[25,79–82]
To have a break	[10,25,77]
Health (digestion, against headache, increase blood pressure)	[24,25,77,81]
Family tradition and culture	[24,25,82]
Habit	[24,81,82]
Price, promotion, value for money	[23,83,84]
Coffee roast, coffee recipe, intensity and taste information	[2,22,80]
Country of origin	[20,80,85,86]
Sustainability (fair-trade, organic)	[23,84–86]
Brand knowledge, packaging, advertising	[83,87–90]
Expert recommendations	[21,91]

3.2. Data Elaboration

Data elaboration followed different phases. First, data elaboration calculated the consumers' level of perception of coffee health benefits. The level of perception was calculated as mean value of the first sub-section items belonging to Section 3, that is, whether consumers agreed that coffee consumption could bring health benefits, reduce diseases, be a functional beverage for human wellness, and have nutritional properties that can improve human health. The mean values of positively versus negatively inclined consumers were cross-checked with the analysis of variance (ANOVA). The levels of perception of positively versus negatively inclined consumers were cross-analyzed with consumers' socio-economic characteristics and coffee consumption habits, and tested using the chi-squared test.

Second, the research identified the existing latent factors in consumers' coffee consumption and purchasing motives, with the support of two factor analyses. Two separate factor analyses were run, one for coffee consumption motives, and one for the coffee purchasing motives in order to highlight possible different habits in the consumers' approaches to coffee. The principal components method (PCA) and Varimax rotation (Eigenvalue criterion being higher than 1) were applied.

Third, the factors were used in the logistic regression (enter method), carried out to explore the relationship between consumers' perceptions of health benefits of coffee and their consumption and purchasing motives. The factor variables were also checked for the multicollinearity analysis, to verify the possibility that one variable is a linear function of the other. Multicollinearity has been tested through tolerance and variable inflation factors (VIFs) [92]. Omnibus tests of model coefficient were analyzed to test the level-of-fit of the model. Model variance with Nagelkerke was considered. Finally, the research calculated the WTP and cross-analyzed values with socio-economic characteristics of the consumers. Data elaboration was carried out with the support of SPSS (version 21).

3.3. Sample

Out of the 250 respondents, the majority were women, and about half had an academic degree (Table 3). There was a majority of people working, and a generally low or medium family income. The age was well distributed, as 55.2% of the respondents are aged younger than or equal to the average age, that is, 40.97 years (maximum age is 85 and minimum age 18).

Table 3. Sample characteristics.

Gender	%
Women	66.4
Men	33.6
Total	100.0
LEVEL OF EDUCATION	
No academic degree	51.0
With academic degree	49.0
Total	100.0
AGE	
Below or equal to average age	55.2
Above average age	44.8
Total	100.0
EMPLOYMENT STATUS	
Working	80.8
Not Working	19.2
Total	100.0
LEVEL OF FAMILY INCOME	
Low and medium income (up to €55,000/year)	87.3
High income (above €55,000/year)	12.7
Total *	100.0

* 39.1% did not respond to this question ("I do not know" or "I do not want to respond").

4. Results

4.1. Consumers Characteristics and Perception of Health Effects of Coffee

A relevant minority of consumers (25%) thought that drinking coffee could have positive effects on health (Table 4). The average value of the perception on coffee health benefits of the positively inclined consumers was fairly high (3.7). The analysis of consumers' socio-economic characteristics, coffee consumption, and purchasing habits of the positively versus the negatively inclined consumers showed interesting elements (Table 4). A higher percentage of men (31%), of younger (30.4%), and of working (27.2%) consumers had a positive perception of the health effects of coffee consumption compared to female, older, and not working consumers. The level of education was not an explanatory characteristic for the perception of health effect of coffee consumption. There were more consumers that tended to drink non-espresso based coffee (36.2%), that consumed from one to two cups of coffee per day (32.5%), that never or rarely drank coffee for breakfast (34.3%), and that bought coffee in big retailer chains (27.9%) that had a positive perception of coffee health benefits. A chi-squared p-value confirmed the results. Other data support that positively inclined consumers tended to drink coffee with other people (28.5%), and that they did not to have coffee as a break (29.4%) or after lunch (28.1%).

These results suggest that consumers positively inclined towards coffee health benefits are more likely to be male, young, and working, tending to appreciate non espresso-based coffee, consume in limited amounts and in social settings, and not usually consuming in the morning. They are more likely to purchase it in common outlets, probably with other food items.

Table 4. Consumers' perceptions of health effect of coffee consumption and consumers' characteristics.

	Negative Perception %	Positive Perception %	Total	ANOVA	p-Value
Total [a]	75.2	24.8	100		
Perception of health effect of coffee (average) [a]	2.29	3.70	2.91	0.000	***
Standard deviations	0.500	0.484	0.762		

Socio-economic characteristics					
	Negative Perception %	Positive Perception %	Total	Pearson's chi-squared	p-Value
Gender					
Men	69.0	31.0	100	0.075	*
Women	78.3	21.7	100		
Age					
Below equal to average age	69.6	30.4	100	0.015	**
Above average age	82.1	17.9	100		
Level of education					
No academic degree	72.0	28.0	100	0.153	
Academic degree	78.4	21.6	100		
Working condition					
Working	72.8	27.2	100	0.047	**
Not working	85.4	14.6	100		
Consumption and purchasing habits					
Type of coffee most frequently drunk [b]					
Espresso	77.8	22.2	100	0.038	**
Non espresso-based coffee	63.8	36.2	100		
Frequency of consumption					
One to two cups of coffee/day	67.5	32.5	100	0.038	**
Three or more cups of coffee/day	78.8	21.3	100		
Companionship in consumption					
On my own	78.7	21.3	100	0.121	
With others	71.5	28.5	100		
Place of consumption					
At home	75.5	24.5	100	0.527	
Out of home	75.0	25.0	100		
Method of preparation most frequently adopted [c]					
Moka pot	76.6	23.4	100	0.409	
Capsules	74.4	25.6	100		
Consumption of caffeine [d]					
Low/medium caffeine consumption	75.7	24.3	100	0.497	
High caffeine consumption	74.8	25.2	100		
Coffee Consumption for breakfast					
Never/rarely	65.7	34.3	100	0.098	*
Often/always	77.1	22.9	100		
Coffee Consumption as a break					
Never/rarely	70.6	29.4	100	0.106	
Often/always	78.4	21.6	100		
Coffee Consumption after lunch					
Never/rarely	71.9	28.1	100	0.228	
Often/always	77.0	23.0	100		
Coffee Consumption after dinner					
Never/rarely	76.0	24.0	100	0.382	
Often/always	73.2	26.8	100		
Place of purchasing					
Big retailer	72.1	27.9	100	0.096	*
Small retailer	82.5	17.5	100		

Note: *, **, *** Significant at $p < 0.10$; $p < 0.05$; $p < 0.01$; [a] Based on the average value of coffee health impact perception. Negative and neutral coffee health impact (below or equal to 3); Positive coffee health impact (above 3). [b] "Espresso" type includes black espresso and *macchiato*, that is, with a small amount of milk; "Other types" include American long coffee (espresso topped with hot water), cappuccinos, decaffeinated coffee, filter coffee, iced coffee, and coffee powder. [c] The moka coffee pot is the most common coffee brewing technique in Italy. This results includes only the moka coffee pot and capsules as they were the most frequently ticked answers (94%). [d] Other sources of caffeine consumption, in addition to coffee, are: tea, energy drinks, coke, other caffeine drinks. Low/medium caffeine consumption has values of 1, 2, 3. High caffeine consumption has values of 4 and 5 in a 5-point Likert scale where 1 is "never" and 5 is "always".

Consumers are better inclined towards a limited number of benefits of coffee consumption (Figure 1). In particular, almost 80% of consumers believe that drinking coffee increases blood pressure, more than half think that it decreases depression and headache, one-third that it decreases the risk of stress and anxiety, one-fourth that it decreases the risk of cardiovascular diseases, and one-fifth that it impacts on women's capability to absorb calcium and minerals and stimulates the reduction of body weight. Consumers do not acknowledge other medically tested effects on pregnant women, diabetes, liver, cancer, neurodegenerative diseases, and pain.

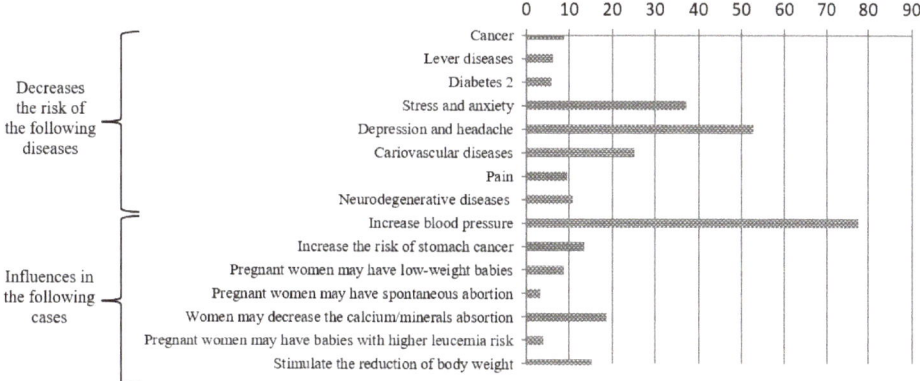

Figure 1. Consumers' perception of health effect of coffee consumption (%). Note: Consumers' response options were "yes"/"no" for each item. Therefore, the figure shows that around 80% of respondents thought that drinking coffee increased blood pressure.

Moreover, 61% of consumers believe that the correct number of cups of coffee per day is between three and four. According to scientific studies, this is the recommended quantity (equivalent to 300–400 milligrams of caffeine per day) [7,26,32]. Therefore, the vast majority has an adequate knowledge of the daily quantity of coffee to be consumed. Around 35% of consumers think that between one and two cups is adequate, values lower than the threshold set by scientists, thereby showing some skepticism towards coffee impact on health. Moreover, 84% of consumers think that the effect is similar in men and women, and 80% that decaffeinated coffee has a similar impact to caffeinated coffee on human health. These results support that consumers have adequate knowledge on the quantity to be consumed, the effects on gender, and the types of coffee, fairly in line with scientific evidence [7,26,32]. There is no evident misconception of the effects of coffee on health.

4.2. Consumers' Perception of Coffee Health Effect and Motives for Coffee Consumption and Purchasing

The two factor analyses on consumers' coffee consumption and purchasing motives identified seven main components (Tables 5 and 6). Four components derive from the factor analysis on the initial 12 items on coffee consumption motives, and three components derive from the factor analysis on the initial 13 items on purchasing motives. The second factor analysis was tested until all identified components had satisfactory internal consistency values. This lead to delete three items. In both factor analyses items were loaded into single factors, with factor loadings above 0.585. The Kaiser–Meyer–Olkin measure of sampling adequacy and Bartlett's test of sphericity were calculated to assess the appropriateness of the data for factor analysis. The Kaiser–Meyer–Olkin index was 0.649 in the coffee consumption motives PCA and 0.660 in the coffee purchasing motives PCA. Bartlett's tests of sphericity were highly significant (0.000). The cumulated variance values explained by the factors were respectively 66.2 and 66.3. Elaboration results confirmed the data appropriateness. The values of the factors were calculated based on the mean of the items loading into the single factors.

Table 5. Factor analysis on motives for coffee consumption and convergent validity and discriminant validity for each construct.

	Habit and Pleasure	Social	Therapeutic	Energy
Awakening and attention				0.880
Physical energy				0.882
Cronbach's alpha 0.742				
Habit	0.669			
Mood and emotion	0.585			
Family tradition and culture	0.693			
Smell	0.814			
Taste	0.786			
Cronbach's alpha 0.771				
To have a break		0.841		
To socialize		0.798		
Cronbach's alpha 0.665				
Digestion			0.651	
Against headache			0.798	
Increase blood pressure			0.717	
Cronbach's alpha 0.633				
Variance explained (%)	21.97	14.12	13.91	13.90
Mean value of factors	3.1	2.7	1.7	2.7
Convergent validity and discriminant validity				
	Habit and Pleasure	Social	Therapeutic	Energy
Habit and pleasure	*0.510*			
Social	0.324	*0.672*		
Therapeutic	0.092	0.187	*0.525*	
Energy	0.273	0.194	0.173	*0.776*
Composite reliability	0.84	0.81	0.77	0.88

Note: Diagonal data (in italics) represent Fornell and Larcker's average variance extracted (AVE). Subdiagonal represent the inter-construct correlations.

The internal consistency and convergent and discriminant validity of each component was verified (Tables 5 and 6). The internal consistency of each set of items was measured using Cronbach's alpha and composite reliability (CR). Alpha component values were from 0.633 to 0.771, and CR values were from 0.77 to 0.88 in the first factor analysis. In the second factor analysis, alpha component values were from 0.675 to 0.836 and CR values were from 0.81 to 0.94. Values were satisfactory and acceptable [93,94]. The average variance extracted (AVE) provides a measure of convergent validity, and ranged from 0.504 to 0.696 in the first factor analysis and from 0.510 and 0.776 in the second factor analysis. These were satisfactory as above the 0.50 threshold [95]. To confirm discriminant validity, the square root of each construct's AVE was calculated to ensure it was greater than its bivariate correlation with other constructs in the model. This led to adequate outcomes. The results confirm the reliability and validity of the research components.

The factors were labeled according to coffee consumption and purchasing motives associated with the statements. Coffee consumption is driven by four main factors. The most important factor is the habit and pleasure of drinking it (3.1). This connects to the organoleptic characteristics that are coffee smell and taste, family traditions and habits, and the emotions and moods created by coffee. The energetic physical and mental awakening power of coffee is as important as its role in having a break during the day and socializing at work (2.7). The fourth motive for drinking coffee is its therapeutic impact, that is, the capability of coffee to help digestion, increase blood pressure, and alleviate headaches (1.7). Coffee purchasing is driven by three main motives. The main driving element is the price, that is promotion and value for money (3.3). Another key aspect is the declared aroma, recipe, level of roasting, and intensity (3.2). The coffee sustainability (1.8) does not strongly influence consumers' coffee purchasing. In synthesis, consumers have a hedonistic approach towards coffee, focused on its taste, smell, and family habits and culture. Their consumer behavior is also driven by utilitarian reasoning, focused on price. In addition, coffee is drunk for its relevant socializing and energetic power.

Table 6. Factor analysis on motives for coffee purchasing and convergent validity and discriminant validity for each construct.

	Price	Sustainability	Aroma
Price	0.902		
Value for money	0.859		
Promotion	0.842		
Cronbach's alpha 0.836			
Coffee recipe			0.663
Coffee roast			0.775
Brand knowledge			0.641
Intensity and taste information			0.752
Cronbach's alpha 0.675			
Country of origin		0.735	
Fair-trade		0.910	
Organic		0.848	
Cronbach's alpha 0.790			
Variance explained (%)	24.21	22.02	20.11
Mean value of factors	3.3	1.8	3.2
Convergent validity and discriminant validity			
	Price	Sustainability	Aroma
Price	*0.517*		
Sustainability	0.069	*0.696*	
Aroma	0.017	0.101	*0.504*
Composite Reliability	0.94	0.88	0.81

Note: Diagonal data (in italics) represent Fornell and Larcker's average variance extracted (AVE). Subdiagonal represent the inter-construct correlations.

There is a statistically significant relationship between consumers' perception of coffee health benefits and motives for coffee consumption and purchasing (Tables 7 and 8). The VIF values were between 1.020 and 1.401, and the lowest tolerance value was 0.714. Therefore, there was no multicollinearity between variables. The significant relation is between the perception that coffee can have health benefits, and the following motives of coffee experience: habit and pleasure (0.017), aroma (0.048), and price (0.058). The significant relation is in some cases an unpredicted direction. If the consumers believe in the coffee health benefits, they tend not to drink it as a habit or for pleasure or consume coffee for its aroma. Moreover, the positively inclined consumers believe price is a motive of coffee purchasing. Results are confirmed by p-values.

These results suggest that if consumers drink coffee for the pleasure of it, out of family and traditional habits, and because of the taste and coffee roasting/recipes, then they are distant from the idea that coffee may have a positive health impact. If their coffee purchasing experience is influenced by the product price, then they are sensitive to coffee's health impact. If coffee purchasing and consumption are not driven by hedonism and traditional routine and are not emotional, then their perception is better inclined towards new features of coffee.

Table 7. Logistic regression on the relationship between consumers' perception of coffee health benefits and motives for coffee consumption and purchasing.

	B	S.E.	Wald	Sig.		Exp(B)	Tolerance	VIF
Habit/pleasure	−1.037	0.433	5.744	0.017	**	0.355	0.980	1.020
Social	−0.359	0.440	0.664	0.415		0.699	0.912	1.097
Energy	−0.510	0.838	0.370	0.543		0.601	0.714	1.401
Price	0.706	0.373	3.585	0.058	*	2.027	0.961	1.041
Sustainability	−0.627	0.631	0.987	0.320		0.534	0.755	1.325
Aroma	−0.816	0.412	3.925	0.048	**	0.442	0.972	1.028
Constant	2.099	1.403	2.236	0.135		8.155		

Dependent variable: level of coffee health benefit perception—(0) negative and neutral (average value below or equal to 3) vs. (1) positive (average value above 3). Note: *, ** significant at $p < 0.10$; $p < 0.05$. Omnibus tests: 0; VIF: between 1.020 and 1.041; Nagelkerke R-square: 0.313. The limited number of consumers with positive perceptions of coffee's health benefits and with consumption behavior driven by therapeutic motives (one consumer) suggests not including the therapeutic component in the regression exercise. VIF: variable inflation factor.

Table 8. Relationship between consumers' perception of coffee health benefits and motives for coffee consumption and purchasing, with chi-squared results

		Consumers Perception of Coffee's Health Benefits (%)		Total	Chi-Squared	
		Negative	Positive			
Habit/pleasure	Negative	63.7	85.4	75.9	0.000	***
	Positive	36.3	14.6	24.1		
Social	Negative	72.2	85.7	76.8	0.022	**
	Positive	27.3	14.3	23.2		
Therapeutic	Negative	76.1	91.7	77.0	0.192	
	Positive	23.9	8.3a	23.0		
Energy	Negative	76.3	72.2	76.0	0.442	
	Positive	23.7	27.8	24.0		
Price	Negative	82.2	71.0	76.2	0.031	**
	Positive	17.8	29.0	23.8		
Sustainability	Negative	76.5	82.6	77.2	0.361	
	Positive	23.5	17.4	22.8		
Aroma	Negative	65.6	87.9	78.5	0.000	***
	Positive	34.4	12.1	21.5		

Note: **, *** significant at $p < 0.05$; $p < 0.01$.

4.3. Consumers' Willingness to Pay a Price Premium for Coffee Health Benefits

The vast majority of consumers (74%) is willing to pay a price premium for coffee with health benefits (Table 9). Given that the average price is around €2.75/brick pack, a €1.03 average price premium is equivalent to +37% (average price is €2.78/250 g brick pack, equivalent to €11/kg) [96]. The price premium is significant. There are variations among the different socio-economic groups of consumers. The highest price premium (between €1.00 and €1.50) would be paid mostly by older (62.9%) and higher income consumers (17.5%). A higher percentage of women (70.4%) are favorable towards fairly high coffee price premiums (between €0.51 and €1.00).

Table 9. Willingness to pay a price premium for coffee with associated health claims (%).

	Yes, I Am Willing to Pay a Price Premium 73.6%		
	From €0.10 to €0.50	From €0.51 to €1.00	From €1.01 to €1.50
All consumers (average €1.03)	17.2	28.4	28.0
Men	33.9	29.6	37.1
Women	66.1	70.4	62.9
Total	100.0	100	100
Below equal to average age	62.4	62.0	37.1
Above average age	37.6	38.0	62.9
Total	100	100	100
Low and medium income	91.7	92.1	82.5
High income	8.3	7.9	17.5
Total	100	100	100

5. Discussion

The debate over coffee's effects on the human body has gone through various stages, with recommendations aimed at promoting or avoiding coffee consumption. The history of coffee started in the 15th century [97]. Its consumption first grew in Arabic countries and then expanded to Persia, Egypt, Syria, and Turkey. It was known as "wine of Araby", and drunk as a substitute for alcohol, which was prohibited according to the Islamic religion. In the 17th century coffee arrived in Europe (e.g., Italy, England, France, Austria). Consumers increasingly drank it in coffee houses that become competitors for pubs, with coffee becoming a substitute for beer and wine. During the 18th century it became common in North America, and then, thanks to the optimal weather, it was cultivated in South America. Brazil is currently the most significant coffee-exporting country. During its long history, coffee has been criticized for various reasons: because it was considered to stimulate critical thinking (Mecca), because it was considered Satanic (Italy), because it was considered as a toxic substance used to bring about death (unsuccessfully) (Sweden), and because it threatened beer consumption and therefore local agricultural production (Prussia) [97,98]. As history shows, coffee consumption and the beliefs in its nutritional properties have always been intertwined. Coffee properties perceptions have often shaped coffee consumption and purchasing habits, including preparation methods, favorite types of coffee, and places of consumption and purchasing.

The present research paper provides valuable insights on consumers' perception over coffee health effects, and profiles coffee consumers' characteristics based on their positive or negative attitudes towards coffee health effects. There are a number of results that highlight consumers' socio-economic characteristics and coffee consumption habits, consumers' motives for coffee consumption and purchasing, and consumers' interest in coffee with associated health claims.

The present research shows that men are more positively inclined towards coffee health benefits as compared to women. Women appear more skeptical, whereas a higher percentage of men already believe that drinking coffee benefits their health. Considering women's general strong propensity towards healthy food [99], coffee with certified health claims may lead women to have a more positive inclination towards it. Moreover, the consumer with a positive attitude towards coffee health benefits is fairly young, works, and has a habit of drinking coffee in social occasions, in limited quantity, and in various preparations, not necessarily espresso. This approach to coffee drinking is in line with the most recent coffee consumption trends. Recent studies support that there is an increasing number of people drinking coffee, with interest in gourmet coffee, new types of coffee (e.g., frozen blended coffee drinks, nitro coffee, and cold brew), out-of-home consumption, and lower appreciation for cafe moka [9]. Moreover consumers believe coffee has some effects on the human body (e.g., blood pressure, depression, headache, stress and anxiety, body weight). This suggests that there are no specific misconceptions over coffee, but consumers are still not fully aware of coffee's nutritional potential and health impacts.

Results on the motives for coffee consumption support that the energy coffee provides is the key health effect consumers aim for. Coffee drinkers expect improved alertness and higher physical and mental performance [24,25,77,78]. There are motives for coffee consumption that differ among the positively and negatively inclined consumers with respect to coffee's health benefits. The positively inclined consumer to a certain extent values coffee for its aroma, pleasure, habits, and socialization. This is a relevant difference compared to past studies that supported taste as the main motive for coffee drinking [25,77–79]. In consumers, coffee evokes feelings of pleasure and comfort during the drinking experience [77–79]. The wide audience of coffee consumers gives particular importance to coffee habit and family traditions that influence preferred occasions, locations, and types of coffee consumption [24,25,82]

Despite the fact that positively inclined consumers drink coffee with others to have a break, socialization is not a key motive. This approach brings a distinguishing interpretation with respect to past studies. These studies suggest that drinking coffee is a way to socialize and be part of a group [25,77,79,82]. In synthesis, the energizing effect is what the consumer aims for. The consumer aims for a functional drink with a clear mental- and body-stimulating function. This is the same consumer objective for soft drinks and energy drinks.

Results on the motives of coffee purchasing support that for the positively inclined consumer, price is a significant attribute. The consumer is influenced by extrinsic coffee attributes. Coffee purchasing is to a certain degree driven by aroma, coffee recipe, brand, information, and emotions, but rather by rational and economic elements. Therefore, for these consumers messages focused on health claims that give value to the money spent may be important for coffee consumption and purchasing. Past studies found that the use of texts, brands, and metaphorical images on coffee packaging moderately influenced product expectations, intrinsic quality perception, and purchase intention [89]. Brand identification is especially important in the coffeehouse market [87–90]. Drinking a specific coffee brand (e.g., Starbucks) represents a status symbol and way of life for consumers [87,88].

Sustainability is one of the most studied subjects in consumer purchasing research on coffee [20]. Present and past research results suggest that aroma, price, and promotions are more important factors as compared to sustainability [85]. Only consumers with a strong attitude towards sustainability gave more importance to the sustainability claims over hedonic attributes and were willing to pay more for sustainably produced coffee [84,86,100].

The present research on consumers' interest in the economic investment over coffee products with health claims further highlights the importance of price in coffee purchasing. Results show that price is an important element for all consumers and that coffee is mostly purchased from large retailers. The importance of price in coffee purchasing shows that coffee is still a rather undifferentiated commodity. Consumers with positive attitudes towards coffee's health benefits give particular importance to price. Moreover, consumers are generally willing to pay higher prices for coffee with health claims. This is suggested for both positively and negatively coffee health-oriented consumers. In particular, women and consumers with higher monetary resources are more favorable towards healthy food. This is consistent with past research results [101–103].

The willingness to pay for coffee with innovative attributes is confirmed by the market expansion of coffee capsules. Capsules have been successful thanks to the low cost of machines, the ease of use, the practicality of packaging, and effective marketing communication campaigns [96,104]. This success was achieved despite the high price, with consumers willing to pay up to five times more than coffee powder brick (around €55/kg for coffee capsules). This market phenomenon has been disruptive for the coffee market. It contributed to stopping the price competition that excessively lowered the price of the powder coffee brick, coffee quality, and the capability for investing in coffee research and development as well as innovations.

6. Conclusions

Consumer attitudes toward food products determine consumption behavior more than knowledge. Attitudes and perceptions influence dietary behavior intentions [105]. Results from the current study on coffee consumers' consumption and purchasing habits can contribute to a better understanding of food lifestyle decisions. The integration of knowledge of nutritional qualities with knowledge of consumers' expectations and perceived food qualities allows for addressing possible misconceptions and more effectively defining food consumption and purchasing behavior recommendations.

There is an expanding consumers' interest for healthy food. Consumers are increasingly aware of the impact food has on body functions [69,71,106]. Coffee consumption has often been negatively criticized for its health effect. Recent studies show that coffee can have positive health effects, but consumers are still cautious on drinking coffee. The coffee image is of a drink with a health impact, but not necessarily positive, and not based on the latest science-based outcomes. Coffee is used for its energetic and therapeutic effects. Together with other energy drinks, it is increasingly used as a substitute for soft drinks. Coffee is a drink with some advantages. It is naturally low in calories if drunk "black", and it is a drink good for socializing. Coffee chains are expanding. Soft drinks companies are increasingly interested in developing their business to include coffee shop chains [107].

The coffee market is very dynamic, and consumers are increasingly interested in artisanal coffee and small coffee breweries. Drinking coffee is already acknowledged as a pleasure. The aspects of aroma, taste, smell, and occasions of consumption are still crucial. However, there is space to improve perceptions of scientifically-based health benefits. To increase awareness and improve knowledge among consumers, coffee marketing strategies could focus more on health benefits and nutritional values of coffee [4,66,108] in addition to the other positive characteristics consumers already associate with coffee. As a result, coffee consumption could be marketed as being pleasant and healthy at the same time.

There are already examples for market trends and innovations focusing on the functional and health aspects of coffee. Ready-to-drink (RTD) coffee (packaged liquid coffee designed to be consumed when opened without any additional steps) is interpreted as a clean functional beverage category and a healthier alternative to soft drinks. The RTD coffee segment is expected to grow due to global trends in the coffee sector: worldwide coffee culture growth, active on-the-go-lifestyle, and investments by major players [109]. Some coffee brands already use health focused strategies for coffee marketing (RTD and ground coffee). RTD cold brew coffee is marketed as a sugar and fat-free alternative to traditional energy drinks [110] or as a probiotic cold brewed coffee supporting digestive and immune health [111]. There are examples for a prebiotic fiber-enriched ground coffees with digestive health benefits [112] and for antioxidant-enriched ground coffees [113].

The discussion whether coffee can be claimed as an actual functional food is ongoing and there is not enough long-term evidence that coffee can prevent disease. Therefore coffee consumption for health reasons requires further scientific evidence before being recommended and promoted [7,28,114].

Limitations and Future Research

There are some study limitations. Results come from a convenience sample, focused on Italian consumers. Future studies may aim for samples with statistical representativeness and compare perceptions of consumers living in different countries. Coffee consumption behavior is related to various countries' consumption traditions and habits, and cross-country analysis may bring a more comprehensive perspective. Furthermore, considering the fast development in coffee consumption habits, future studies may focus the analysis on consumers that specifically favor coffee consumption out-of-home or specific coffee types preparations, such as filter, capsules, and powder. Future studies may also test consumers' WTP for different combinations of coffees with associated health claims such as disease reduction and health-promoting effects. Finally, future studies may explore coffee consumption motives within the dietary lifestyle, so as to provide sound information on the food behavior of coffee consumers for nutritionists and doctors.

Author Contributions: The research reported in this paper is the result of the cooperation between authors. The specific author contributions are: Conceptualization, A.S.; Methodology, A.S.; Software, A.S.; Validation, A.S. and B.R.; Formal Analysis, A.S.; Data Curation, A.S.; Writing—Original Draft Preparation, Review & Editing, B.R. for Sections 1 and 2, A.S. for Sections 3–6; Supervision, A.S.

Funding: This research received no external funding.

Conflicts of Interest: The authors declare no conflict of interest.

References

1. International Coffee Organization (ICO). *Coffee Market Report, December 2018*; ICO: London, UK, 2018; Available online: http://www.ico.org/Market-Report-18-19-e.asp (accessed on 11 February 2019).
2. Euromonitor International. *Coffee in 2018: The New Era of Coffee Everywhere*; Euromonitor International: London, UK, 2018.
3. Guimarães, E.R.; Leme, P.H.; De Rezende, D.C.; Pereira, S.P.; Dos Santos, A.C. The brand new Brazilian specialty coffee market. *J. Food Prod. Mark.* **2019**, *25*, 49–71. [CrossRef]
4. Corso, M.; Kalschne, D.; Benassi, M. Consumer's Attitude Regarding Soluble Coffee Enriched with Antioxidants. *Beverages* **2018**, *4*, 72. [CrossRef]
5. Ciaramelli, C.; Palmioli, A.; Airoldi, C. Coffee variety, origin and extraction procedure: Implications for coffee beneficial effects on human health. *Food Chem.* **2019**, *278*, 47–55. [CrossRef] [PubMed]
6. Messina, G.; Zannella, C.; Monda, V.; Dato, A.; Liccardo, D.; De Blasio, S.; Valenzano, A.; Moscatelli, F.; Messin, A.; Cibelli, G.; et al. The Beneficial Effects of Coffee in Human Nutrition. *Biol. Med.* **2015**, *7*, 240:1–240:5. [CrossRef]
7. Poole, R.; Kennedy, O.J.; Roderick, P.; Fallowfield, J.A.; Hayes, P.C.; Parkes, J. Coffee consumption and health: Umbrella review of meta-analyses of multiple health outcomes. *BMJ* **2017**, *359*, j5024. [CrossRef] [PubMed]
8. *World Health Organization Global Action Plan for the Prevention and Control of Noncommunicable Diseases: 2013–2020*; WHO: Geneva, Switzerland, 2013; ISBN 978-92-4-150623-6.
9. Auffermann, K. *From Brew Boomers to the Gourmet Generation: National Coffee Drinking Trends 2017*; National Coffee Association of USA: New York, NY, USA, 2017; Available online: https://nationalcoffee.blog/2017/03/28/from-basic-boomers-to-specialty-snowflakes-national-coffee-drinking-trends-2017/ (accessed on 11 February 2019).
10. Institute for Scientific Information on Coffee (ISIC). *Roundtable Report. The Good Things in Life: Coffee as Part of a Healthy Diet and Lifestyle*; ISIC: Worcestershire, UK, 2016; Available online: https://www.coffeeandhealth.org/wp-content/uploads/2016/03/Roundtable-report_Coffee-as-part-of-a-healthy-diet.pdf (accessed on 11 February 2019).
11. Ludwig, I.A.; Clifford, M.N.; Lean, M.E.J.; Ashihara, H.; Crozier, A. Coffee: Biochemistry and potential impact on health. *Food Funct.* **2014**, *5*, 1695–1717. [PubMed]
12. Stalmach, A.; Clifford, M.N.; Williamson, G.; Crozier, A. Phytochemicals in Coffee and the Bioavailability of Chlorogenic Acids. In *Teas, Cocoa and Coffee*; Crozier, A., Ashihara, H., Tomás-Barbéran, F., Eds.; Wiley-Blackwell: Oxford, UK, 2011; pp. 143–168. ISBN 978-1-4443-4709-8.
13. Svilaas, A.; Sakhi, A.K.; Andersen, L.F.; Svilaas, T.; Ström, E.C.; Jacobs, D.R.; Ose, L.; Blomhoff, R. Intakes of Antioxidants in Coffee, Wine, and Vegetables Are Correlated with Plasma Carotenoids in Humans. *J. Nutr.* **2004**, *134*, 562–567. [CrossRef]
14. Elhussein, E.A.A.; Kurtulbaş, E.; Bilgin, M.; Birteksöz Tan, A.S.; Hacıoğlu, M.; Şahin, S. Screening of the most consumed beverages and spices for their bioactive non-nutrient contents. *Food Meas.* **2018**, *12*, 2289–2301. [CrossRef]
15. Pellegrini, N.; Serafini, M.; Colombi, B.; Del Rio, D.; Salvatore, S.; Bianchi, M.; Brighenti, F. Total Antioxidant Capacity of Plant Foods, Beverages and Oils Consumed in Italy Assessed by Three Different In Vitro Assays. *J. Nutr.* **2003**, *133*, 2812–2819. [CrossRef]

16. Richelle, M.; Tavazzi, I.; Offord, E. Comparison of the Antioxidant Activity of Commonly Consumed Polyphenolic Beverages (Coffee, Cocoa, and Tea) Prepared per Cup Serving. *J. Agric. Food Chem.* **2001**, *49*, 3438–3442. [CrossRef]
17. Casal, S.; Oliveira, M.B.P.P.; Alves, M.R.; Ferreira, M.A. Discriminate Analysis of Roasted Coffee Varieties for Trigonelline, Nicotinic Acid, and Caffeine Content. *J. Agric. Food Chem.* **2000**, *48*, 3420–3424. [CrossRef]
18. Gloess, A.N.; Schönbächler, B.; Klopprogge, B.; D'Ambrosio, L.; Chatelain, K.; Bongartz, A.; Strittmatter, A.; Rast, M.; Yeretzian, C. Comparison of nine common coffee extraction methods: Instrumental and sensory analysis. *Eur. Food Res. Technol.* **2013**, *236*, 607–627. [CrossRef]
19. Parras, P. Antioxidant capacity of coffees of several origins brewed following three different procedures. *Food Chem.* **2007**, *102*, 582–592. [CrossRef]
20. Samoggia, A.; Riedel, B. Coffee consumption and purchasing behavior review: Insights for further research. *Appetite* **2018**, *129*, 70–81. [CrossRef]
21. Quintão, R.T.; Brito, E.P.Z.; Belk, R.W. The taste transformation ritual in the specialty coffee market. *Rev. Adm. Empresas* **2017**, *57*, 483–494. [CrossRef]
22. Ornelas, S.; Vera, J. Ground Roasted Coffee Consumers' Ability to Determine Actual Quality: The Use of Attributes and the Role of Education Level in Mexico. *J. Food Prod. Mark.* **2019**, *25*, 72–91. [CrossRef]
23. Bissinger, K.; Leufkens, D. Ethical food labels in consumer preferences. *Br. Food J.* **2017**, *119*, 1801–1814. [CrossRef]
24. Aguirre, J. Culture, health, gender and coffee drinking: A Costa Rican perspective. *Br. Food J.* **2016**, *118*, 150–163. [CrossRef]
25. Sousa, A.G.; Machado, L.M.M.; da Silva, E.F.; da Costa, T.H.M. Personal characteristics of coffee consumers and non-consumers, reasons and preferences for foods eaten with coffee among adults from the Federal District, Brazil. *Food Sci. Technol.* **2016**, *36*, 432–438. [CrossRef]
26. Grosso, G.; Godos, J.; Galvano, F.; Giovannucci, E.L. Coffee, Caffeine, and Health Outcomes: An Umbrella Review. *Annu. Rev. Nutr.* **2017**, *37*, 131–156. [CrossRef]
27. Nawrot, P.; Jordan, S.; Eastwood, J.; Rotstein, J.; Hugenholtz, A.; Feeley, M. Effects of caffeine on human health. *Food Addit. Contam.* **2003**, *20*, 1–30. [CrossRef]
28. Wikoff, D.; Welsh, B.T.; Henderson, R.; Brorby, G.P.; Britt, J.; Myers, E.; Goldberger, J.; Lieberman, H.R.; O'Brien, C.; Peck, J.; et al. Systematic review of the potential adverse effects of caffeine consumption in healthy adults, pregnant women, adolescents, and children. *Food Chem. Toxicol.* **2017**, *109*, 585–648. [CrossRef]
29. Jeszka-Skowron, M.; Zgoła-Grześkowiak, A.; Grześkowiak, T. Analytical methods applied for the characterization and the determination of bioactive compounds in coffee. *Eur. Food Res. Technol.* **2015**, *240*, 19–31. [CrossRef]
30. Loomis, D.; Guyton, K.Z.; Grosse, Y.; Lauby-Secretan, B.; El Ghissassi, F.; Bouvard, V.; Benbrahim-Tallaa, L.; Guha, N.; Mattock, H.; Straif, K. Carcinogenicity of drinking coffee, mate, and very hot beverages. *Lancet Oncol.* **2016**, *17*, 877–878. [CrossRef]
31. Freeman, A.M.; Morris, P.B.; Aspry, K.; Gordon, N.F.; Barnard, N.D.; Esselstyn, C.B.; Ros, E.; Devries, S.; O'Keefe, J.; Miller, M.; et al. A Clinician's Guide for Trending Cardiovascular Nutrition Controversies. *J. Am. Coll. Cardiol.* **2018**, *72*, 553–568. [CrossRef]
32. EFSA Panel on Dietetic Products, Nutrition and Allergies (NDA) Scientific Opinion on the safety of caffeine. *EFSA J.* **2015**, *13*, 4102:1–4102:120. [CrossRef]
33. Gunter, M.J.; Murphy, N.; Cross, A.J.; Dossus, L.; Dartois, L.; Fagherazzi, G.; Kaaks, R.; Kühn, T.; Boeing, H.; Aleksandrova, K.; et al. Coffee Drinking and Mortality in 10 European Countries: A Multinational Cohort Study. *Ann. Intern. Med.* **2017**, *167*, 236–247. [CrossRef]
34. Ding, M.; Bhupathiraju, S.N.; Satija, A.; van Dam, R.M.; Hu, F.B. Long-Term Coffee Consumption and Risk of Cardiovascular Disease. *Circulation* **2014**, *129*, 643–659. [CrossRef]
35. Wu, J.; Ho, S.C.; Zhou, C.; Ling, W.; Chen, W.; Wang, C.; Chen, Y. Coffee consumption and risk of coronary heart diseases: A meta-analysis of 21 prospective cohort studies. *Int. J. Cardiol.* **2009**, *137*, 216–225. [CrossRef] [PubMed]
36. Kim, B.; Nam, Y.; Kim, J.; Choi, H.; Won, C. Coffee Consumption and Stroke Risk: A Meta-analysis of Epidemiologic Studies. *Korean J. Fam. Med.* **2012**, *33*, 356–365. [CrossRef]

37. Liebeskind, D.S.; Sanossian, N.; Fu, K.A.; Wang, H.-J.; Arab, L. The coffee paradox in stroke: Increased consumption linked with fewer strokes. *Nutr. Neurosci.* **2016**, *19*, 406–413. [CrossRef]
38. Lopez-Garcia, E.; Orozco-Arbeláez, E.; Leon-Muñoz, L.M.; Guallar-Castillon, P.; Graciani, A.; Banegas, J.R.; Rodríguez-Artalejo, F. Habitual coffee consumption and 24-h blood pressure control in older adults with hypertension. *Clin. Nutr. ESPEN* **2016**, *35*, 1457–1463. [CrossRef] [PubMed]
39. Ranheim, T.; Halvorsen, B. Coffee consumption and human health—Beneficial or detrimental?—Mechanisms for effects of coffee consumption on different risk factors for cardiovascular disease and type 2 diabetes mellitus. *Mol. Nutr. Food Res.* **2005**, *49*, 274–284. [CrossRef]
40. Jiang, X.; Zhang, D.; Jiang, W. Coffee and caffeine intake and incidence of type 2 diabetes mellitus: A meta-analysis of prospective studies. *Eur. J. Nutr.* **2014**, *53*, 25–38. [CrossRef] [PubMed]
41. Huxley, R. Coffee, Decaffeinated Coffee, and Tea Consumption in Relation to Incident Type 2 Diabetes Mellitus: A Systematic Review with Meta-analysis. *Arch. Intern. Med.* **2009**, *169*, 2053–2063. [CrossRef]
42. Zhang, Y.; Lee, E.T.; Cowan, L.D.; Fabsitz, R.R.; Howard, B.V. Coffee consumption and the incidence of type 2 diabetes in men and women with normal glucose tolerance: The Strong Heart Study. *Nutr. Metab. Cardiovasc. Dis.* **2011**, *21*, 418–423. [CrossRef] [PubMed]
43. Carlström, M.; Larsson, S.C. Coffee consumption and reduced risk of developing type 2 diabetes: A systematic review with meta-analysis. *Nutr. Rev.* **2018**, *76*, 395–417. [CrossRef] [PubMed]
44. Larsson, S.C.; Wolk, A. Coffee Consumption and Risk of Liver Cancer: A Meta-Analysis. *Gastroenterology* **2007**, *132*, 1740–1745. [CrossRef] [PubMed]
45. Setiawan, V.W.; Wilkens, L.R.; Lu, S.C.; Hernandez, B.Y.; Le Marchand, L.; Henderson, B.E. Association of coffee intake with reduced incidence of liver cancer and death from chronic liver disease in the US multiethnic cohort. *Gastroenterology* **2015**, *148*, 118–125. [CrossRef]
46. Bravi, F.; Bosetti, C.; Tavani, A.; Bagnardi, V.; Gallus, S.; Negri, E.; Franceschi, S.; La Vecchia, C. Coffee drinking and hepatocellular carcinoma risk: A meta-analysis. *Hepatology* **2007**, *46*, 430–435. [CrossRef] [PubMed]
47. Saab, S.; Mallam, D.; Cox, G.A.; Tong, M.J. Impact of coffee on liver diseases: A systematic review. *Liver Int.* **2014**, *34*, 495–504. [CrossRef]
48. Liu, Q.-P.; Wu, Y.-F.; Cheng, H.-Y.; Xia, T.; Ding, H.; Wang, H.; Wang, Z.-M.; Xu, Y. Habitual coffee consumption and risk of cognitive decline/dementia: A systematic review and meta-analysis of prospective cohort studies. *Nutrition* **2016**, *32*, 628–636. [CrossRef]
49. Santos, C.; Costa, J.; Santos, J.; Vaz-Carneiro, A.; Lunet, N. Caffeine Intake and Dementia: Systematic Review and Meta-Analysis. *J. Alzheimer Dis.* **2010**, *20*, 187–204. [CrossRef]
50. Hernán, M.A.; Takkouche, B.; Caamaño-Isorna, F.; Gestal-Otero, J.J. A meta-analysis of coffee drinking, cigarette smoking, and the risk of Parkinson's disease: Coffee, Smoking, and PD. *Ann. Neurol.* **2002**, *52*, 276–284. [CrossRef] [PubMed]
51. Qi, H.; Li, S. Dose-response meta-analysis on coffee, tea and caffeine consumption with risk of Parkinson's disease: Coffee, tea and caffeine and PD risk. *Geriatr. Gerontol. Int.* **2014**, *14*, 430–439. [CrossRef]
52. Hussain, A.; Tabrez, E.S.; Mavrych, V.; Bolgova, O.; Peela, J.R. Caffeine: A Potential Protective Agent Against Cognitive Decline in Alzheimer's Disease. *Crit. Rev. Eukaryot. Gene Expr.* **2018**, *28*, 67–72. [CrossRef]
53. Palacios, N.; Gao, X.; McCullough, M.L.; Schwarzschild, M.A.; Shah, R.; Gapstur, S.; Ascherio, A. Caffeine and risk of Parkinson's disease in a large cohort of men and women. *Mov. Disord.* **2012**, *27*, 1276–1282. [CrossRef] [PubMed]
54. Nehlig, A. Effects of coffee/caffeine on brain health and disease: What should I tell my patients? *Pract. Neurol.* **2016**, *16*, 89–95. [CrossRef]
55. Smit, H.J.; Rogers, P.J. Effects of low doses of caffeine on cognitive performance, mood and thirst in low and higher caffeine consumers. *Psychopharmacology* **2000**, *152*, 167–173. [CrossRef] [PubMed]
56. Haskell, C.F.; Kennedy, D.O.; Wesnes, K.A.; Scholey, A.B. Cognitive and mood improvements of caffeine in habitual consumers and habitual non-consumers of caffeine. *Psychopharmacology* **2005**, *179*, 813–825. [CrossRef]
57. Wang, L.; Shen, X.; Wu, Y.; Zhang, D. Coffee and caffeine consumption and depression: A meta-analysis of observational studies. *Aust. N. Z. J. Psychiatry* **2016**, *50*, 228–242. [CrossRef] [PubMed]

58. Tse, W.S.; Chan, C.C.S.; Shiu, S.Y.K.; Chung, P.Y.A.; Cheng, S.H. Caffeinated coffee enhances co-operative behavior in the Mixed Motive Game in healthy volunteers. *Nutr. Neurosci.* **2009**, *12*, 21–27. [CrossRef] [PubMed]
59. International Agency for Research on Cancer (IARC). Working Group on the Evaluation of Carcinogenic Risks to Humans. In *Drinking Coffee, Mate, and Very Hot Beverages*; IARC Monographs on the Evaluation of Carcinogenic Risks to Humans: Lyon, France, 2016; Volume 16.
60. Zhang, Z.; Hu, G.; Caballero, B.; Appel, L.; Chen, L. Habitual coffee consumption and risk of hypertension: A systematic review and meta-analysis of prospective observational studies. *Am. J. Clin. Nutr.* **2011**, *93*, 1212–1219. [CrossRef] [PubMed]
61. Peck, J.D.; Leviton, A.; Cowan, L.D. A review of the epidemiologic evidence concerning the reproductive health effects of caffeine consumption: A 2000–2009 update. *Food Chem. Toxicol.* **2010**, *48*, 2549–2576. [CrossRef]
62. Lyngsø, J.; Ramlau-Hansen, C.H.; Bay, B.; Ingerslev, H.J.; Hulman, A.; Kesmodel, U.S. Association between coffee or caffeine consumption and fecundity and fertility: A systematic review and dose-response meta-analysis. *Clin. Epidemiol.* **2017**, *9*, 699–719. [CrossRef]
63. Lee, D.R.; Lee, J.; Rota, M.; Lee, J.; Ahn, H.S.; Park, S.M.; Shin, D. Coffee consumption and risk of fractures: A systematic review and dose–response meta-analysis. *Bone* **2014**, *63*, 20–28. [CrossRef] [PubMed]
64. Heaney, R. Effects of caffeine on bone and the calcium economy. *Food Chem. Toxicol.* **2002**, *40*, 1263–1270. [CrossRef]
65. Hallström, H.; Byberg, L.; Glynn, A.; Lemming, E.W.; Wolk, A.; Michaëlsson, K. Long-term Coffee Consumption in Relation to Fracture Risk and Bone Mineral Density in Women. *Am. J. Epidemiol.* **2013**, *178*, 898–909. [CrossRef]
66. Corso, M.; Benassi, M. Packaging Attributes of Antioxidant-Rich Instant Coffee and Their Influence on the Purchase Intent. *Beverages* **2015**, *1*, 273–291. [CrossRef]
67. Saliba, A.J.; Moran, C.C. The influence of perceived healthiness on wine consumption patterns. *Food Qual. Prefer.* **2010**, *21*, 692–696. [CrossRef]
68. Yoo, Y.J.; Saliba, A.J.; MacDonald, J.B.; Prenzler, P.D.; Ryan, D. A cross-cultural study of wine consumers with respect to health benefits of wine. *Food Qual. Prefer.* **2013**, *28*, 531–538. [CrossRef]
69. Samoggia, A. Wine and health: Faraway concepts? *Br. Food J.* **2016**, *118*, 946–960. [CrossRef]
70. Trondsen, T.; Braaten, T.; Lund, E.; Eggen, A. Consumption of seafood—The influence of overweight and health beliefs. *Food Qual. Prefer.* **2004**, *15*, 361–374. [CrossRef]
71. Mogendi, J.B.; De Steur, H.; Gellynck, X.; Makokha, A. Consumer evaluation of food with nutritional benefits: A systematic review and narrative synthesis. *Int. J. Food Sci. Nutr.* **2016**, *67*, 355–371. [CrossRef]
72. Smith, R. Regulation (EC) No 764/2008 of the European Parliament and of the Council. In *Core EU Legislation*; Macmillan Education UK: London, UK, 2015; pp. 183–186, ISBN 978-1-137-54501-5.
73. Breidert, C. *Estimation of Willingness-To-Pay Theory, Measurement, Application*; Deutscher Universitäts-Verlag/GWV Fachverlage GmbH, Wiesbaden: Wiesbaden, Germany, 2006; ISBN 978-3-8350-9244-0.
74. Samoggia, A.; Nicolodi, S. Consumer's Perception of Fruit Innovation. *J. Int. Food Agribus. Mark.* **2017**, *29*, 92–108. [CrossRef]
75. Prata, N.; Bell, S.; Weidert, K.; Gessessew, A. Potential for Cost Recovery: Women's Willingness to Pay for Injectable Contraceptives in Tigray, Ethiopia. *PLoS ONE* **2013**, *8*, e64032. [CrossRef] [PubMed]
76. Andersen, S.; Harrison, G.W.; Lau, M.I.; Rutström, E.E. Elicitation using multiple price list formats. *Exp. Econ.* **2009**, *12*, 365–366. [CrossRef]
77. Spinelli, S.; Dinnella, C.; Masi, C.; Zoboli, G.P.; Prescott, J.; Monteleone, E. Investigating preferred coffee consumption contexts using open-ended questions. *Food Qual. Prefer.* **2017**, *61*, 63–73. [CrossRef]
78. Labbe, D.; Ferrage, A.; Rytz, A.; Pace, J.; Martin, N. Pleasantness, emotions and perceptions induced by coffee beverage experience depend on the consumption motivation (hedonic or utilitarian). *Food Qual. Prefer.* **2015**, *44*, 56–61. [CrossRef]
79. Bhumiratana, N.; Adhikari, K.; Chambers, E. The development of an emotion lexicon for the coffee drinking experience. *Food Res. Int.* **2014**, *61*, 83–92. [CrossRef]
80. van der Merwe, K.; Maree, T. The behavioural intentions of specialty coffee consumers in South Africa: Behavioural intentions of coffee consumers. *Int. J. Consum. Stud.* **2016**, *40*, 501–508. [CrossRef]

81. Ágoston, C.; Urbán, R.; Király, O.; Griffiths, M.D.; Rogers, P.J.; Demetrovics, Z. Why Do You Drink Caffeine? The Development of the Motives for Caffeine Consumption Questionnaire (MCCQ) and Its Relationship with Gender, Age and the Types of Caffeinated Beverages. *Int. J. Ment. Health Addict.* **2018**, *16*, 981–999. [CrossRef]
82. Richelieu, A.; Korai, B. The consumption experience of Tim Hortons' coffee fans. *Qual. Mark. Res. Int. J.* **2014**, *17*, 192–208. [CrossRef]
83. Huang, H.-C.; Chang, Y.-T.; Yeh, C.-Y.; Liao, C.-W. Promote the price promotion: The effects of price promotions on customer evaluations in coffee chain stores. *Int. J. Contemp. Hosp. Manag.* **2014**, *26*, 1065–1082. [CrossRef]
84. Cailleba, P.; Casteran, H. Do Ethical Values Work? A Quantitative Study of the Impact of Fair Trade Coffee on Consumer Behavior. *J. Bus. Ethics* **2010**, *97*, 613–624. [CrossRef]
85. Van Loo, E.J.; Caputo, V.; Nayga, R.M.; Seo, H.-S.; Zhang, B.; Verbeke, W. Sustainability labels on coffee: Consumer preferences, willingness-to-pay and visual attention to attributes. *Ecol. Econ.* **2015**, *118*, 215–225. [CrossRef]
86. Klimas, C.A.; Webb, E. Comparing stated and realized preferences for shade-grown vs. conventionally grown coffee. *Int. J. Consum. Stud.* **2018**, *42*, 76–92. [CrossRef]
87. Tumanan, M.A.R.; Lansangan, J.R.G. More than just a cuppa coffee: A multi-dimensional approach towards analyzing the factors that define place attachment. *Int. J. Hosp. Manag.* **2012**, *31*, 529–534. [CrossRef]
88. Smith Maguire, J.; Hu, D. Not a simple coffee shop: Local, global and glocal dimensions of the consumption of Starbucks in China. *Soc. Identities* **2013**, *19*, 670–684. [CrossRef]
89. Fenko, A.; de Vries, R.; van Rompay, T. How Strong Is Your Coffee? The Influence of Visual Metaphors and Textual Claims on Consumers' Flavor Perception and Product Evaluation. *Front. Psychol.* **2018**, *9*, 53. [CrossRef]
90. Kim, S.-H.; Lee, S. Promoting customers' involvement with service brands: Evidence from coffee shop customers. *J. Serv. Mark.* **2017**, *31*, 733–744. [CrossRef]
91. Giacalone, D.; Fosgaard, T.R.; Steen, I.; Münchow, M. "Quality does not sell itself": Divergence between "objective" product quality and preference for coffee in naïve consumers. *Br. Food J.* **2016**, *118*, 2462–2474. [CrossRef]
92. Kutner, M.H.; Nachtsheim, C.; Neter, J. *Applied Linear Regression Models*; McGraw-Hill/Irwin: Boston, MA, USA; New York, NY, USA, 2004; ISBN 978-0-07-238691-2.
93. Bagozzi, R.P.; Yi, Y. On the Evaluation of Structural Equation Models. *J. Acad. Mark. Sci.* **1988**, *16*, 74–94. [CrossRef]
94. DeVellis, R.F. *Scale Development: Theory and Applications*; Applied Social Research Methods Series; Sage: Newbury Park, CA, USA, 1991; ISBN 978-0-8039-3775-8.
95. Fornell, C.; Larcker, D.F. Evaluating Structural Equation Models with Unobservable Variables and Measurement Error. *J. Mark. Res.* **1981**, *18*, 39. [CrossRef]
96. Brem, A.; Maier, M.; Wimschneider, C. Competitive advantage through innovation: The case of Nespresso. *Eur. J. Innov. Manag.* **2016**, *19*, 133–148. [CrossRef]
97. National Coffee Association USA (NCA). The History of Coffee. Available online: http://www.ncausa.org/about-coffee/history-of-coffee (accessed on 8 February 2019).
98. Grigg, D. The worlds of tea and coffee: Patterns of consumption. *GeoJournal* **2002**, *57*, 283–294. [CrossRef]
99. Samoggia, A.; Bertazzoli, A.; Hendrixson, V.; Glibetic, M.; Arvola, A. Women's Income and Healthy Eating Perception. In *Advances in Gender Research*; Segal, M.T., Demos, V., Eds.; Emerald Group Publishing Limited: Bingley, UK, 2016; Volume 22, pp. 165–191. ISBN 978-1-78635-054-1.
100. Sörqvist, P.; Hedblom, D.; Holmgren, M.; Haga, A.; Langeborg, L.; Nöstl, A.; Kågström, J. Who Needs Cream and Sugar When There Is Eco-Labeling? Taste and Willingness to Pay for "Eco-Friendly" Coffee. *PLoS ONE* **2013**, *8*, e80719. [CrossRef]
101. Ruggeri, A.; Arvola, A.; Samoggia, A.; Hendrixson, V. Food behaviours of Italian consumers at risk of poverty. *Br. Food J.* **2015**, *117*, 2831–2848. [CrossRef]
102. Lassen, A.D.; Lehmann, C.; Andersen, E.W.; Werther, M.N.; Thorsen, A.V.; Trolle, E.; Gross, G.; Tetens, I. Gender differences in purchase intentions and reasons for meal selection among fast food customers—Opportunities for healthier and more sustainable fast food. *Food Qual. Prefer.* **2016**, *47*, 123–129. [CrossRef]

103. Dammann, K.W.; Smith, C. Food-Related Environmental, Behavioral, and Personal Factors Associated with Body Mass Index among Urban, Low-Income African-American, American Indian, and Caucasian Women. *Am. J. Health Promot.* **2011**, *25*, e1–e10. [CrossRef]
104. Gandia, R.M.; Sugano, J.Y.; de Barros Vilas Boas, L.H.; Mesquita, D.L. Beverage capsule consumption: A laddering study. *Br. Food J.* **2018**, *120*, 1250–1263. [CrossRef]
105. Ajzen, I.; Fishbein, M. *Understanding Attitudes and Predicting Social Behavior*; Prentice-Hall: Upper Saddle River, NJ, USA, 1980; ISBN 978-0-13-936443-3.
106. Deloitte Touche Tohmatsu Limited. *Health & Wellness Progress Report*; Deloitte Touche Tohmatsu Limited: London, UK, 2018; Available online: https://www2.deloitte.com/global/en/pages/consumer-business/articles/health-wellness.html (accessed on 11 February 2019).
107. Arthur, R. Coca-Cola Completes Costa Acquisition: "Our Vision is to Use Costa's Platform to Expand in the Growing Coffee Category". Available online: https://www.beveragedaily.com/article/2019/01/03/coca-cola-completes-costa-coffee-acquisition (accessed on 11 February 2019).
108. National Coffee Association USA (NCA). Coffee at a Crossroad: 3 Industry Trends to Watch in 2019. 30 January 2019. Available online: https://nationalcoffee.blog/2019/01/30/coffee-at-a-crossroad-3-industry-trends-to-watch-in-2019/ (accessed on 5 March 2019).
109. Barry, M. *Top Ready-To-Drink Coffee Trends in 2018*; Euromonitor International: London, UK, 2018; Available online: https://go.euromonitor.com/webinar-hdsd-2018-HD-RTD-Coffee-2018.html (accessed on 28 February 2019).
110. Point Blank Home Page. Available online: https://pointblankcoldbrew.com/ (accessed on 28 February 2019).
111. Jus by Julie Probiotic Cold Brew Coffee. Available online: https://www.jusbyjulie.com/products/probiotic-cold-brew-coffee (accessed on 28 February 2019).
112. Brioni's Coffee Healthy Morning Coffee. Available online: http://www.brionis.com/healthy-morning/ (accessed on 28 February 2019).
113. Hawaii Coffee Company Antioxidant Taster Pack. Available online: https://www.hawaiicoffeecompany.com/p/specials/all-products/antioxidant-taster-pack (accessed on 28 February 2019).
114. Guallar, E. Coffee gets a clean bill of health. *BMJ* **2017**, *359*, j5356. [CrossRef] [PubMed]

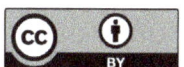

© 2019 by the authors. Licensee MDPI, Basel, Switzerland. This article is an open access article distributed under the terms and conditions of the Creative Commons Attribution (CC BY) license (http://creativecommons.org/licenses/by/4.0/).

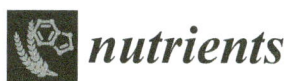

Article

Caffeine Intake During Pregnancy and Neonatal Anthropometric Parameters

Regina Wierzejska *, Mirosław Jarosz and Barbara Wojda

Department of Nutrition and Dietetics, Clinic of Metabolic Diseases and Gastroenterology, Institute of Food and Nutrition, 02-903 Warsaw, Poland; jarosz.zaklad@izz.waw.pl (M.J.); bwojda@izz.waw.pl (B.W.)
* Correspondence: rwierzejska@izz.waw.pl; Tel.: +48-22-550-97-47; Fax: +48-22-842-11-03

Received: 6 March 2019; Accepted: 3 April 2019; Published: 9 April 2019

Abstract: Caffeine is a psychoactive substance that may affect the normal course of pregnancy, therefore its intake during that time should not exceed 200 mg/day. The aim of this study was to evaluate caffeine intake among pregnant women from the Warsaw region. The study was conducted among 100 pregnant women who delivered at the Department of Obstetrics, Gynecology and Oncology, Medical University of Warsaw. Caffeine intake from coffee, tea, and energy drinks was measured using a questionnaire. Direct interviewing was used, with all interviews conducted by the same dietitian. Multiple regression analysis was used to investigate the relationship between caffeine intake and anthropometric measurements of the newborns. Mean caffeine intake among pregnant women was 68 ± 51 mg/day. Only 2% of the respondents exceeded the safe dose of 200 mg. Tea (mostly black) was the source of 63% of all caffeine. No relationships were found between caffeine intake and neonatal weight, length, or head and chest circumference ($p > 0.05$). Caffeine intake in our study population was relatively low and did not negatively affect fetal growth.

Keywords: caffeine; coffee; tea; energy drinks; pregnancy; newborn

1. Introduction

Caffeine, being a component of many popular products (tea and coffee), is widely consumed by pregnant women [1,2]. The half-life of caffeine is significantly prolonged in the body of a pregnant woman [3,4], due to decreased activity of the liver enzyme that is responsible for caffeine metabolism (by one-third in the first trimester of pregnancy and by half in the second trimester of pregnancy) [5]. The caffeine-induced increase in catecholamine concentrations (adrenaline, dopamine, and serotonin) interferes with placental blood flow and hampers transplacental nutrient transport to the fetus [6,7]. Caffeine and its metabolites easily cross the placental barrier [2,3,8], and caffeine excretion is delayed due to the immaturity of the fetal liver [2,9].

The impact of caffeine on the course of pregnancy and the development of the fetus is largely dependent on maternal intake and, supposedly, also on the speed of caffeine metabolism in the mother's body [3,10]. Until recently, most experts believed that daily maternal intake of caffeine should not exceed 300 mg [9–11], although recent recommendations of the European Food Safety Authority (EFSA) and the American Institute of Medicine have limited the amount to 200 mg/day [12,13].

High maternal caffeine intake may lead to a miscarriage, premature birth, or low-birth neonatal weight but, despite extensive research, the evidence remains inconclusive [2,14]. The results of three meta-analyses, published between 2014 and 2016, of studies on caffeine intake and the risk for miscarriage seem to be the most unambiguous so far. According to these sources, a 100–150 mg increase in daily caffeine intake results in an elevated (by 7–19%) risk for miscarriage [14–16]. The risk increases by 40% among women who consume large amounts of caffeine (350–699 mg/day) as compared to small amounts (<50 mg) [14]. Nevertheless, research limitations of the abovementioned studies as far as methodology is concerned and lack of randomized trials, which yield the most credible results, need to be emphasized. As for premature birth, a meta-analysis of the available studies revealed no relationship between caffeine intake during pregnancy and the duration of pregnancy [11], nor has such a negative correlation been confirmed by a meta-analysis of studies on the risk for central nervous system defects in the fetus [17,18]. However, a relationship between maternal coffee intake and the risk for leukemia in the offspring has been suggested by meta-analyses of clinical case-control trials on the safety of coffee consumption [18,19].

The effects of maternal caffeine intake on the emotional development of their children remains yet another matter. While some authors found no evidence for the link between maternal caffeine intake (even over 300 mg/day) and the development of attention-deficit hyperactivity disorder (ADHD) in children aged 4–11 years [20–22], other researchers are less optimistic. A study from Denmark found that maternal consumption of ≥8 cups of coffee/day in the second trimester results in hyperexcitability in their children [23]. Noteworthy, caffeine citrate remains the gold standard in the treatment of apnea in premature newborns [24,25]. No adverse side effects have ever been reported [26], and some authors even observed a positive effect of such therapy on the psychomotor development of the affected children at the age of 18–22 months [27].

In light of a limited amount of data from Poland on caffeine intake during pregnancy, the aim of our study was to evaluate the level of maternal caffeine intake and its effect on neonatal anthropometric parameters.

2. Material and Methods

2.1. Study Design

The study was conducted among 100 pregnant women, who delivered at the Department of Obstetrics, Gynecology and Oncology, Medical University of Warsaw. The women presented at the hospital on weekdays (Monday–Friday), in the morning, during four months of 2014 and 2015. Approximately 20% of the women did not consent to participate in the study. The exclusion criteria were the following: non-Polish nationality, multiple gestation, advanced stage of the delivery, chronic maternal diseases before pregnancy, and threatened course of labor. A written informed consent was obtained from all participants. The local ethics committee approved of the study (no. 10/162/KB/2014). Maternal characteristics are presented in Table 1.

2.2. Data Collection

Caffeine intake from coffee and tea, which according to the available literature constitute the main sources of caffeine in the diet of pregnant women [1,3,22,28], were evaluated. Energy drinks were also included in the analysis, predominantly to investigate maternal attitudes to their consumption during pregnancy. Dietary caffeine intake from coffee and tea was investigated using a questionnaire, along with the type of coffee and the way of preparing infusions, since the brewing method is largely the factor behind caffeine content. Direct interviewing (face-to-face) was used and all interviews were conducted by the same dietitian (the main author of the manuscript) in order to ensure data homogeneity. The 'Photo Album of Meals and Products' was used to precisely evaluate portion size. Mean caffeine content values in coffee and tea brews were taken from our earlier analysis (Table 2) [28]. Neonatal data (sex, weight, length, Apgar score at 5 min., head and chest circumference) were obtained from the hospital medical records. The anthropometric measurements were taken by the midwives immediately upon delivery. Weight was measured using a physician beam scale. The remaining measurements were taken with the use of a tape measure. The total neonatal length was measured from the vertex of the head to the soles (with the feet kept vertical at 90 degrees). The occipital-frontal head circumference (tape was placed on the maximum protrusion of the occiput and supraorbital ridges) and the chest circumference (tape was placed horizontally on the sternum and lower tip of the shoulder blade) were measured.

2.3. Statistical Analysis

The normal distribution of all studied parameters was checked using the Kolmogorov–Smirnov test. The Mann–Whitney test was used to compare the distribution of caffeine intake between independent groups (education, age, place of residence, smoking, gestational diabetes, and pregnancy-induced hypertension). A multivariate logistic regression model was used to investigate a relationship between caffeine intake and other factors (calcium intake, use of dietary supplements, pre-pregnancy body mass index (BMI), weight gain during pregnancy, smoking, gestational diabetes, maternal age and education, gravidity, professional activity during pregnancy, and sex of the neonate) versus neonatal weight, length, head and chest circumference lower than the median. Only term deliveries (94 newborns) were included into the analysis. Using the method of step elimination with 0.1 level for staying in the model, statistically significant factors were selected at a significance level of 5%. The relation of statistically significant factors was expressed by the odds ratio (OR) and the 95% confidence interval (95% CI).

Table 1. Maternal and neonatal characteristics.

Maternal Characteristics	
Number of Women	100
age (in years) mean ± SD	30.0 ± 4.4
education	
higher (%)	66
other (%)	34
place of residence	
Warsaw (%)	58
other (%)	42
parity	
primipara (%)	42
multipara (%)	58
premature birth (%)	6
pre-pregnancy BMI (mean) ± SD	22.7 ± 3.8
gestational diabetes (%)	11
pregnancy-induced hypertension (%)	9
smoking during pregnancy (%)	15
professionally active during pregnancy (%)	58
daily calcium consumption—from milk and dairy products (mg) median (min–max)	598 (69–1872)
supplementation with vitamin/mineral preparations (%)	89
Neonatal Characteristics	
number of newborns	94
gestational age (weeks) mean ± SD	39.4 ± 1.0
neonatal weight (g) median (min–max)	3530 (2390–4650)
LBW neonates (<2500 g), n (%)	1 (1.1)
macrosomia (>4000 g), n (%)	19 (20.2)
neonatal length (cm) median (min–max)	56 (50–60)
neonatal head circumference (cm) median (min–max)	35 (32.5–38.0)
neonatal chest circumference (cm) median (min–max)	34 (29–38)
Apgar score (points) mean ± SD	9.9 ± 0.1

Table 2. Caffeine content in coffee and tea brews used to evaluate caffeine intake by the pregnant women.

Product	Portion Size (mL)	Caffeine Content (mg)
brewed coffee (boiling water poured over ground coffee in a cup):		
1-teaspoon brew	160	36
2-teaspoon brew	160	74
instant coffee:		
1-teaspoon brew	160	61
2-teaspoon brew	160	117
black tea:		
1-min brew	200	22
5-min brew	200	33
green tea:		
1-min brew	200	22
5-min brew	200	33

3. Results

3.1. Caffeine Intake

Mean caffeine intake among the pregnant women from our study was 68 ± 51 mg/day. A vast majority of the women (79%) consumed <100 mg of caffeine, while the remaining 19% and 2% of the respondents consumed 100–200 mg and >200 mg/day, respectively. None of the subjects exceeded the dose of 300 mg of caffeine/day.

Tea was the source of 63% (43 mg) of total caffeine, and the remaining 37% came from coffee. Only 2 (2%) out of all respondents declared sporadic use of energy drinks, and for this reason these products were not included in evaluation of total caffeine intake.

Black tea supplied 4-fold more caffeine than green tea (34 ± 33 mg and 9 ± 26 mg, respectively). No statistically significant differences were found between caffeine intake and maternal age, education, place of inhabitance, smoking, gestational diabetes mellitus, or pregnancy-induced hypertension.

3.2. Caffeine Exposure and Neonatal Anthropometric Parameters

Maternal caffeine intake was not linked with neonatal anthropometric parameters (weight, length, head and chest circumference) ($p > 0.05$). Neonatal characteristics are presented in Table 1. Maternal weight gain during pregnancy was the parameter that turned out to be related to neonatal length. Pregnant women with too low weight gain are at a 3-fold higher risk for giving birth to infants with lower than median length for term neonates as compared to women with either recommended or excessive weight gain (Table 3).

Table 3. Analysis of the influence of maternal caffeine intake and other factors on the risk for neonatal length below the median.

N = 94	OR (95% CI)	p-Value
Caffeine intake: >100 mg/day vs. ≤100 mg/day	2.52 (0.86; 7.40)	0.092
Calcium intake: >611 mg/day vs. ≤611 mg/day		>0.1
Supplementation with vitamin/mineral preparations		>0.1
Pre-pregnancy BMI: underweight vs. normal overweight/obesity vs. normal		>0.1
Gestational weight gain: too low vs. recommended and excessive	3.01 (1.08; 8.3)	0.034

Table 3. *Cont.*

N = 94	OR (95% CI)	p-Value
Smoking		>0.1
Gestational diabetes		>0.1
Age (years): >30 vs. ≤30		>0.1
Education: secondary vs. higher	0.38 (0.15; 1.00)	0.051
Gravidity: primiparas vs. multiparas		>0.1
Professional activity during pregnancy		>0.1
Neonatal sex		>0.1

BMI: body mass index.

3.3. Coffee, Tea, and Energy Drinks Consumption

Tea and/or coffee brews were very popular in the diet of pregnant women. Only 10% of the respondents declared complete abstinence. Coffee was consumed by 43% of the women, including 1 subject who consumed only decaffeinated coffee. Instant coffee was the most popular drink (31%), and only 2% of the respondents consumed coffee from a coffee maker (Table 4). Daily consumption of coffee was declared by 32% of the women, mostly 1 cup/day (26%), and only 1 subject drank 3 cups of coffee/day. Mean coffee consumption in the entire study population was 74 ± 117 mL/day. All women consumed light coffee brews (i.e., 1 teaspoon of coffee per cup).

Tea consumption was reported by 80% of the respondents, including 72% who consumed tea every day, while the remaining women drank tea several times a week or less (Table 4). The amount of tea consumption varied between 2 cups (26%), 1 cup (21%), 3 cups (15%), or 4–8 cups (10%) a day. Mean tea consumption in the entire study population was 346 ± 379 mL/day. The vast majority of the women consumed only black tea (60%), mainly tea bags (90% of tea drinkers), whereas only 10% used tea leaves. As for brew strength, 84% of the tea bag drinkers declared that they preferred light- or medium-intensity brews (up to 1 min), and only 16% brewed the tea longer.

Table 4. Coffee and tea consumption among pregnant women.

	Number of Women (%)
Coffee	43
instant	31
brewed	12
in a cup	10
in a coffee maker	2
Consumption Frequency	
every day	32
3–4 times a week	4
1–2 times a week	8
2–3 times a month	1

Table 4. *Cont.*

	Number of Women (%)
Tea	80
black	60
green	6
black and green	14
Consumption Frequency	
every day	72
3–4 times a week	5
1–2 times a week	2
2–3 times a month	1

4. Discussion

In our study, we detected a small caffeine intake among the investigated population, significantly below 100 mg/day. Bearing in mind that, according to the literature, coffee and tea are the main sources of that component in the diet of pregnant women (80–90%) [1,22], it seems possible to conclude that the amount consumed is at a safe level, even taking into account consumption of other products with caffeine content.

To the best of our knowledge, only two studies on caffeine intake during pregnancy have been conducted in Poland so far, and both report optimistic findings. Mean daily caffeine intake was 91 mg/day according to the first study (conducted between 2005–2007) and 50 mg/day according to the second study (conducted between 2014–2015) [28,29]. The current result (68 mg from coffee, tea, and energy drinks) confirmed that consumption of caffeinated products by women in Poland during pregnancy is reasonable and non-excessive. Also, other data revealed that 73% of the Polish pregnant women declared an awareness of the potentially negative impact of coffee on the developing fetus [30]. Until recently, the amount of over 300 mg of caffeine/day was considered excessive and such consumption was reported for 1.6% of the investigated women [28]. Lately however, the so-called 'safe' dose of caffeine was significantly lowered (to 200 mg), but still only 2% of our study population and 1.4% of the subjects in the study of Błaszczyk-Bębenek et al. [29] exceeded the recommended dose. Mean caffeine intake among pregnant women in the US, Great Britain, and Sweden has been estimated at 58–125 mg, 159 mg, and 215 mg per day, respectively [9,31,32]. Very high (mean 258 mg/day) caffeine intake was observed in Japan, where over 67% of pregnant women consume over 200 mg/day [3]. In contrast, a surprisingly low (median 44–62 mg/day) caffeine intake among pregnant women was reported in Norway [1], whose inhabitants are well-known coffee lovers [2].

A relatively low caffeine intake in our study may be the result of a decision to reduce coffee consumption during pregnancy. In studies by Jarosz et al. [28], and by Wyka et al. [30], 26% and 19% of the study population, respectively, chose not to drink coffee during pregnancy. Similar findings have been reported by authors from other countries, where reduced tea and coffee consumption was the most common modification in the diet of pregnant women [33]. In our study, 43% of the respondents declared coffee consumption, which is consistent with the national data (39–52% of women) [28,30,34]. Espresso, which contains more caffeine than other coffee brews [1,35], has seldom been consumed by pregnant women in Poland, which might also account for the low caffeine intake we detected. Tea, whose consumption was declared by 80% of the respondents in this study and 93% in another study, is decidedly more popular and continues to be the main source of caffeine in the diet of pregnant women from Poland [28]. In Poland, black tea is the most popular drink and the main source of daily caffeine intake (44–59% according to the earlier studies [28,29] and 50% according to the current study), and only a small amount is derived from green tea (5–16% according to the earlier studies [28,29] and 13% according to the current study). Tea is also the main source of caffeine in Great Britain [9] and Japan [22], although in Japan, most caffeine in the diet of pregnant women comes from green tea (75%), and only some from black tea (4%). In contrast, coffee remains the main caffeine source in the Scandinavian countries, the US, and Canada [1,3,28,36]. In our study, we found that pregnant women avoid energy drinks, which is consistent with reports from Western European countries, where only 1–2% of total caffeine content in the diet of pregnant women is supplied by energy drinks [9,12,28].

The results of the Care Study Group from Great Britain were the reason why EFSA lowered the safety threshold (to 200 mg) for daily intake of caffeine during pregnancy. The study revealed that caffeine intake over 200 mg/day results in a 60–70 g decrease in neonatal weight [9]. In our study, we found no relationship between neonatal anthropometric parameters and caffeine intake. Importantly, mean caffeine intake was significantly below the permissible dose (i.e., 200 mg/day). No relationship between neonatal anthropomorphic parameters and caffeine intake in Poland was found in our previous study as well, where mean caffeine intake was <100 mg, which is similar to the findings in the present study [28]. According to the latest reports in the literature, in particular a study from Norway, daily caffeine intake of <200 mg increases the risk for small-for-gestational-age infant by 16% [37]. In a study from Ireland, a daily increase in caffeine intake by 100 mg resulted in a decrease in neonatal weight (by 72 g), length (by 0.3 cm), and head circumference (by 0.12 cm) [38]. On the other hand, a study from Brazil revealed no relationship between high caffeine intake (≥300 mg) and low-birth-weight (LBW) neonates [39]. In light of the recent meta-analyses, Rhee et al. in their meta-analysis of eight cohort and four case-control studies concluded that high maternal intake of caffeine increases the risk for LBW neonate by 38% [7], while Greenwood et al., in their meta-analysis of 26 cohort and 27 case-control studies, found that increased caffeine intake (by 100 mg) results in higher risk (by 7%) for LBW neonate [15]. Some experts are of the opinion that neonates born to non-smoking mothers who consume ≥300 mg of caffeine/day, but only those who metabolize caffeine fast (i.e., AA genotype), are at higher risk for delivering infants with decreased birth size [40].

Several limitations of the present study might have biased the final results, chief among them a small sample size, which was the result of the number of deliveries at the clinic, but also the fact that it was a pilot study. It was a preliminary study to recognize the attitudes of pregnant women to coffee consumption after the introduction of a coffee cup into the graphic representation of the nutrition guidelines (food pyramid) in Poland. Also, we collected data on maternal caffeine intake on the day of the delivery, so the study was retrospective in nature. Nonetheless, drinking coffee and tea is a common component of many individuals' eating habits and it should not be problematic to recall the frequency of their consumption, even from the time perspective. Also, caffeine intake might have been different throughout the pregnancy, although various studies reported lack of significant differences between caffeine intake and pregnancy trimesters [9,39]. Furthermore, the questionnaire did not include information about other sources of caffeine, such as soft drinks, but many authors have previously reported that coffee and tea are the sources of over 80% of the caffeine in the diets of pregnant women [1,22,38]. Our data included information on types of coffee (e.g., instant, brewed), as well as the intensity of tea and coffee brews, which to a large extent is the decisive factor for determining caffeine content in a drink and allows for a precise evaluation of the intake.

5. Conclusions

Caffeine intake among our study population was relatively low, which resulted from low coffee consumption. Tea, due to its higher popularity during pregnancy, constituted the main source of caffeine. No relationship was found between such caffeine intake and neonatal anthropometric parameters.

Author Contributions: R.W. conceived the idea for the study. R.W. and M.J. contributed to the design of the research. R.W. and B.W. collected the data. R.W. analyzed the data and wrote the paper. All authors edited and approved the final version of the manuscript.

Funding: This research received no external funding.

Acknowledgments: The authors wish to express their sincere gratitude to the management and personnel of the Department of Obstetrics, Gynecology and Oncology, Medical University of Warsaw for their assistance in the project.

Conflicts of Interest: The authors declare no conflict of interest.

References

1. Sengpiel, V.; Elind, E.; Bacelis, J.; Nilsson, S.; Grove, J.; Myhre, R.; Haugen, M.; Meltzer, H.M.; Alexander, J.; Jacobsson, B.; Brantsaeter, A.L. Maternal caffeine intake during pregnancy is associated with birth weight but not with gestational length: Results from a large prospective observational cohort study. *BMC Med.* **2013**, *11*, 42. [CrossRef]
2. Temple, J.L.; Bernard, C.; Lipshultz, S.E.; Czachor, J.D.; Westphal, J.A.; Mestre, M.A. The safety of ingested caffeine: A comprehensive review. *Front. Psychiatry* **2017**, *26*, 80. [CrossRef] [PubMed]
3. Okubo, H.; Miyake, Y.; Tanaka, K.; Sasaki, S.; Hirota, Y. Maternal total caffeine intake, mainly from Japanese and Chinese tea, during pregnancy was associated with risk of preterm birth: The Osaka Maternal and Child Health Study. *Nutr. Res.* **2015**, *35*, 309–316. [CrossRef]
4. Yu, T.; Campbell, S.C.; Stockmann, C.; Tak, C.; Schoen, K.; Clark, E.A.; Varner, M.W.; Spigarelli, M.G.; Sherwin, C.M. Pregnancy-induced changes in the pharmacokinetics of caffeine and its metabolites. *J. Clin. Pharmacol.* **2016**, *56*, 590–596. [CrossRef] [PubMed]
5. Tsutsumi, K.; Kotegawa, T.; Matsuki, S.; Tanaka, Y.; Ishii, Y.; Kodama, Y.; Kuranari, M.; Miyakawa, I.; Nakano, S. The effect of pregnancy on cytochrome P4501A2, xanthine oxidase, and N-acetyltransferase activities in humans. *Clin. Pharmacol. Ther.* **2001**, *70*, 121–125. [CrossRef] [PubMed]
6. Grosso, L.M.; Bracken, M.B. Caffeine metabolism, genetics and perinatal outcomes: A review of exposure assessment considerations during pregnancy. *Ann. Epidemiol.* **2005**, *15*, 460–466. [CrossRef]
7. Rhee, J.; Kim, R.; Kim, Y.; Tam, M.; Lai, Y.; Keum, N.; Oldenburg, C.E. Maternal caffeine consumption during pregnancy and risk of low birth weight: A dose-response meta-analysis of observational studies. *PLoS ONE* **2015**, *10*. [CrossRef]
8. Wierzejska, R.; Jarosz, M.; Siuba, M.; Sawicki, W. Comparison of maternal and fetal blood levels of caffeine and its metabolite. A pilot study. *Ginekol. Pol.* **2014**, *85*, 500–503. [CrossRef] [PubMed]
9. Care Study Group. Maternal caffeine intake during pregnancy and risk of fetal growth restriction: A large prospective observational study. *BMJ* **2008**, *337*. [CrossRef]
10. Nawrot, P.; Jordan, S.; Eastwood, J.; Rotstein, J.; Hugenholtz, A.; Feeley, M. Effects of caffeine on human health. *Food Addit. Contam.* **2003**, *20*, 1–30. [CrossRef] [PubMed]
11. Maslova, E.; Bhattacharya, S.; Lin, S.; Michels, K.B. Caffeine consumption during pregnancy and risk of preterm birth: A meta-analysis. *Am. J. Clin. Nutr.* **2010**, *92*, 1120–1130. [CrossRef] [PubMed]
12. EFSA Panel on Dietetic Products Nutrition and Allergies. Scientific opinion on the safety of caffeine. *EFSA J.* **2015**, *13*, 4–102.
13. Institute of Medicine. *Caffeine in Food and Dietary Supplements: Examining Safety*; National Academies Press: Washington, DC, USA, 2014.
14. Chen, L.W.; Wu, Y.; Neelakantan, N.; Chong, M.F.; Pan, A.; van Dam, R.M. Maternal caffeine intake during pregnancy and risk of pregnancy loss: A categorical and dose-response meta-analysis of prospective studies. *Public Health Nutr.* **2016**, *19*, 1233–1244. [CrossRef] [PubMed]
15. Greenwood, D.C.; Thatcher, N.J.; Ye, J.; Garrard, L.; Keogh, G.; King, L.G.; Cade, J.E. Caffeine intake during pregnancy and adverse birth outcomes: A systematic review and dose-response meta-analysis. *Eur. J. Epidemiol.* **2014**, *29*, 725–734. [CrossRef] [PubMed]
16. Li, J.; Zhao, H.; Song, J.M.; Zhang, J.; Tang, Y.L.; Xin, C.M. A meta-analysis of risk of pregnancy loss and caffeine and coffee consumption during pregnancy. *Int. J. Gynaecol. Obstet.* **2015**, *130*, 116–122. [CrossRef]
17. Li, Z.X.; Gao, Z.L.; Wang, J.N.; Guo, Q.H. Maternal coffee consumption during pregnancy and neural tube defects in offspring: A meta-analysis. *Fetal Pediatr. Pathol.* **2016**, *35*, 1–9. [CrossRef]
18. Poole, R.; Kennedy, O.J.; Roderick, P.; Fallowfield, J.A.; Hayes, P.C.; Parkes, J. Coffee consumption and health: Umbrella review of meta-analyses of multiple health outcomes. *BMJ* **2017**, *22*, 359. [CrossRef] [PubMed]

19. Thomopoulos, T.P.; Ntouvelis, E.; Diamantaras, A.A.; Tzanoudaki, M.; Baka, M.; Hatzipantelis, E.; Kourti, M.; Polychronopoulou, S.; Sidi, V.; Stiakaki, E.; et al. Maternal and childhood consumption of coffee, tea and cola beverages in association with childhood leukemia: A meta-analysis. *Cancer Epidemiol.* **2015**, *39*, 1047–1059. [CrossRef]
20. Del-Ponte, B.; Santos, I.S.; Tovo-Rodriques, L.; Anselmi, L.; Munhoz, T.N.; Matijasevich, A. Caffeine consumption during pregnancy and ADHD at the age of 11 years: A birth cohort study. *BMJ Open* **2016**, *6*. [CrossRef]
21. Klebanoff, M.A.; Keim, S.A. Maternal caffeine intake during pregnancy and child cognition and behavior at 4 and 7 years of age. *Am. J. Epidemiol.* **2015**, *15*, 1023–1032. [CrossRef]
22. Miyake, Y.; Tanaka, K.; Okubo, H.; Sasaki, S.; Arakawa, M. Maternal caffeine intake in pregnancy is inversely related to childhood peer problems in Japan: The Kyushu Okinawa Maternal and Child Health Study. *Nutr. Neurosci.* **2018**, *13*, 1–8. [CrossRef] [PubMed]
23. Hvolgaard Mikkelsen, S.; Obel, C.; Olsen, J.; Niclasen, J.; Bech, B.H. Maternal caffeine consumption during pregnancy and behavioral disorders in 11-year-old offspring: A Danish National Birth Cohort Study. *J. Pediatr.* **2017**, *189*, 120–127. [CrossRef] [PubMed]
24. Boraszewska-Kornacka, M.; Bober-Olesińska, K. Use of caffeine in neonatology. *Stand. Med. Pediatr.* **2017**, *14*, 364–367.
25. Goryniak, A.; Szczęśniak, A.; Śleboda, D.; Dołęgowska, B. Apnea of prematurity—characteristic and treatment. *Postępy Biochem.* **2017**, *63*, 151–154.
26. Zhao, Y.; Tian, X.; Liu, G. Clinical effectiveness of different doses of caffeine for primary apnea in preterm infants. *Zhonghua Er Ke Za Zhi Chin. J. Pediatrics* **2016**. [CrossRef]
27. Gupte, A.S.; Gupta, D.; Ravichandran, S.; Ma, M.M.; Chouthai, N.S. Effect of early caffeine on neurodevelopmental outcome of very low-birth weight newborns. *J. Matern. Fetal Neonatal Med.* **2016**, *29*, 1233–1237. [CrossRef]
28. Jarosz, M.; Wierzejska, R.; Siuba, M. Maternal caffeine intake and its effect on pregnancy outcomes. *Eur. J. Obstet. Gynecol. Reprod. Biol.* **2012**, *160*, 156–160. [CrossRef] [PubMed]
29. Błaszczyk-Bębenek, E.; Piórecka, B.; Kopytko, M.; Chadzińska, Z.; Jagielski, P.; Schlegel-Zawadzka, M. Evaluation of Caffeine Consumption among Pregnant Women from Southern Poland. *Int. J. Environ. Res. Public Health* **2018**, *15*, 2373. [CrossRef] [PubMed]
30. Wyka, J.; Misiarz, M.; Malczyk, E.; Zołoteńka-Synowiec, M.; Całyniuk, B.; Smółka, B.; Mazurek, D. Assessment of consumption of alcohol, coffee and cigarettes smoking among pregnant women. *Bromat. Chem. Toksykol.* **2015**, *3*, 578–582.
31. Clausson, B.; Granath, F.; Ekbom, A.; Lundgren, S.; Nordmark, A.; Signorello, L.B.; Cnattingius, S. Effect of caffeine exposure during pregnancy on birth weight and gestational age. *Am. J. Epidemiol.* **2002**, *155*, 429–436. [CrossRef]
32. Frary, C.D.; Johnson, R.K.; Wang, M.Q. Food sources and intakes of caffeine in the diets of persons in the United States. *J. Am. Diet. Assoc.* **2005**, *105*, 110–113. [CrossRef] [PubMed]
33. Hillier, S.E.; Olander, E.K. Women's dietary changes before and during pregnancy: A systematic review. *Midwifery* **2017**, *49*, 19–31. [CrossRef]
34. Pieszko, M.; Ciesielska-Piotrowicz, J.; Skotnicka, M.; Małgorzewicz, S. Behaviour health pregnant women with secondary and higher education – preliminary studies. *Pediatr. Med. Rodz.* **2017**, *13*, 94–102. [CrossRef]
35. Sanchez, J.M. Methylxanthine content in commonly consumed foods in Spain and determination of its intake during consumption. *Foods* **2017**, *6*, 109. [CrossRef] [PubMed]
36. Bakker, R.; Steegers, E.; Obradov, A.; Raat, H.; Hofman, A.; Jaddoe, V.W. Maternal caffeine intake from coffee and tea, fetal growth and risks of adverse birth outcomes: The Generation R Study. *Am. J. Clin. Nutr.* **2010**, *91*, 1691–1698. [CrossRef]
37. Modzelewska, D.; Bellocco, R.; Elfvin, A.; Brantsæter, A.L.; Meltzer, H.M.; Jacobsson, B.; Sengpiel, V. Caffeine exposure during pregnancy, small for gestational age birth and neonatal outcome—results from the Norwegian Mother and Child Cohort Study. *BMC Pregnancy Childbirth* **2019**, *19*. [CrossRef] [PubMed]
38. Chen, L.W.; Fitzgerald, R.; Murrin, C.M.; Mehegan, J.; Kelleher, C.C.; Phillips, C.M. Associations of maternal caffeine intake with birth outcomes: Results from the Lifeways Cross Generation Cohort Study. *Am. J. Clin. Nutr.* **2018**, *108*, 1301–1308. [CrossRef] [PubMed]

39. Vitti, F.P.; Grandi, C.; Cavalli, R.C.; Simões, V.M.F.; Batista, R.F.L.; Cardoso, V.C. Association between caffeine consumption in pregnancy and low birth weight and preterm birth in the birth Cohort of Ribeirão Preto. *Rev. Bras. Ginecol. Obstet.* **2018**, *40*, 749–756. [CrossRef]
40. Sasaki, S.; Limpar, M.; Sata, F.; Kobayashi, S.; Kishi, R. Interaction between maternal caffeine intake during pregnancy and CYP1A2 C164A polymorphism affects infant birth size in the Hokkaido study. *Pediatr. Res.* **2017**, *82*, 19–28. [CrossRef]

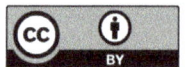

© 2019 by the authors. Licensee MDPI, Basel, Switzerland. This article is an open access article distributed under the terms and conditions of the Creative Commons Attribution (CC BY) license (http://creativecommons.org/licenses/by/4.0/).

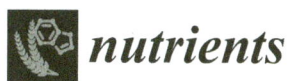

Article

Determination of Urinary Caffeine Metabolites as Biomarkers for Drug Metabolic Enzyme Activities

Hyeong Jun Kim [1,†], Min Sun Choi [1,†], Shaheed Ur Rehman [2,3], Young Seok Ji [1], Jun Sang Yu [1], Katsunori Nakamura [4] and Hye Hyun Yoo [1,*]

1. Institute of Pharmaceutical Science and Technology and College of Pharmacy, Hanyang University, Ansan-si, Gyeonggi-do 15588, Korea
2. Department of Pharmacy, COMSATS Institute of Information Technology, Abbottabad 22060, Pakistan
3. Hygiene House Healthcare Center (HHHC), Bannu 28100, Pakistan
4. Department of Pharmacy, Ryukyu University Hospital, Okinawa 903-0215, Japan
* Correspondence: yoohh@hanyang.ac.kr; Tel.: +82-31-400-5804
† Hyeong Jun Kim and Min Sun Choi equally contributed to this work.

Received: 2 July 2019; Accepted: 15 August 2019; Published: 19 August 2019

Abstract: Caffeine is commonly taken via the daily dietary consumption of caffeine-containing foods. The absorbed caffeine is metabolized to yield various metabolites by drug-metabolizing enzymes, and measuring the levels of each caffeine metabolite can provide useful information for evaluating the phenotypes of those enzymes. In this study, the urinary concentrations of caffeine and its 13 metabolites were determined, and the phenotypes of drug metabolic enzymes were investigated based on the caffeine metabolite ratios. Human urine samples were pretreated using solid phase extraction, and caffeine and its metabolites were analyzed using liquid chromatography-tandem mass spectrometry. Based on the urinary caffeine metabolite concentrations, the caffeine metabolite ratios were calculated for six human subjects at specified time points after caffeine intake. Variations in urinary metabolite levels among individuals and time points were reported. In addition, the resultant enzyme activities showed different patterns, depending on the metabolite ratio equations applied. However, some data presented a constant metabolite ratio range, irrespective of time points, even at pre-dose. This suggests the possibility of urinary caffeine metabolite analysis for routine clinical examination. These findings show that urinary caffeine and the metabolite analysis would be useful in evaluating metabolic phenotypes for personalized medicine.

Keywords: caffeine; metabolites; phenotyping; CYP450; NAT; xanthine oxidase

---

1. Introduction

Caffeine, an alkaloid of the methylxanthine class, is the world's most widely consumed psychoactive substance. As a naturally occurring substance, caffeine is found in the leaves, fruits, or seeds of more than 60 plant species. Caffeine is popularly and extensively taken via the daily dietary consumption of caffeine-containing beverages or foods [1,2].

In the liver, caffeine is subjected to a series of metabolic reactions to yield a mixture of N-methylated xanthines, uric acids, and an acetylated uracil, as its metabolites [3]. There are various metabolic enzymes involved in each caffeine metabolic pathway (Figure 1). These enzymes include N-acetyltransferase 2 (NAT2), xanthine oxidase (XO), and cytochrome P450—particularly 1A2 (CYP1A2) and 2A6 (CYP2A6)—which are of prime interest and must be phenotypically evaluated because of their roles in metabolizing various xenobiotics [4–6]. These four enzymes involved in caffeine metabolism display genetic polymorphism, and their metabolizing activities can vary in individuals [4–6]. Accordingly, inter-individual variability can be observed in caffeine and its metabolite levels, or their ratios in biological fluids or tissues. In this context, measuring the levels of caffeine and each caffeine metabolite can provide useful information for evaluating the phenotypes of drug-metabolizing enzymes. Furthermore, caffeine is popularly, and even routinely, consumed worldwide as various types of foods, such that caffeine or its metabolites are likely to be detected in urine. Due to these aspects, the measurement of urinary caffeine metabolite levels can be an advantageous marker for the phenotyping of individual drug-metabolizing activities.

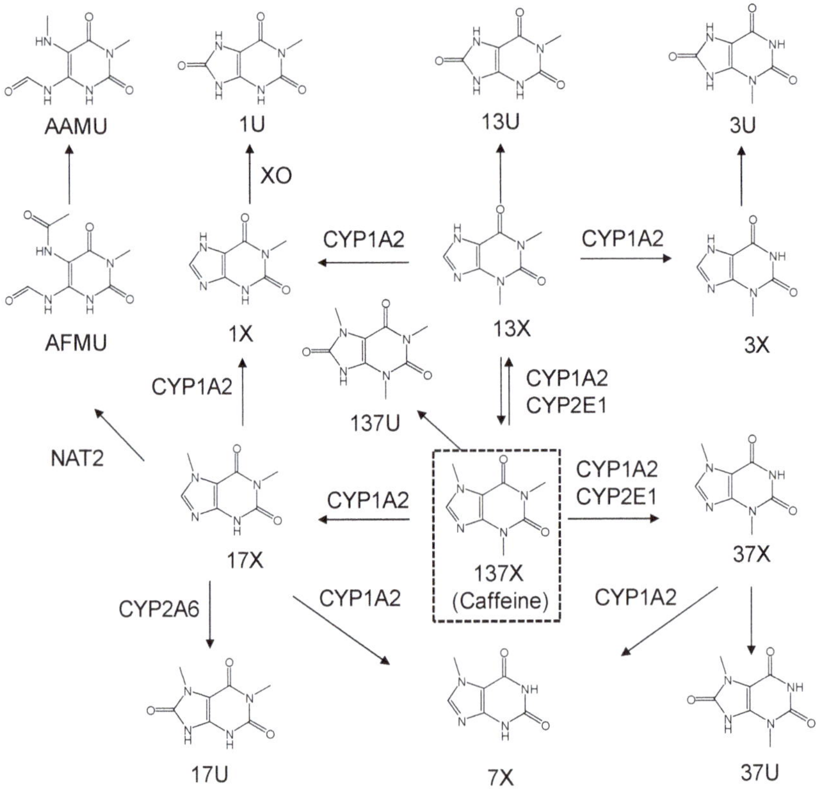

Figure 1. The metabolic pathway of caffeine.

Several analytical methods have been reported for measuring caffeine and its metabolites in urine using high-performance liquid chromatography (HPLC) or high-performance liquid chromatography-tandem mass spectrometry (LC-MS/MS) [7–16]. Based on such analytical methods, the phenotyping of CYP1A2, CYP2A6, NAT2, or XO enzyme activity has been investigated by measuring urinary caffeine and its metabolites in subjects receiving a regulated dietary caffeine intake and in uncontrolled subjects [7,9,10,12,13,17–20]. However, each study evaluated the enzyme phenotypes based on different metabolite ratio equations for a limited population, and information on the feasibility of those methods is still insufficient for general, practical application.

In this study, the urinary concentrations of caffeine and its metabolites were determined using LC-MS/MS analysis. The resulting concentration data was applied to various caffeine metabolite ratio equations to determine the phenotypes of each drug metabolic enzyme. The feasibility of phenotyping the drug-metabolizing enzyme based on urinary caffeine metabolite ratios was examined.

2. Materials and Methods

2.1. Chemicals and Reagents

Chemicals including, 1-methylxanthine (1X), 3-methylxanthine (3X), 7-methylxanthine (7X), 1,3-dimethylxanthine (theophylline, 13X), 1,7-dimethylxanthine (paraxanthine, 17X), 3,7-dimethylxanthine (theobromine, 37X), 1,3,7-trimethylxanthine (caffeine, 137X), 1-methyluric acid (1U), 1,3-dimethyluric acid (13U), 1,7-dimethyluric acid (17U), 3,7-dimethyluric acid (37U), and 1,3,7-trimethyluric acid (137U), and acetic acid were provided by Sigma-Aldrich (St. Louis, MO, USA). The following chemicals were procured from Santa Cruz (Dallas, TX, USA): 5-acetylamino-6-amino-3-methyluracil (AAMU), 5-acetylamino-6-formylamino-3-methyluracil (AFMU) and internal standards (IS) including 1-methylxanthine-2,4,5,6-13C4 (1X*), 1,3,9-15N3, and 1-methyluricacid-2,4,5,6-13C4,1,3,9-15N3 (1U*). HPLC-grade acetonitrile was purchased from J. T. Baker (Philipsburg, NJ, USA). Water was prepared using a Milli-Q purification system (Millipore, Bedford, MA, USA). All other chemicals used were of analytical grade and used as received. All the standard solutions and mobile phases were passed through a 0.22-µm membrane filter before use.

2.2. Human Urine Specimens

The study protocol and consent forms were approved by the Institutional Review Board of the Hanyang University, and all the participants provided written informed consent to participate in the study. The eligibility criteria for the study included physically healthy ethnic Korean adult men (19 years of age or older) who signed written informed consent. Participants were excluded if they were being treated for acute disease or other diseases or who needed treatment, or were receiving any medication that might affect the metabolism or excretion of caffeine. Urine samples were collected from 6 volunteers prior to the consumption of a caffeine-containing drink (120 mg of caffeine intake), and 1 h, 2 h, 4 h, 6 h, 8 h, and 10 h after the drink. Blank urine samples were obtained from healthy volunteers who had not consumed any methyl xanthine-containing food or beverage for the last 24 h. The urine samples were collected in clear 15-mL centrifuge tubes. All the study procedures were conducted in compliance with the principles of Declaration of Helsinki and Korean Good Clinical Practice guidelines (IRB HYG-16-193-2).

2.3. Urine Sample Preparation and Standard Samples

For the LC–MS/MS analysis, 100 µL of urine was added to 10 mL of 0.1% acetic acid with IS. Then, 1 mL of diluted mixture was passed through pre-activated Sep-Pak C18 cartridges (96-well type OASIS HLB extraction cartridge, Waters). The cartridge was washed with 1 mL of 0.1% formic acid two times, and then eluted with 1 mL of methanol. The eluate was dried under nitrogen gas. The residue was resolved in 0.1% acetic acid/acetonitrile (90:10, 100 µL), and a 5-µL aliquot was injected into the HPLC column for LC-MS/MS analysis. The analyte mixture was dissolved in MeOH at a concentration of 1 mg/mL and diluted to a series of working standard solutions. A 5-µL aliquot of each working standard solution was spiked to 95 µL of human blank urine. Then, the spiked samples were pretreated as described above. The concentrations of QC samples for each analyte are provided as supplementary data (Table S1).

2.4. Method Validation

The developed method was validated according to the US Food and Drug Administration (FDA) guidelines as mentioned in the "Guidance for Industry, Bioanalytical Method Validation, 2018" [21].

2.4.1. Selectivity, Linearity, and LLOQ

The selectivity of the method was assessed by comparing multiple reaction monitoring (MRM) chromatograms between a blank sample and a standard spiked mixture. Lower limits of quantitation

(LLOQs) for each analyte were determined considering the concentration level found in human urine samples, and evaluated for accuracy and precision. The calibration curves were prepared using the samples at concentration ranges depending on their LLOQ. The calibration curves were generated by plotting the peak area ratios of the analytes/IS versus the concentrations in the standard spiked samples. The linear correlation coefficient (r^2) for all the calibration curves should be greater than 0.99.

2.4.2. Precision and Accuracy

To assess the intra-day precision and accuracy, QC samples were analyzed, in triplicate, at different concentration levels ($n = 3$) on the same day. In case of inter-day assays, the precision and accuracy were assessed by determining the QC samples over three consecutive days. The accuracy was measured as a deviation of the calculated mean value from the nominal mean value, which should be within 15% of the nominal value except for LLOQ, which should not exceed 20% of the nominal value. The precision was determined at each concentration level, in terms of percent relative standard deviation (%RSD), which should not exceed 15% of the nominal concentration, except for the LLOQ, where it should not deviate by more than 20%.

2.4.3. Matrix Effect and Recovery

The matrix effect was evaluated by comparing the spiked QC samples at low, middle, and high concentrations in the blank, to the same QC sample in 0.1% acetic acid. The recovery was determined by comparing the reaction of the extracted sample, to which the analyte is added, and the biological sample after extraction.

2.4.4. Stability

Stability was evaluated for the QC samples under various conditions such as freeze-and-thaw, short-term, long-term, and processed sample stability. For the freeze-and-thaw stability test, three aliquots of the QC samples were stored at −20 °C for 24 h and thawed at room temperature. When completely thawed, the samples were refrozen for 24 h under the same condition, and this was repeated three times. For short-term stability, the QC samples were maintained at room temperature for 12 h, and then analyzed. For long-term stability, the QC samples were stored at −20 °C for 7 days, and then analyzed. The post-preparative stability was evaluated by analyzing the QC samples placed in the autosampler for 24 h at 4 °C.

2.5. LC-MS/MS Analysis

The LC-MS/MS system consisted of a Shiseido SP LC SP3202 binary pump HPLC system (Tokyo, Japan) and TSQ Quantum™ Access MAX Triple Quadrupole Mass Spectrometer (Thermo Fisher Scientific, Waltham, MA, USA), equipped with an electrospray ionization (ESI) source. Chromatographic separation was achieved on a Kinetex C18 column (3.0 × 100 mm, 2.6 µm; Phenomenex, Torrance, CA, USA) at a temperature of 40 °C. The HPLC mobile phases consisted of two solvents: (A) 0.1% acetic acid and (B) acetonitrile in 0.1% acetic acid. A linear gradient program was used with a flow rate of 0.2 mL/min. The initial mobile phase was set at 15% of solvent B and gradually increased to 90% in 3 min, kept at 90% for 1 min, and then followed by re-equilibrium for 3 min. Electrospray ionization (ESI) was performed in both positive and negative ion mode, with nitrogen as the nebulizing agent, spray voltage, sheath gas pressure, and aux gas pressure at optimal values of 3000, 60, and 20 (arbitrary units), respectively. The capillary temperature was 350 °C. Multiple reaction monitoring (MRM) detection was employed. The precursor–product ion pairs used in MRM mode are provided as supplementary data (Table S2).

2.6. Metabolic Ratio Calculation

The urinary caffeine and its metabolite concentrations were measured using the LC-MS/MS analysis. The resulting data were evaluated using the equations for the metabolic ratio calculation. The molar urinary ratios specific for each drug-metabolizing enzyme were calculated referring to the equations previously reported [4,10,17,18,20]. Thus, a higher metabolic ratio indicates a higher enzyme activity.

3. Results

3.1. LC-MS/MS

Caffeine, 1X, 7X, 17X, 37X, 13U, 17U, 37U, 137U, AAMU, and 1X* were ionized to yield the protonated molecular ions ($[M+H]^+$) at m/z 195.2, 167.1, 167.0, 181.2, 181.2, 197.2, 197.1, 197.1, 211.2, 199.2, and 174.1, respectively. Additionally, 3X, 13X, 1U, AFMU, and 1U* were ionized to yield the deprotonated molecular ions ($[M-H]^-$) at m/z 164.9, 179.1, 181.1, 225.1, and 188.1, respectively. Ion polarity switching was applied for the simultaneous detection of protonated and deprotonated ions. Water and acetonitrile were used as the mobile phase solutions; to increase the response of 1U, 0.1% acetic acid was added to both mobile phase solvents. Using the gradient elution, all the analytes were eluted within 5 min. The representative LC-MS/MS extracted ion chromatograms are provided in the supplementary data (Figure S1).

3.2. Method Validation

The calibration curves for each analyte were linear over each corresponding, selected concentration range, with correlation coefficient (r2) values greater than 0.99. The linear ranges for caffeine and its metabolites are presented in the supplementary data (Table S2). The LLOQ values for all analytes ranged from 10 ng/mL to 166 ng/mL with an accuracy of approximately 91.4% to 114.0% and a precision of ≤16.3%.

The intra-day precision was less than 16.4%, while the accuracy (as a percentage of relative error values) was within the range of ±11.9% at the tested QC concentrations. The inter-day assay also showed satisfactory accuracy and reproducibility, with a precision of less than 11.4%, and an accuracy within the range of ±14.0% at the tested QC levels. These results are summarized in Table 1.

The matrix effect was negligible for caffeine and its metabolites, except for 1X, 137U, and AAMU, which seemed to be affected by it. However, they showed acceptable RSD criteria (within ±15%). For recovery evaluation, caffeine and all its metabolites were stable and well recovered (%RSD, <10.6) from samples. The matrix effect and recovery data are provided in the supplementary data (Tables S3 and S4).

In all the tested conditions, caffeine and its metabolites were shown to be stable, with acceptable recovery (RSD within ±15%), except for the long-term stability of AAMU and AFMU (Table S5). The accuracy and RSD values were within ±12.4% and ±9.4% for freeze-and-thaw stability, within ±11.6% and ±9.7% for short-term stability, within ±12.3% and ±10.8% for long-term stability, and within ±12.1% and ±8.2% for processed sample stability. Meanwhile, the long-term stability of AAMU was 323.4%, and that of AFMU was 47.2%. AFMU is known to be spontaneously converted to AAMU, and the present results may reflect this phenomenon. According to Nyeki et al. [22], the conversion of AFMU into AAMU is not only subjected to nonenzymatic hydrolysis in urine, but is also NAT2 phenotype-dependent. Nevertheless, it would be better to analyze urine samples immediately after voiding to minimize errors in calculating the metabolite ratio for enzyme phenotyping.

Table 1. Intra-day and inter-day accuracy (A) and precision for the determination of caffeine and its metabolites

Analyte	Intra-Day Assay (n = 5)									Inter-Day Assay (n = 5)								
	LLOQ		Low QC		Middle QC		High QC		LLOQ		Low QC		Middle QC		High QC			
	A (%)	RSD (%)	A (%)	RSD (%)	A (%)	RSD (%)	A (%)	RSD (%)	A (%)	RSD (%)	A (%)	RSD (%)	A (%)	RSD (%)	A (%)	RSD (%)		
137U	106.3	3.0	115.0	1.1	104.2	1.1	108.7	0.9	108.6	8.1	113.0	3.5	104.7	5.9	106.3	1.9		
13X	102.4	16.3	94.0	4.9	100.4	5.2	101.5	4.1	91.4	10.8	91.2	4.5	94.3	6.7	96.0	11.0		
17X	109.0	3.3	112.4	2.4	101.8	2.5	101.1	9.6	109.4	3.0	110.0	3.8	108.6	4.0	100.4	1.7		
37X	102.5	4.6	105.2	3.8	98.2	3.6	99.4	5.2	106.5	7.4	100.8	4.1	104.9	3.3	101.5	2.6		
17U	102.6	2.0	102.9	9.9	86.6	1.6	95.7	4.7	106.4	11.4	90.5	6.8	87.0	2.0	95.0	3.3		
AFMU	103.4	8.1	96.8	4.8	98.9	1.8	89.1	5.5	95.0	5.6	92.5	3.9	95.6	4.0	89.1	2.2		
AAMU	111.9	7.7	107.4	5.6	105.3	4.5	101.0	7.0	106.0	6.8	106.6	5.6	103.0	2.7	107.4	4.1		
1U	104.3	3.3	101.0	1.9	102.8	7.3	88.7	2.4	114.0	6.3	105.2	6.8	107.5	7.8	88.1	1.8		
13U	104.7	11.4	96.4	9.7	113.3	1.1	108.0	2.3	110.9	4.7	99.3	9.3	114.3	0.5	111.7	2.6		
1X	104.4	6.0	108.7	5.8	101.9	1.3	102.2	7.2	106.0	7.0	100.7	10.3	101.0	3.7	96.8	6.2		
3X	101.7	12.9	101.5	3.9	102.4	9.1	104.3	5.9	97.0	2.9	97.2	9.4	98.2	7.8	107.7	4.3		
37U	96.3	6.1	97.1	5.1	102.7	11.7	101.9	1.7	102.4	4.2	100.0	6.3	97.4	8.3	100.0	5.5		
7X	108.6	2.1	103.4	7.7	98.7	2.0	101.0	7.2	103.3	6.3	106.1	3.7	100.2	9.6	97.2	6.3		
137X	92.8	8.7	107.3	3.9	103.7	9.9	103.5	6.6	93.4	7.4	108.9	8.4	110.1	3.0	105.5	9.5		

LLOQ: lower limits of quantitation, %RSD: percent relative standard deviation. QC: quality control.

3.3. Enzyme Phenotyping Based on Urinary Caffeine Metabolite Ratio

The urinary caffeine metabolite levels in the six subjects are as shown in Figure 2. When the six urine samples were analyzed, the targeted caffeine metabolites were successfully detected in most of the samples. The urinary concentration ranges of each metabolite were tabulated in Table 2. The measured metabolite concentrations exhibited large variations among individuals and time points. However, the concentration ranges were generally consistent with previously reported values [8].

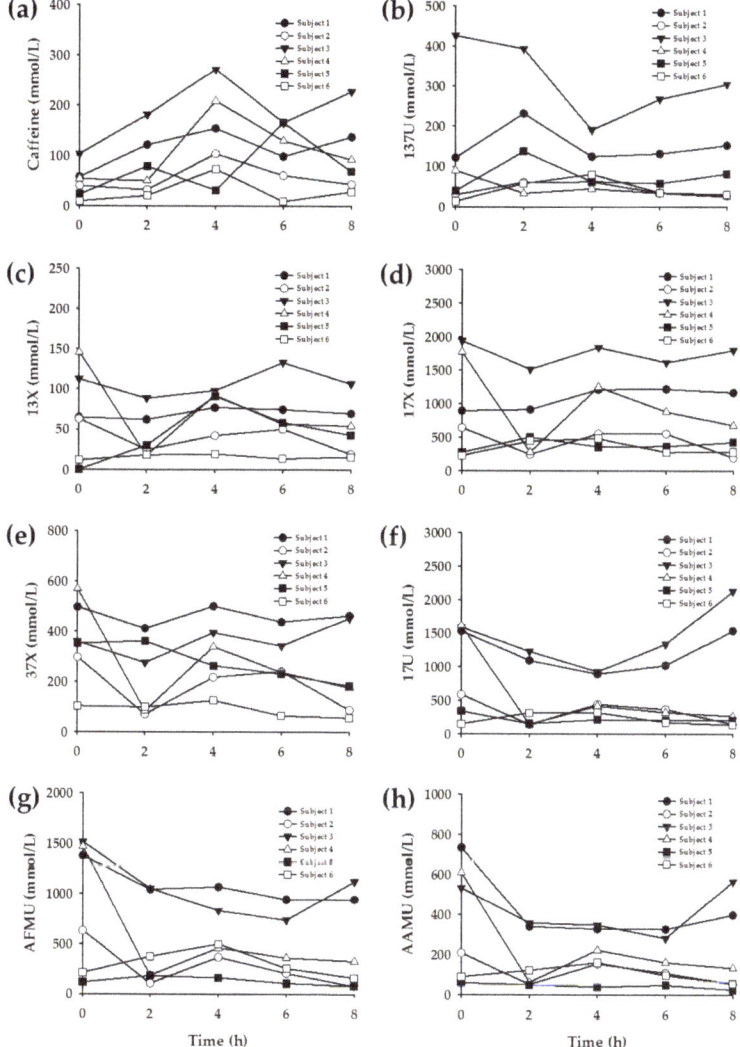

Figure 2. *Cont.*

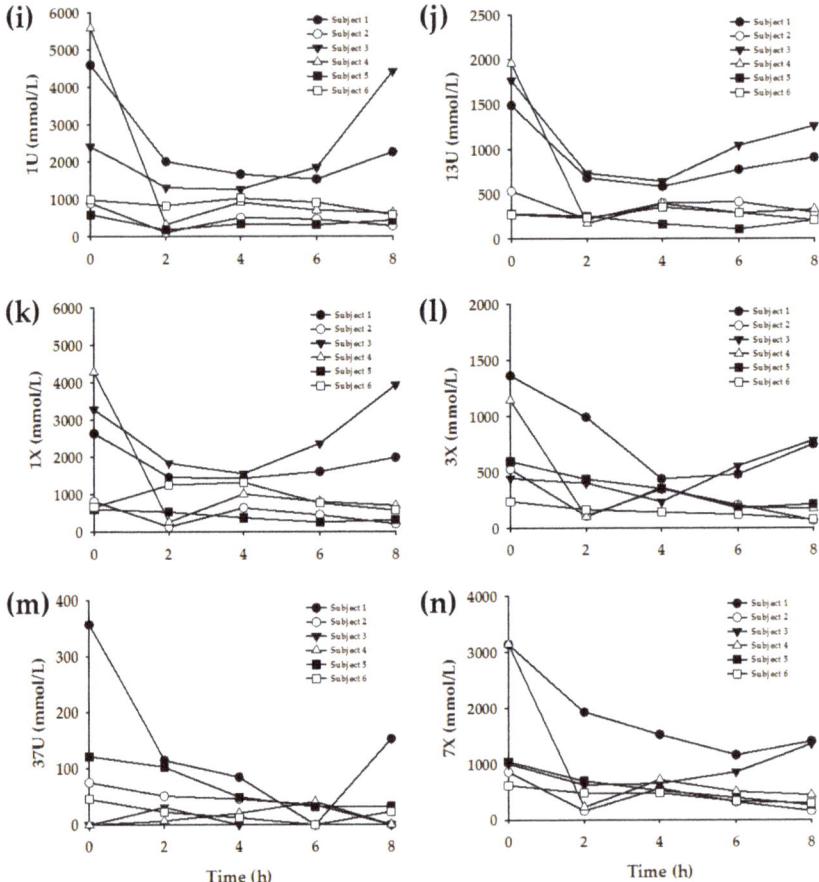

Figure 2. Urinary concentration levels of caffeine and its metabolites in six subjects. (**a**) caffeine, (**b**) 1,3,7-trimethyluric acid (137U), (**c**) 1,3-dimethylxanthine (13X), (**d**) 1,7-dimethylxanthine (17X), (**e**) 3,7-dimethylxanthine (37X), (**f**) 1,7-dimethyluric acid (17U), (**g**) 5-acetylamino-6-formylamino-3-methyluracil (AFMU), (**h**) 5-acetylamino-6-amino-3-methyluracil (AAMU), (**i**) 1-methyluric acid (1U), (**j**) 1,3-dimethyluric acid (13U), (**k**) 1-methylxanthine (1X), (**l**) 3-methylxanthine (3X), (**m**) 3,7-dimethyluric acid (37U), and (**n**) 7X.

Table 2. Urinary concentration ranges of caffeine and its metabolites.

Metabolite	Concentration Range (µM)	Metabolite	Concentration Range (µM)
137U	13.9–426.3	1U	104.5–5577.5
13X	0–145.9	13U	104.6–1957.9
17X	191.8–1941.3	1X	126.3–4273.4
37X	54.9–569.3	3X	65.2–1362.3
17U	131.6–2127.2	37U	0–357.2
AFMU	76.8–1514.9	7X	154.3–3145.5
AAMU	26.1–735.0	137X (caffeine)	8.7–271.7

Subsequently, enzyme-specific metabolite ratios were calculated based on the urinary concentration data. Referring to the extant literature, the urinary metabolite concentrations were applied to various equations to yield enzyme-specific metabolite ratios (Table 3). Figures 3–6 display the plots for each enzyme activity in individuals, which is expressed as the metabolite ratio. The metabolite ratio patterns varied between individuals and time points, depending on the equations applied, even for identical enzymes.

Table 3. Equations of caffeine metabolic ratios used for enzyme-specific activities.

Enzyme		Equation	Reference
CYP1A2	(a)	(AFMU + 1X + 1U + 17X + 17U)/137X	[4,17,18]
	(b)	(17X + 17U)/137X	[4]
	(c)	17X/137X	[4]
	(d)	(AAMU + 1X + 1U)/17U	[4]
	(e)	(AFMU + 1X + 1U)/17U	[4]
	(f)	(AFMU + 1X + 1U)/17X	[4]
	(g)	(AAMU + AFMU + 1X + 1U)/17U	[4]
CYP2A6	(a)	17U/(AFMU + 1U + 1X + 17X + 17U)	[4]
	(b)	17X/17U	[4]
NAT2	(a)	(AAMU + AFMU)/(AAMU + AFMU + 1X + 1U)	[4,10,20]
	(b)	AAMU/(AAMU + 1X + 1U)	[4]
	(c)	AFMU/(AFMU + 1X + 1U)	[4]
	(d)	AFMU/1X	[4]
XO	(a)	1U/1X + 1U	[4,20]
	(b)	1U/1X	[4]

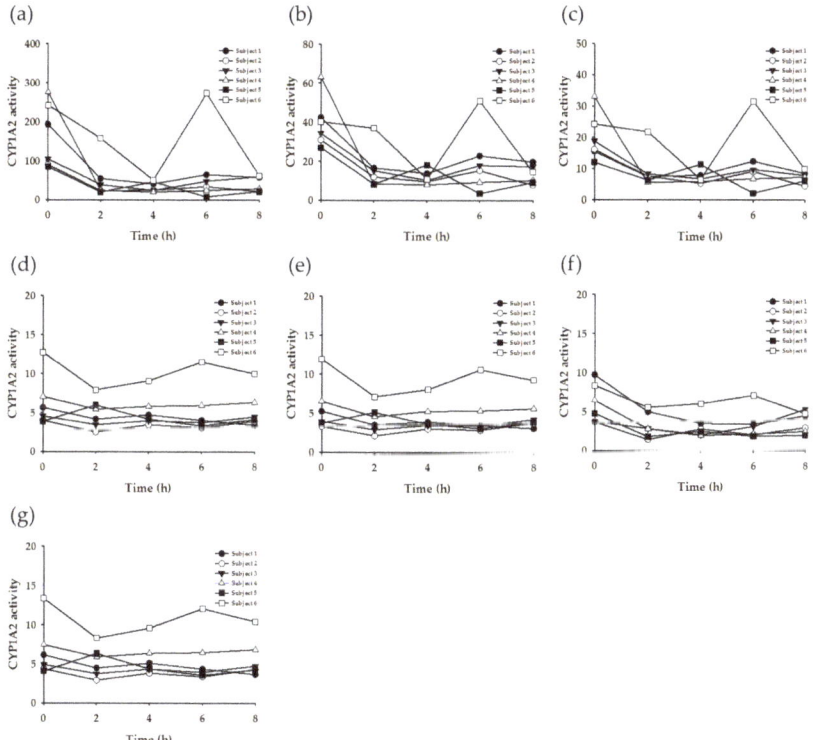

Figure 3. Plots of metabolite ratio for CYP1A2. The metabolic ratio equations used are as follows: (**a**) (AFMU + 1X + 1U + 17X + 17U)/137X, (**b**) (17X + 17U)/137X, (**c**) 17X/137X, (**d**) (AAMU + 1X + 1U)/17U, (**e**) (AFMU + 1X + 1U)/17U, (**f**) (AFMU+1X+1U)/17X, (**g**) (AAMU+AFMU+1X+1U)/17U.

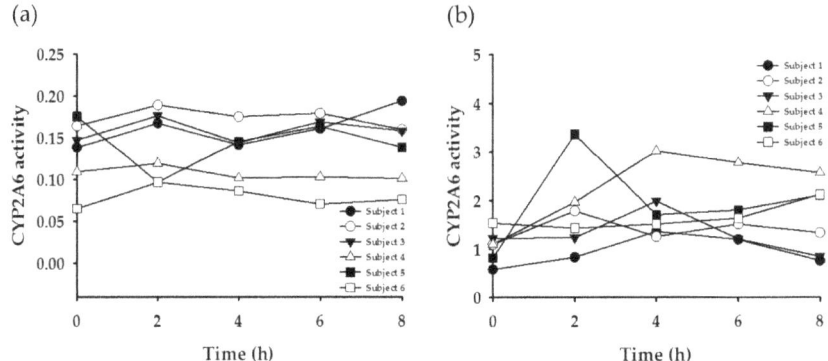

Figure 4. Plots of metabolite ratio for CYP2A6. The metabolic ratio equations used are as follows: (**a**) 17U/(AFMU + 1U + 1X + 17X + 17U), (**b**) 17X/17U.

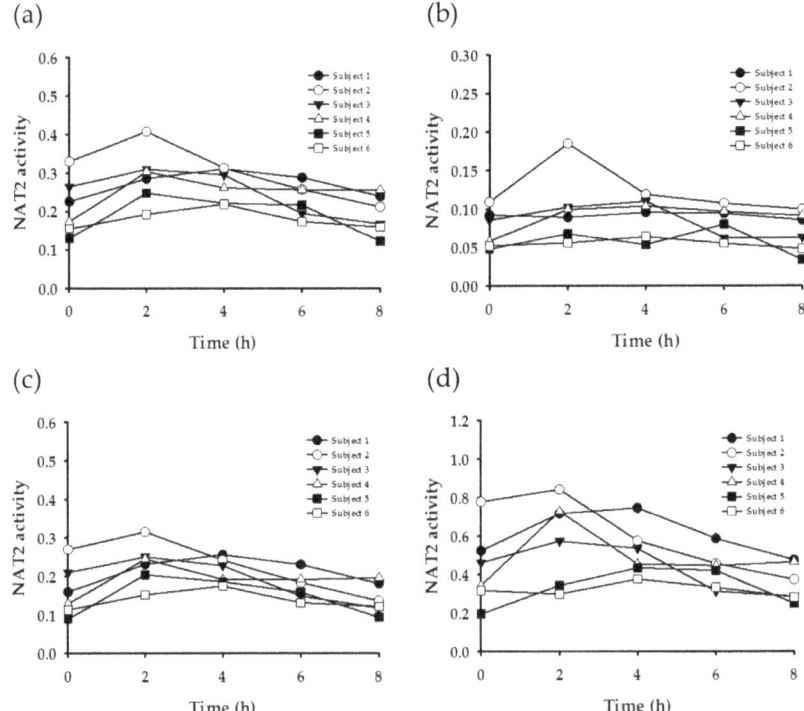

Figure 5. Plots of metabolite ratio for NAT2. The metabolic ratio equations used are as follows: (**a**) (AAMU+AFMU)/(AAMU+AFMU+1X+1U), (**b**) AAMU/(AAMU+1X+1U), (**c**) AFMU/(AFMU+1X+1U), (**d**) AFMU/1X.

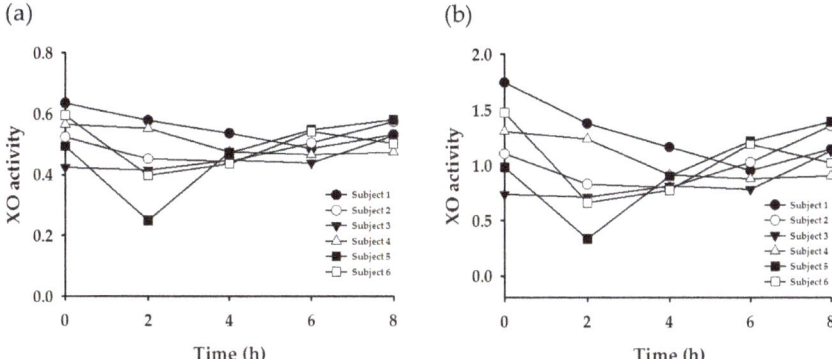

Figure 6. Plots of metabolite ratio for XO. The metabolic ratio equations used are as follows: (a) 1U/1X + 1U, (b) 1U/1X.

To investigate the CYP1A2 phenotypes, seven equations were tested. The resulting metabolic ratio plots are shown in Figure 3. Figure 3a–c exhibited a considerable difference between pre-dose (0 h) and post-dose data. The metabolic ratio patterns of Subject #6 were generally different from those of other subjects.

To investigate the CYP2A6 phenotypes, two equations were tested (Figure 4). Figure 4a generally showed constant metabolite ratio patterns within individuals (except for Subject #5) over all of the time points. However, Figure 4b showed a larger variation according to time. The order of the metabolite ratio values for all six subjects (i.e., the relative metabolic activity) was not consistent between two plots.

NAT2 activity was tested with four different equations. Three equations (Figure 5a–c) generated similar metabolite ratio patterns, whereas the other (Figure 5d) showed a large variation between individuals and time points.

The XO activity was evaluated using two equations. The metabolite ratio plots are shown in Figure 6. The resultant patterns were generally similar between the two plots, but the variation was larger in plot (b).

4. Discussion

This study measured the urinary concentrations of caffeine and its 13 metabolites for 8 h, including a pre-dose time point, using LC-MS/MS. The metabolic ratios for phenotyping the drug metabolizing enzymes were calculated based on the various equations previously reported. Subsequently, the resulting metabolic ratios or patterns were compared, and their validity and feasibility were investigated.

The resulting urinary caffeine concentration data showed a relatively obvious increase and decrease pattern across time, which indicated the absorption and elimination of caffeine after oral intake. Meanwhile, the changes in caffeine metabolite concentration levels, according to time points, were not as evident as those of caffeine. However, caffeine metabolites also showed a weak pattern of slow increase after caffeine intake, on excluding the data at pre-dose. Most metabolites showed the highest concentrations at pre-dose, which was presumably due to the urine concentration. Thus, the urine was diluted in post-dose samples, as the urine was frequently collected (i.e., at 2-h intervals) after caffeine intake; meanwhile, at pre-dose, the caffeine metabolites, which resulted from usual dietary caffeine intake, could be detected at higher concentrations in relatively concentrated urine.

The most diverse equations have been suggested to determine the enzyme activity of CYP1A2 in previous research. This study applied seven equations to yield the metabolite ratio. Among them, three equations (Figure 3a–c) showed a significant difference between pre-dose (0 h) and post-dose data, and the within-individual variation was large according to the time points. Meanwhile, the other four plots showed a more constant ratio pattern within individuals. The caffeine (137X) concentration was included in the former three equations (Table 3: Equations CYP1A2-(a), (b), and (c)). Accordingly, the activity showed a large difference in the results between pre-dose and post-dose. However, the other equations showed relatively constant results over time, even between pre-dose and post-dose measurements, as those equations did not involve caffeine concentration. Generally, the CYP1A2 activity of Subject #6 appeared to be higher than that of the other subjects, but plot F (Figure 2f) did not exhibit this tendency. These findings suggest that Equations CYP1A2-(d), (e), and (g) (Table 3) may be more appropriate for determining the CYP1A2 phenotype.

Acetylation is a primary route for the biotransformation of many hydrazine drugs, which is mediated by NAT [4]. The polymorphism of NAT (in particular, NAT2) is responsible for the inter-individual variability in the acetylation of drugs. Thus, the population can be categorized into rapid acetylators and slow acetylators, according to their NAT2 phenotypes [6]. Such acetylation polymorphism is reported to vary among ethnic groups [6]. It is known that rapid acetylators are dominant in the Korean population [23]. In the present study, when the metabolite ratios were calculated by the equation (AFMU + AAMU)/(AFMU + AAMU + 1X + 1U) (corresponding to Figure 4a) and evaluated by the criteria reported by Jetter et al. [10,20], the six subjects tested in this study were determined to be rapid acetylators. This seems to be reasonable based on the generally recognized facts on acetylation polymorphism in Koreans. However, when evaluated by the criteria based on other equations, such as AFMU/(AFMU + 1U + 1X) or AAMU/(AAMU + 1U + 1X) [7,13,24], these six subjects were shown to be slow acetylators. Therefore, to determine the phenotypes exactly, comprehensive genotyping data is necessary.

Meanwhile, the time point for sample collection may affect the metabolic ratio results, as the rate of metabolic reaction may be different depending on each metabolic pathway. Jetter et al. (2009) reported that the timing of urine collection can affect XO phenotyping results [20]. However, this study's data, generated from the same equation [1U/(1U + 1X)] (Figure 5a), did not show a significant variation according to the urine collection time, except in Subject #5. This suggests the possibility that spot urine samples, under normal dietary conditions, can be used for XO phenotyping.

Recently, research on polymorphism and personalized medicine has been extensive. Genotyping and phenotyping for drug metabolizing enzymes are vital strategies for characterizing the polymorphism of drug-metabolizing enzymes in individuals for personalized medicine. However, evaluating the phenotype is more critical than evaluating the genotype in some enzymes. For example, XO is a form of xanthine oxidoreductase, which is a type of enzyme that generates reactive oxygen species [25]. These enzymes catalyze the oxidation of hypoxanthine to xanthine and can further catalyze the oxidation of xanthine to uric acid. Xanthine oxidase plays a crucial role in many drug metabolic processes, such as thiopurine drugs, containing 6-mercaptopurine, allopurinol, and uric acid, etc. [26–29]. Xanthine oxidase is important in gout patients, because XO produces uric acid, which is a crucial factor in gout. In addition, xanthine oxidase is involved in the catabolism of xenobiotics; for example, it converts a prodrug (mercaptopurine) into the active form 6-thioinosine-5′triphosphate [30]. About 20 genetic variants are reported, and each XO variant may differ in its enzymatic activity [20]; however, decreased enzyme activity is shown only in 4% or fewer volunteers [31]. Thus, it would be difficult to explain the cause of the variations in XO activity on the basis of genetic polymorphisms alone [20]. Therefore, it is meaningful to establish an optimized method for assessing the activity of the drug-metabolizing enzymes, including XO, for phenotyping.

Meanwhile, it has been recognized that differences in the activity of enzymes involved in nicotine metabolism are partly responsible for inter-individual variation in lung cancer risk among smokers [32–35]. CYP2A6 is a principal enzyme in nicotine metabolism, and CYP2A6-mediated C-oxidase activity has been reported to correlate with exposure to carcinogens by smoking [32–35]. Many reports have demonstrated that CYP2A6 variants that exert reduced enzymatic activity are associated with lower lung cancer risk [32–35]. However, these genetic polymorphisms are reported to account for only a portion of the variation in CYP2A6 activity [4]. Therefore, the phenotyping of CYP2A6 activity could be more appropriate for estimating lung cancer risk related to nicotine metabolism. In this context, the urinary caffeine metabolite ratio is a useful biomarker for predicting the risk of lung cancer.

The limitations of this study are its small sample size, the lack of genotyping data, and that this data was obtained from a single set of experiments. Nevertheless, this study enables the evaluation of phenotyping results by demonstrating the caffeine metabolite ratio plots generated from different phenotyping equations. In addition, the data obtained at different time points, including the pre-dose and post-dose suggests the possibility that the enzyme phenotyping for CYP1A2, CYP2A6, NAT2, and XO can be conducted as a routine urine test, without the administration of drugs.

5. Conclusions

Caffeine is popularly present in a wide variety of foods and beverages, and is extensively consumed via the daily diet. By measuring the exposure to caffeine in biological samples, such as the urine, the extent of caffeine consumption could be directly indicated. However, caffeine can be also used as a biomarker to indicate the activities of drug-metabolizing enzymes. This study demonstrated the possibility that enzyme phenotyping based on urinary caffeine metabolite ratios can be routinely used under general dietary conditions. This suggests a possibility for urinary caffeine metabolite analysis as a routine clinical examination. Urinary caffeine and its metabolite analysis would be useful in evaluating drug metabolic phenotypes for personalized medicine.

Supplementary Materials: The following are available online at http://www.mdpi.com/2072-6643/11/8/1947/s1, Figure S1: Representative LC-MS/MS extracted ion chromatograms for caffeine and its metabolites in human urine at 2 h after administration of caffeine-containing drink, Table S1: Concentrations of quality control standards for caffeine and its metabolites, Table S2: Calibration range, retention time and multiple reactions monitoring data for caffeine and its metabolites, Table S3: Matrix effect data for caffeine and its metabolites, Table S4: Recovery data for caffeine and its metabolites, Table S5: Stability of caffeine and its metabolites in various conditions.

Author Contributions: Conceptualization, H.H.Y. and K.N.; methodology, H.J.K.; validation, H.J.K.; investigation, H.J.K., Y.S.J., J.S.Y and M.S.C.; data curation, M.S.C.; writing—original draft preparation, H.J.K. and S.U.R.; writing—review and editing, H.H.Y. and M.S.C.; supervision, H.H.Y.; funding acquisition, H.H.Y.

Funding: This research was supported by the National Research Foundation of Korea funded by the Korean government (NRF-2017R1A2B4001814).

Conflicts of Interest: The authors declare no conflict of interest.

References

1. Ashihara, H.; Sano, H.; Crozier, A. Caffeine and related purine alkaloids: Biosynthesis, catabolism, function and genetic engineering. *Phytochemistry* **2008**, *69*, 841–856. [CrossRef] [PubMed]
2. Butt, M.S.; Sultan, M.T. Coffee and its consumption: Benefits and risks. *Crit. Rev. Food Sci. Nutr.* **2011**, *51*, 363–373. [CrossRef] [PubMed]
3. Juliano, L.M.; Ferre, S.; Griffiths, R.R. The pharmacology of caffeine. In *The ASAM Principles of Addiction Medicine*, 5th ed.; Wolters Kluwer Health Adis (ESP): Alphen aan den Rijn, The Netherlands, 2014.
4. Hakooz, N.M. Caffeine metabolic ratios for the in vivo evaluation of CYP1A2, N-acetyltransferase 2, xanthine oxidase and CYP2A6 enzymatic activities. *Curr. Drug Metab.* **2009**, *10*, 329–338. [CrossRef] [PubMed]
5. Kot, M.; Daniel, W.A. Caffeine as a marker substrate for testing cytochrome P450 activity in human and rat. *Pharmacol. Rep.* **2008**, *60*, 789–797. [PubMed]
6. Miners, J.O.; Birkett, D.J. The use of caffeine as a metabolic probe for human drug metabolizing enzymes. *Gen. Pharmacol.* **1996**, *27*, 245–249. [CrossRef]
7. Begas, E.; Kouvaras, E.; Tsakalof, A.; Papakosta, S.; Asprodini, E.K. In vivo evaluation of CYP1A2, CYP2A6, NAT-2 and xanthine oxidase activities in a Greek population sample by the RP-HPLC monitoring of caffeine metabolic ratios. *Biomed. Chromatogr.* **2007**, *21*, 190–200. [CrossRef] [PubMed]
8. Caubet, M.S.; Comte, B.; Brazier, J.L. Determination of urinary 13C-caffeine metabolites by liquid chromatography-mass spectrometry: The use of metabolic ratios to assess CYP1A2 activity. *J. Pharm. Biomed. Anal.* **2004**, *34*, 379–389. [CrossRef]

9. Chung, W.G.; Kang, J.H.; Park, C.S.; Cho, M.H.; Cha, Y.N. Effect of age and smoking on in vivo CYP1A2, flavin-containing monooxygenase, and xanthine oxidase activities in Koreans: Determination by caffeine metabolism. *Clin. Pharmacol. Ther.* **2000**, *67*, 258–266. [CrossRef] [PubMed]
10. Jetter, A.; Kinzig-Schippers, M.; Illauer, M.; Hermann, R.; Erb, K.; Borlak, J.; Wolf, H.; Smith, G.; Cascorbi, I.; Sorgel, F.; et al. Phenotyping of N-acetyltransferase type 2 by caffeine from uncontrolled dietary exposure. *Eur. J. Clin. Pharmacol.* **2004**, *60*, 17–21. [CrossRef]
11. Marchei, E.; Pellegrini, M.; Pacifici, R.; Palmi, I.; Pichini, S. Development and validation of a high-performance liquid chromatography-mass spectrometry assay for methylxanthines and taurine in dietary supplements. *J. Pharm. Biomed. Anal.* **2005**, *37*, 499–507. [CrossRef]
12. Nordmark, A.; Lundgren, S.; Cnattingius, S.; Rane, A. Dietary caffeine as a probe agent for assessment of cytochrome P4501A2 activity in random urine samples. *Br. J. Clin. Pharmacol.* **1999**, *47*, 397–402. [CrossRef] [PubMed]
13. Rybak, M.E.; Pao, C.I.; Pfeiffer, C.M. Determination of urine caffeine and its metabolites by use of high-performance liquid chromatography-tandem mass spectrometry: Estimating dietary caffeine exposure and metabolic phenotyping in population studies. *Anal. Bioanal. Chem.* **2014**, *406*, 771–784. [CrossRef]
14. Schneider, H.; Ma, L.; Glatt, H. Extractionless method for the determination of urinary caffeine metabolites using high-performance liquid chromatography coupled with tandem mass spectrometry. *J. Chromatogr. B Analyt. Technol. Biomed. Life Sci.* **2003**, *789*, 227–237. [CrossRef]
15. Thevis, M.; Opfermann, G.; Krug, O.; Schanzer, W. Electrospray ionization mass spectrometric characterization and quantitation of xanthine derivatives using isotopically labelled analogues: An application for equine doping control analysis. *Rapid Commun. Mass Spectrom.* **2004**, *18*, 1553–1560. [CrossRef] [PubMed]
16. Weimann, A.; Sabroe, M.; Poulsen, H.E. Measurement of caffeine and five of the major metabolites in urine by high-performance liquid chromatography/tandem mass spectrometry. *J. Mass Spectrom.* **2005**, *40*, 307–316. [CrossRef]
17. Aklillu, E.; Carrillo, J.A.; Makonnen, E.; Hellman, K.; Pitarque, M.; Bertilsson, L.; Ingelman-Sundberg, M. Genetic polymorphism of CYP1A2 in Ethiopians affecting induction and expression: Characterization of novel haplotypes with single-nucleotide polymorphisms in intron 1. *Mol. Pharmacol.* **2003**, *64*, 659–669. [CrossRef]
18. Carrillo, J.A.; Benitez, J. Caffeine metabolism in a healthy Spanish population: N-acetylator phenotype and oxidation pathways. *Clin. Pharmacol. Ther.* **1994**, *55*, 293–304. [CrossRef]
19. De Kesel, P.M.; Lambert, W.E.; Stove, C.P. Paraxanthine/Caffeine Concentration Ratios in Hair: An Alternative for Plasma-Based Phenotyping of Cytochrome P450 1A2? *Clin. Pharmacokinet.* **2015**, *54*, 771–781. [CrossRef]
20. Jetter, A.; Kinzig, M.; Rodamer, M.; Tomalik-Scharte, D.; Sorgel, F.; Fuhr, U. Phenotyping of N-acetyltransferase type 2 and xanthine oxidase with caffeine: When should urine samples be collected? *Eur. J. Clin. Pharmacol.* **2009**, *65*, 411–417. [CrossRef]
21. Bioanalytical Method Validation: Guidance for Industry. Available online: https://www.fda.gov/downloads/drugs/guidances/ucm070107.pdf (accessed on 19 August 2018).
22. Nyeki, A.; Buclin, T.; Biollaz, J.; Decosterd, L.A. NAT2 and CYP1A2 phenotyping with caffeine: Head-to-head comparison of AFMU vs. AAMU in the urine metabolite ratios. *Br. J. Clin. Pharmacol.* **2003**, *55*, 62–67. [CrossRef] [PubMed]
23. Kang, T.S.; Jin, S.K.; Lee, J.E.; Woo, S.W.; Roh, J. Comparison of genetic polymorphisms of the NAT2 gene between Korean and four other ethnic groups. *J. Clin. Pharm. Ther.* **2009**, *34*, 709–718. [CrossRef] [PubMed]
24. Rihs, H.P.; John, A.; Scherenberg, M.; Seidel, A.; Bruning, T. Concordance between the deduced acetylation status generated by high-speed: Real-time PCR based NAT2 genotyping of seven single nucleotide polymorphisms and human NAT2 phenotypes determined by a caffeine assay. *Clin. Chim. Acta* **2007**, *376*, 240–243. [CrossRef] [PubMed]
25. Ardan, T.; Kovaceva, J.; Cejkova, J. Comparative histochemical and immunohistochemical study on xanthine oxidoreductase/xanthine oxidase in mammalian corneal epithelium. *Acta Histochem.* **2004**, *106*, 69–75. [CrossRef] [PubMed]
26. de Araujo, M.; Franco, Y.E.M.; Alberto, T.G.; Messias, M.C.F.; Leme, C.W.; Sawaya, A.; Carvalho, P.O. Kinetic study on the inhibition of xanthine oxidase by acylated derivatives of flavonoids synthesised enzymatically. *J. Enzyme Inhib. Med. Chem.* **2017**, *32*, 978–985. [CrossRef] [PubMed]

27. Kitamura, S.; Sugihara, K.; Ohta, S. Drug-metabolizing ability of molybdenum hydroxylases. *Drug Metab. Pharmacokinet.* **2006**, *21*, 83–98. [CrossRef] [PubMed]
28. Pacher, P.; Nivorozhkin, A.; Szabo, C. Therapeutic effects of xanthine oxidase inhibitors: Renaissance half a century after the discovery of allopurinol. *Pharmacol. Rev.* **2006**, *58*, 87–114. [CrossRef] [PubMed]
29. Pritsos, C.A. Cellular distribution, metabolism and regulation of the xanthine oxidoreductase enzyme system. *Chem. Biol. Interact.* **2000**, *129*, 195–208. [CrossRef]
30. Choughule, K.V.; Barnaba, C.; Joswig-Jones, C.A.; Jones, J.P. In vitro oxidative metabolism of 6-mercaptopurine in human liver: Insights into the role of the molybdoflavoenzymes aldehyde oxidase, xanthine oxidase, and xanthine dehydrogenase. *Drug Metab. Dispos.* **2014**, *42*, 1334–1340. [CrossRef] [PubMed]
31. Aklillu, E.; Carrillo, J.A.; Makonnen, E.; Bertilsson, L.; Ingelman-Sundberg, M. Xanthine oxidase activity is influenced by environmental factors in Ethiopians. *Eur. J. Clin. Pharmacol.* **2003**, *59*, 533–536. [CrossRef]
32. Park, S.L.; Murphy, S.E.; Wilkens, L.R.; Stram, D.O.; Hecht, S.S.; Le Marchand, L. Association of CYP2A6 activity with lung cancer incidence in smokers: The multiethnic cohort study. *PLoS ONE* **2017**, *12*, e0178435. [CrossRef] [PubMed]
33. Soeroso, N.N.; Zain-Hamid, R.; Sinaga, B.Y.M.; Sadewa, A.H.; Syafiuddin, T.; Syahruddin, E.; Tann, G.; Mutiara, E. Genetic Polymorphism of CYP2A6 and Its Relationship with Nicotine Metabolism in Male Bataknese Smokers Suffered from Lung Cancer in Indonesia. *Open Access Maced. J. Med. Sci.* **2018**, *6*, 1199–1205. [CrossRef] [PubMed]
34. Tanner, J.A.; Henderson, J.A.; Buchwald, D.; Howard, B.V.; Nez Henderson, P.; Tyndale, R.F. Variation in CYP2A6 and nicotine metabolism among two American Indian tribal groups differing in smoking patterns and risk for tobacco-related cancer. *Pharmacogenet. Genom.* **2017**, *27*, 169–178. [CrossRef] [PubMed]
35. Yuan, J.M.; Nelson, H.H.; Carmella, S.G.; Wang, R.; Kuriger-Laber, J.; Jin, A.; Adams-Haduch, J.; Hecht, S.S.; Koh, W.P.; Murphy, S.E. CYP2A6 genetic polymorphisms and biomarkers of tobacco smoke constituents in relation to risk of lung cancer in the Singapore Chinese Health Study. *Carcinogenesis* **2017**, *38*, 411–418. [CrossRef] [PubMed]

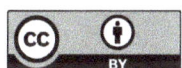

© 2019 by the authors. Licensee MDPI, Basel, Switzerland. This article is an open access article distributed under the terms and conditions of the Creative Commons Attribution (CC BY) license (http://creativecommons.org/licenses/by/4.0/).

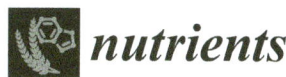

Article

The Effects of High Peripubertal Caffeine Exposure on the Adrenal Gland in Immature Male and Female Rats

Ki-Young Ryu [1] and Jaesook Roh [2,*]

[1] Department of Obstetrics and Gynecology, College of Medicine, Hanyang University, Seoul 133-791, Korea; drryuky@hanyang.ac.kr
[2] Dept. of Anatomy and Cell Biology, College of Medicine, Hanyang University, Seoul 133-791, Korea
* Correspondence: rohjaesook@hanyang.ac.kr; Tel.: +82-2-2220-0609

Received: 3 April 2019; Accepted: 24 April 2019; Published: 26 April 2019

Abstract: The consumption of high levels of dietary caffeine has increased in children and adolescents. Human and animal studies have shown that chronic intake of high doses of caffeine affects serum glucocorticoid levels. Given that glucocorticoids play a role in peripubertal organ growth and development, chronic high doses of caffeine during puberty might impair maturation of the adrenal glands. To evaluate any effects of caffeine exposure on growing adrenal glands, 22-day-old male ($n = 30$) and female Sprague Dawley rats ($n = 30$) were divided into three groups ($n = 10$/group); group 1 received tap water (control) and groups 2 and 3 received water containing 120 and 180 mg/kg/day caffeine, respectively, via gavage for 4 weeks. At the end of the experiment, adrenal glands were weighed and processed for histological analysis. Relative adrenal weights increased in both groups of caffeine-fed males and females, whereas absolute weights were decreased in the females. In the female caffeine-fed groups the adrenal cortical areas resembled irregularly arranged cords and the medullary area was significantly increased, whereas no such effects were seen in the male rats. Our results indicate that the harmful effects of caffeine on the adrenal glands of immature rats differ between females and males. Although female rats seemed to be more susceptible to damage based on the changes in the microarchitecture of the adrenal glands, caffeine affected corticosterone production in both female and male rats. In addition, increased basal adrenocorticotropic hormone levels in caffeine-fed groups may reflect decreased cortical function. Therefore, caffeine may induce an endocrine imbalance that disturbs the establishment of the hypothalamo–pituitary adrenal axis during puberty, thereby leading to abnormal stress responses.

Keywords: adrenal gland; caffeine; corticosterone; puberty; rat; sex-difference

1. Introduction

Energy drinks have become a popular source of caffeine, and most of them contain between three and five times the amount of caffeine found in other soft drinks [1]. Caffeine intake has been increasing rapidly in children and adolescents due to regular consumption of energy drinks [2,3], but the majority of studies on caffeine effects have been conducted in adults.

It is known that chronic stress alters the thickness of the cortical and medullary areas and the secretory response to adrenocorticotropic hormone (ACTH) in rats [4]. In addition, a number of xenobiotics produce hypertrophic or atrophic changes in the cortex or medulla [5]. Moreover, caffeine has also been viewed as causing stress [6,7]. This suggests that it could induce morphological changes in the adrenal glands. Clinical and experimental studies suggest that caffeine affects the function and morphology of the adrenal glands. For instance, prenatal exposure of rats to caffeine inhibits glucocorticoid production and reduces the size of the adrenal cortical zone in male offspring; it also leads to a disorganized arrangement of cells and cellular swelling [8,9]. In contrast, in adult humans and animals, high doses of caffeine elevate glucocorticoid levels in a stress-like pattern of endocrine responses [6,7]. Most studies have focused on prenatal exposure, because the adrenal gland plays a pivotal role in the regulation of intrauterine homeostasis and fetal development [10]. Since children have immature adrenal glands with cortical and medullary areas of significantly increased thickness [11,12], their responses to stressors may differ from those at other stages of life. However, it is not known whether caffeine consumption affects the morphometric characteristics of the adrenal glands during puberty.

Data on the effects of caffeine on the adrenal gland during puberty are sparse and conflicting [6,13]. Because puberty is a critical period for the completion of adrenal zonation and the establishment of pituitary responsiveness to corticotrophin-releasing hormone [11,12], its vulnerability to insults seems to be greater than that of adults. In addition, corticosterone release in response to stress is more delayed in immature animals than in adults, but more prolonged [14]. Therefore, the responses of children and adolescents to caffeine exposure might differ from those of adults. Although glucocorticoid secretion under stress is a beneficial response, constant prolonged secretion due to chronic stressful episodes may lead to dysregulation of the hypothalamic–pituitary–adrenal axis and cause pathologic conditions [15].

There is much concern about the impact on human health of environmental chemicals that are able to interfere with the endocrine system, particularly those that affect steroidogenesis. Previously, we showed that caffeine acts as an endocrine disruptor of the reproductive system in both immature male and female rats owing to its effects on sex hormone levels [16,17]. In addition, some of the effects of caffeine on gonadal sex steroid production in immature rats are sex specific [16,17]. In addition, sex differences in susceptibility to caffeine during both gestation and lactation have been reported in the offspring of rats [18]. Therefore, the aim of the present study was to investigate the effects of high doses of caffeine exposure during puberty on the growth and secretory activity of the adrenal cortex, and to identify sex-specific differences in susceptibility between immature male and female rats. After exposing the rats to caffeine, their adrenal glands were weighed, and histological analyses were performed. In addition, serum corticosterone and ACTH levels were analyzed to identify any effects of caffeine on adrenal cortical hormone production.

2. Materials and Methods

2.1. Animal

Sixty immature male and female Sprague Dawley rats were obtained at 17 days of age along with their mothers from Samtako Biokorea (Kyunggi, South Korea) and were allowed to acclimate under controlled humidity (40–50%), temperature (22–24 °C), and light conditions (12 h light-dark cycle). Animal care was consistent with institutional guidelines, and the Hanyang University Animal Care and Use Committee approved all procedures involving animals (HY-IACUC-2013-0110A). All animals were housed individually the day after weaning at 21 days of age and were fed standard rat chow ad libitum. The experiment was started when the rats were 22 days old, as postnatal days (PD) 22–25 are considered the beginning of sexual maturation in rats [19].

2.2. Experimental Design

Ten animals were assigned to each of three groups based on their mean body weights to obtain an even distribution. Caffeine (Sigma-Aldrich, St. Louis, MO, USA) was dissolved in distilled water (10 mL/kg) at concentrations calculated to deliver 120 and 180 mg/kg body weight/day (these caffeine groups are designated CF1 and CF2, respectively) and administered by gavage to ensure complete consumption of the established daily dose in the morning (9 to 11 a.m.). The control group (CT) received distilled water daily for 4 weeks. The choice of dose levels was based on the literature, coupled with range finding studies to avoid sub-lethal effects at the highest dose [10,16].

Animals were examined for any treatment-related clinical signs and weighed daily. Body weight was measured to the nearest 0.1 g with an electronic scale (Dretec Corp., Seoul, South Korea) and recorded from the day before the start of feeding of caffeine for the four weeks of treatment. All the animals were killed 24 h after their last treatment, using established protocols and ethical procedures. Terminal blood samples were collected by heart puncture, and sera were stored at −70 °C.

2.3. Weighing the Adrenal Glands

The adrenals were dissected and cleaned of fat and connective tissue. They were then weighed to the nearest 0.001 g with an electronic scale (Adventurer™ electronic balance, AR1530, OHAUS Corp., Parsippany, NJ, USA) and their gross morphology was evaluated. Then, both adrenals were fixed in 10% buffered formalin (pH 7) for histological analysis.

2.4. Histological Analysis of the Adrenal Glands

Immediately after removal, both adrenals from each animal were processed for paraffin embedding and sectioning. Serial sections of 5 μm thickness were cut from the mid-portion of the adrenals and stained with hematoxylin and eosin. All histomorphometric evaluations were performed by the same trained and blinded examiner using an image analysis system (Leica LAS software, Heidelberg, Germany) coupled to a light microscope (DM4000B, Leica, Heidelberg, Germany) with final magnifications of 100× or 200×. Ten serial sections were traced for each adrenal gland, and the areas of the cortex and medulla in the same sections were measured and mean values calculated. In addition, four serial sections per animal were traced for each adrenal, and numbers of cortical cells, foamy cells, dilated sinusoids, and cell cords of zona fasciculata were counted within the same defined region (0.307277 mm^2) at 200-fold magnification. For convenience, we considered sinusoids as dilated when their widths were wider than those of cell cords, and the cell cord was defined as at least six cells being regularly aligned and spanning the longitudinal diameter of the zone. The mean value of 5 measurements per section was calculated for each adrenal and combined to obtain a mean value per animal. And then the mean value was calculated for each group.

2.5. Hormone Measurement

Corticosterone and ACTH levels were analyzed in serum samples using commercially available enzyme-linked immunosorbent assay (ELISA) kits (for corticosterone, KGE009, R&D Systems, Inc., Minneapolis, MN, USA) (for ACTH, CSB-E06875r, Cusabio Biotech Co., Ltd., Wuhan, China). The intra- and inter-assay coefficients of variance for corticosterone and ACTH were less than 15%, and the limit of detection was 0.1 ng/mL for corticosterone and 1.25 pg/mL for ACTH under the conditions of our test. Absorbance was read at 450 nm within 15 min against a blanking well in an ELISA Reader (Bio-Rad, Hercules, CA, USA). All samples were run in duplicate.

2.6. Statistical Analysis

Data for each group are expressed as means with standard deviations (SD). All data were analyzed using SPSS version 10.0 for Windows (SPSS Inc., Chicago, IL, USA) The distributions of body weight, adrenal weight and area, hormone levels, and histological data were analyzed for normality using the Shapiro–Wilk test. Then one-way ANOVA (analysis of variance) or the Kruskal–Wallis test was used to compare the control and caffeine groups in both male and female rats. Adrenal weights and cortical or medullary areas were compared in male and female rats by the Mann–Whitney U-test or unpaired t-tests. In all cases, significant differences were followed by post-hoc analysis (Tukey or Dunnett's test). Significance was accepted at $p < 0.05$.

3. Results

3.1. Body Weight Change

The body weights of the rats were checked at the beginning of the experiment, and no difference between the groups was observed (CT, 54.86 g; CF1, 54.8 g; CF2, 53.44 g in female rats) (CT, 53.05 g; CF1, 52.7 g; CF2, 52.64 g in male rats). Throughout the experimental period, there were no treatment-related undue clinical toxicity indicators such as ungroomed appearance, decreased fecal output, altered fecal consistency, or excess salivation. The data are summarized in Figure 1. The body weights of all animals increased continuously during the experiment. After 4 weeks, the body weights of the female and male rats had increased by approximately 3.7- and 4.6-fold, respectively, whereas in the caffeine-fed female and male rats, body weights were 0.8-fold of the control. One-way ANOVA revealed that both caffeine doses reduced body-weight increase in female and male rats, starting from about the first week of exposure (females, F = 15.1, 24.5, 23.9, and 16.8 for 1st, 2nd, 3rd, and 4th week, $p < 0.0001$) (post hoc Tukey analysis, $p < 0.0001$ vs. CT in females) (males, F = 32.7, 48.4, 65.1, and 67.9, for 1st, 2nd, 3rd, and 4th week, $p < 0.0001$) (post hoc Tukey analysis, $p < 0.0001$ vs. CT in males). However, no differential effect of the different caffeine doses was detected.

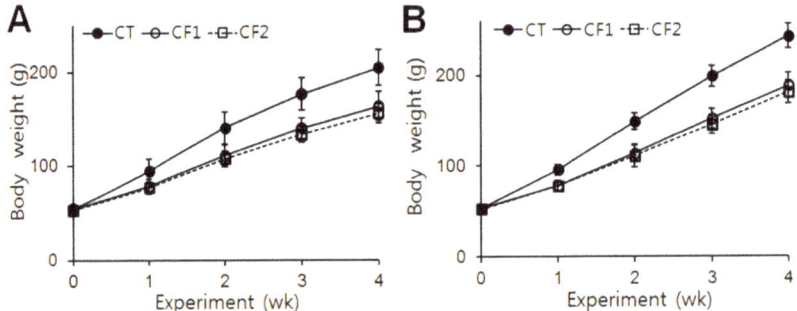

Figure 1. Effects of exposure to caffeine on body weight in immature female and male rats. Average body weights in (**A**) the female groups and (**B**) the male groups in each week of the four-week study period. Both caffeine doses reduced the body-weight changes of the female and male rats, starting from about the first week of exposure ($p < 0.05$ vs. CT in females, $p < 0.001$ vs. CT in males). However, no differential effect of the different caffeine doses was detected. Values are means ± S.D. (n = 10/group). Filled circles, CT (control); open circles, CF1, 120 mg caffeine; open squares, CF2 180 mg caffeine.

3.2. Adrenal Gland Weights

The weights of the adrenals of the control rats after four weeks are summarized in Figure 2. Absolute adrenal weight was analyzed with the Kruskall–Wallis test and one-way ANOVA in female and male rats, respectively, and there were no differences between the control and caffeine-fed groups (Figure 2A). Adrenal gland weight relative to body weight was analyzed by one-way ANOVA followed by the Tukey test. Relative weight increased in a dose-related manner in the caffeine-fed male rats (F = 33.4, $p < 0.0001$) ($p < 0.0001$ vs. CT; 1.3- and 1.4-fold of the controls in the CF1 and CF2, respectively) (Figure 2B). Relative weight also slightly increased in the caffeine-fed female rats (approximately 1.1- and 1.2-fold of the controls in the CF1 and CF2, respectively), but significance was not attained (Figure 2B). These results show that the reductions in absolute adrenal weight due to caffeine exposure were not proportional to body weight in the female rats. On the other hand, male rats had significantly increased adrenal weight relative to their body weights by caffeine exposure, although absolute weights were not different between groups. Similar data were obtained from an analysis of individual adrenal glands. The unpaired t-test was used to compare female and male rats. Both absolute and relative weights were significantly greater in female rats than in male rats (absolute weights: females- 29.1 ± 1.2, 26.2 ± 1.0, 25.9 ± 4.3 mg; males- 22.5 ± 1.9, 22.5 ± 1.8, 23.9 ± 2.6 mg in CT, CF1, CF2, respectively) (relative weight: females- 14.3 ± 1.1, 16.1 ± 1.4, 16.7 ± 3.0 mg/100g body weight; males- 9.3 ± 0.8, 12.0 ± 1.1, 13.2 ± 1.5 mg/100 g body weight in CT, CF1, CF2, respectively).

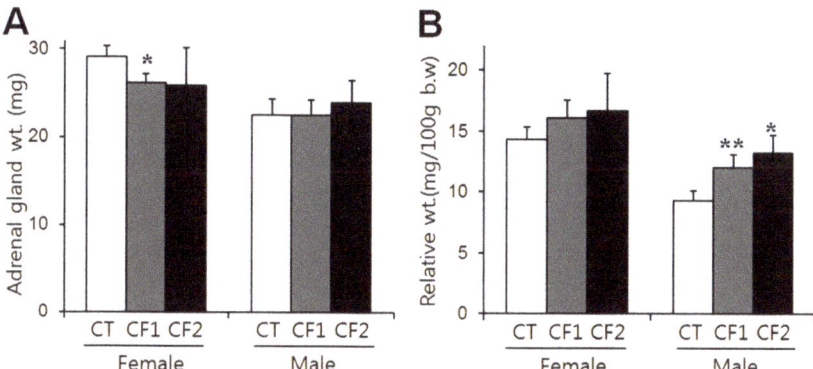

Figure 2. The effect of caffeine on the weights of the adrenal glands in the control and caffeine-fed groups at the end of the experiment. (**A**) Absolute adrenal weights (mg) and (**B**) adrenal weights relative to body weight (mg/100 g body weight). In the female rats, absolute adrenal weight was significantly reduced in CF1 compared to the control, whereas there was no difference between the control and caffeine-fed groups in the male rats. Relative adrenal weight increased in a dose-related manner in the caffeine-fed male rats. Values are expressed as means ± S.D. CT, control; CF1, 120 mg caffeine; CF2, 180 mg caffeine. * $p < 0.05$ vs. CT, ** $p < 0.01$ vs. CT.

3.3. Histological Findings

Because caffeine exposure induced changes in the relative weights of adrenal glands, histological analyses were performed to define whether the weight changes were accompanied by histological changes. Adrenal cortical and medullary areas were measured from the maximum cross-sectional area of each animal, and cortex ratios were calculated as the ratios of the cortical area to total area. Difference between the CT and caffeine-fed groups were analyzed by one-way ANOVA, and between male and female rats by unpaired t-tests. In the caffeine-fed females, both cortical and medullary areas increased relative to the controls, but the latter increased more than the former; as a consequence, there was a significant reduction in the cortical area ratio (post hoc Dunnett's test, $p < 0.01$, CT vs. CF1) (Figure 3A–C). Along with this, a reduced number of cells and cell cords, and increased dilated blood sinusoids particularly in the zona fasciculata were observed in the caffeine-fed females (Table 1), and representative sections are shown in Figure 4A (middle and lower panel). These abnormalities were more obvious as the caffeine dose increased (post hoc Dunnett's test, $p < 0.05$, CT vs. CF2 for cortical cell numbers) (Tukey test, $p < 0.001$, CF2 vs. CT or CF1 for dilated sinusoids). In addition, foamy swellings of cortical cells were significantly more common in the caffeine-fed females (Tukey test, $p < 0.05$, CT vs. CF2), suggesting that the fatty change results from impaired steroidogenesis rather than hypertrophic changes (Table 1) (Figure 4A, lower panel). There was no increase in the number of cell divisions in the image which suggests cell proliferation in the cortex and the medulla in females, despite the increased areas of the cortex and medulla in the caffeine treated groups. On the other hand, no treatment-related differences in cortical (One-way ANOVA; $F = 1.45$, $p = 0.25$ for cortical area; $F = 0.73$, $p = 0.49$ for cortical ratio) or medulla areas (Kruskall–Wallis test; $p = 0.979$) were observed in the male rats (Figure 3). However, histological analysis of the cortical areas revealed a reduced number of cells ($F = 233.3$, $p < 0.001$), disorganized cell cords ($F = 8.78$, $p < 0.01$), dilatation of blood sinusoids ($F = 148.3$, $p < 0.001$), and cytoplasmic vacuolation ($F = 13.39$, $p < 0.005$), especially in CF2, similar to the female rat treatment groups (Table 1) (Figure 4B, lower panel). Overall, negative influences of caffeine on adrenal histology are most likely dependent on dose-level.

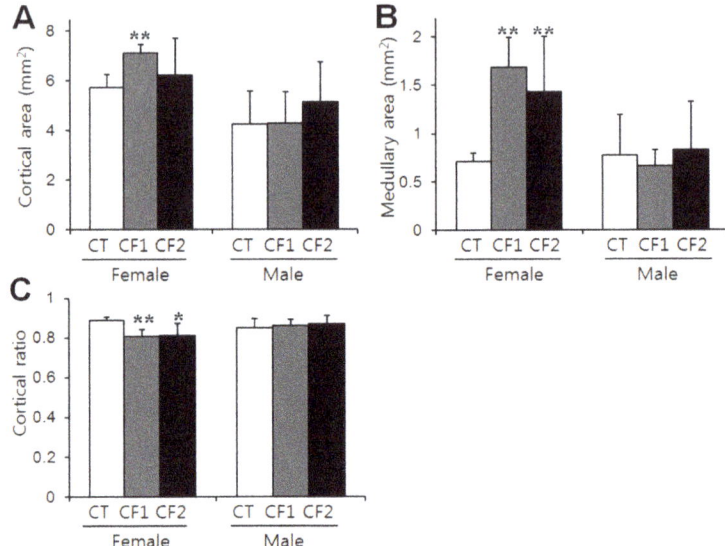

Figure 3. The effect of caffeine on adrenal histology. Whole visual fields in ten consecutive sections of each adrenal gland were evaluated to measure cortical and medullary areas at 40- and 100-fold magnification. Adrenal (**A**) cortical and (**B**) medullary areas were measured from the maximum cross-sectional area of each animal, and (**C**) cortex ratios were calculated as ratios of the cortical area to total area. In the caffeine-fed females, medullary areas increased significantly more than cortical areas; as a consequence, the proportion of the cortical area was significantly reduced. No treatment-related differences in cortical or medulla areas were observed in the male rats. Values represent means ± S.D. of both adrenal glands in groups of ten rats. CT, control; CF1, 120 mg caffeine-fed; CF2, 180 mg caffeine-fed. * $p < 0.05$ vs. CT, ** $p < 0.01$ vs. CT.

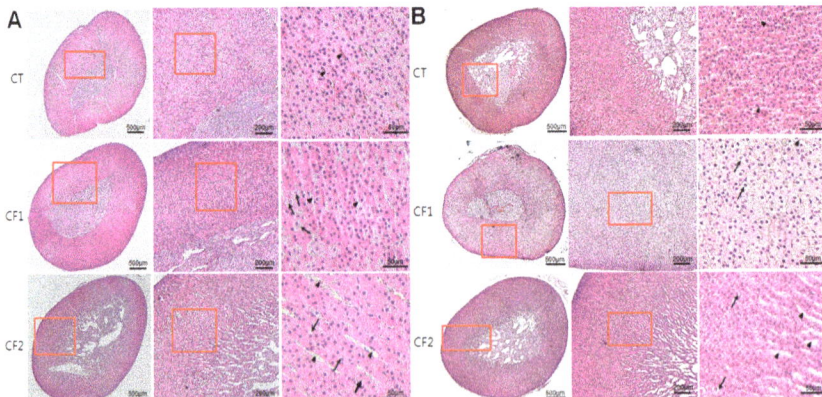

Figure 4. Representative sections of the adrenal glands of control and caffeine-fed rats at the end of caffeine exposure, stained with hematoxylin and eosin. Sections (40, 100, 200× sequentially from the left) from (**A**) the female and (**B**) male groups. In the caffeine-fed females, a reduced number of cells and dilated blood sinusoids were observed, particularly in the zona fasciculata. In addition, in CF1 the cells in the cortex appeared to have foamy swellings. Similarly, a reduced number of cells, disorganized cell cords, and dilatation of some blood sinusoids were observed in the caffeine-fed males. Arrowheads and arrows indicate sinusoids and cells with foamy cytoplasm, respectively. CT, control; CF1, 120 mg caffeine-fed; CF2, 180 mg caffeine-fed.

Table 1. Histomorphometric findings of the adrenal glands in the control and caffeine-fed groups.

Group	Female			Male		
	CT	CF1	CF2	CT	CF1	CF2
Cortical cells	522 ± 29	505 ± 23	356 ± 79 *	936 ± 42	480 ± 31 **	585 ± 19 **,†
Dilated blood sinusoids (ZF)	4 ± 0.3	5 ± 0.8	12 ± 2.1 **,‡	0.8 ± 1.0	1.3 ± 1.0	12 ± 1.3 **,‡
Foamy swelling of cortical cell	15 ± 7.5	25 ± 5.5	27 ± 5.3 *	35 ± 14.9	76 ± 7.9 *	62 ± 10.8 *
Cell cords	24 ± 3.5	15 ± 2.1 *	11 ± 3.7 **	56 ± 18.4	25 ± 1.9	43 ± 3.5 †

Values are expressed as mean ± SD of ten rats per group. The data for the number of cells, dilated sinusoids, foamy cells, or cell cords represent the mean value of 20 measurements from four serial sections per animal counted within the same defined region (0.307277 mm^2) at a 200-fold magnification. * $p < 0.05$, ** $p < 0.001$ vs. CT; † $p < 0.05$, ‡ $p < 0.001$ vs. CF1. CT, control; CF1, 120 mg caffeine; CF2, 180 mg caffeine; ZF, zona fasciculata.

3.4. Serum Corticosterone and ACTH Concentrations

Serum levels of corticosterone after four weeks of exposure were reduced by approximately 40% and 60% of the control levels in the caffeine-fed female and male rats, respectively. One-way ANOVA revealed a substantial effect of caffeine in both female and male rats (females, $F = 21.76$, $p = 0.001$; males, $F = 9.31$, $p = 0.005$). Post hoc analysis found that adolescent caffeine consumption significantly reduced basal corticosterone (females, CT, 43.1 ± 7.6 ng/mL; CF1, 17.4 ± 6.6 ng/mL; CF2, 18.4 ± 2.9 ng/mL) ($p < 0.01$ vs. CT) (males, CT, 41.4 ± 13.8 ng/mL; CF1, 26.0 ± 10.6 ng/mL; CF2, 27.0 ± 13.7 ng/mL) ($p < 0.05$ vs. CT) (T 5A). On the other hand, serum levels of ACTH were significantly different in the caffeine-fed female and male rats compared to their respective control levels (females, $F = 5.021$, $p = 0.017$; males, $F = 3.913$, $p = 0.032$). Although a statistical significance was attained only in the CF2 for female rats ($p < 0.01$ vs. CT) and the CF1 for male rats ($p < 0.05$ vs. CT), caffeine consumption increased ACTH levels compared to the control levels in both female and male rats (females, CT, 2.1 ± 1.5 pg/mL; CF1, 4.6 ± 3.6 pg/mL; CF2, 6.1 ± 2.3 pg/mL) (males, CT, 2.1 ± 0.8 pg/mL; CF1, 3.4 ± 1.2 pg/mL; CF2, 2.9 ± 1.3 pg/mL) (Figure 5B).

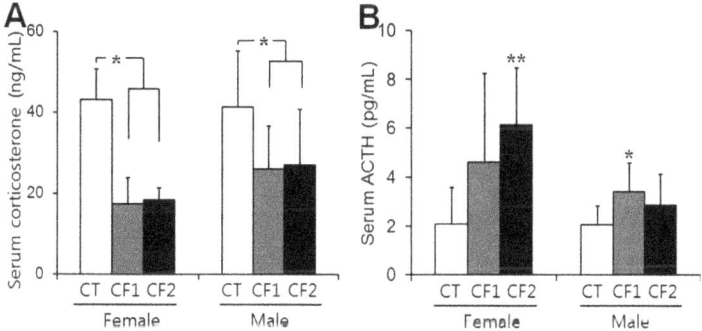

Figure 5. The effects of caffeine on serum corticosterone and ACTH levels in the control and caffeine-fed female and male rats. (**A**) Serum levels of corticosterone were reduced by approximately 40% and 60% of the controls, respectively, in the caffeine-fed female and male rats. (**B**) Serum levels of ACTH were significantly increased in the caffeine-fed female and male rats compared to the controls. Data are means ± S.D. of ten rats per group. CT, control; CF1, 120 mg caffeine-fed; CF2, 180 mg caffeine-fed. * $p < 0.05$, ** $p < 0.01$ vs. CT.

4. Discussion

We have shown that chronic high doses of caffeine during puberty have harmful effects on the adrenal cortex and on corticosterone production, accompanied by the sex-specific histomorphometric changes. To the best of our knowledge, this study is the first to compare the effects of caffeine on the adrenal glands in peripubertal female and male rats.

Increased body size is one of the major physical changes characterizing normal pubertal development. Most human and animal data support a possible influence of caffeine on body size, although some discrepancies exist between studies [1,20,21]. Previously, we demonstrated that peripubertal caffeine exposure reduced body weight gain in immature male and female rats [16,17]. Like others, we observed a significant reduction in body weight gain in the caffeine-fed groups after only one week, and these reductions persisted throughout the experimental period of four weeks in both female and male rats (Figure 1). Although food intake was not examined in this study, our previous reports showed that caffeine exposure decreases food intake in immature rats [16,17] which might contribute to the body weight reduction.

The adrenal gland is the earliest and fastest-developing organ [22,23] and concentrates caffeine more than any other organ [24], suggesting that there could be a high risk of caffeine toxicity to this organ. It has been reported that prenatal exposure to caffeine significantly restricts growth of the adrenals, particularly of the cortical area [9,10]. As puberty is another crucial phase for neuroendocrine transformation, including adrenal cortical maturation [25], it could be anticipated that peripubertal exposure to caffeine would reduce growth of the adrenals. During puberty, mean absolute adrenal weight increased 1.4-fold, whereas relative adrenal weight declined by half by late puberty because of the different growth rates of adrenal glands and overall body weight [26]. Therefore, differences in body weight between rats are not associated with proportional differences in adrenal gland weight in either sex [27]. In agreement with this, the reduction in absolute weights of the adrenals was not proportional to the reduction in body weight (Figures 1 and 2A). On the other hand, we observed a reduction in the absolute weights of the adrenals in the caffeine-fed females, but not in the males (Figure 2A). Considering that the adrenals of females are heavier than those of males at the same age [26], the fast growth of the adrenal glands in females may render them more susceptible to insults. It has also been reported that pubertal caffeine exposure increases the relative weight of adrenals in immature male rats [13] and we indeed noted dose-dependent increases in relative adrenal weights following exposure of both male and female rats to caffeine, although the effect was only statistically significant in the males (Figure 2B). The relative adrenal weights of females were significantly higher overall than those of males, but caffeine treatment increased the relative adrenal weights in males, but not in females. Because caffeine exposure did not change the absolute adrenal weight in male rats, the reduced body weights resulted in increased relative weights, especially in males. Since caffeine exposure reduced body weight gain in both males and females (Figure 1), the increased relative weights of the adrenals indicate that a certain amount of adrenal mass may be preserved regardless of any body weight reduction.

On the other hand, prenatal caffeine exposure has been reported to reduce adrenal cortical area by half in male rat offspring [9]. However, we observed no difference in adrenal cortical or medullary area between caffeine-fed and control males (Figure 3), whereas in the caffeine-fed females, cortical and medullary areas increased in spite of the reduced absolute weights of the adrenals. Sex differences in adrenal weight clearly appear in the course of adrenal maturation from 50 days of age onward, due mainly to the marked increase of the zona fasciculata in female rats [28]. Further research is needed to see whether these sex differences disappear or increase after removal of caffeine.

Considering that absolute adrenal weights reflect the increase in cortical weight during puberty [26], the increased medullary area may not contribute much to adrenal weight. The decreased adrenal weights may be related to the histological alterations in the cortex such as the abnormally dilated intercellular spaces and decreased cellularity. Damage to the adrenal medulla due to various substances is rare compared to damage to the cortex, and chronic toxic effects in the medulla can lead to hypertrophic lesions in rats [29]. If medullary hypertrophy is seen as another index of stress, our results suggest that caffeine-induced stress is more common in female rats than in males. Further study is needed to clarify sex difference in the caffeine-induced secretory responses of the medulla.

Given that cortical zonation is completed during puberty [11], pubertal caffeine exposure may cause cellular damage to the changing adrenal glands regardless of the size of the cortical area. The zona fasciculata is most frequently affected by noxious compounds [29], and chemically-induced toxicity causes impaired steroidogenesis, leading to excess steroid precursors and cytoplasmic vacuolation in the adrenal cortical cells of the zona fasciculata [29]. Similarly, we observed histological distortion of the adrenal cortex including cloudy swellings and some vacuolation within the cells of the zona fasciculata, dilation of some blood sinusoids, and more dilated intercellular spaces in the cortex in the caffeine-fed groups, particularly the females (Figure 4A) (Table 1), consistent with previous data on caffeine exposure of adult and fetal animals [8–10]. During puberty, there is marked expansion of the zona fasciculata [26], which constitutes the main bulk of the adrenal cortex. The adrenal cortex (zona fasciculata) is responsible for the synthesis of glucocorticoids, and their synthesis can be stimulated by stress in response to multiple environmental factors [22]. Caffeine intake also induces endocrine alterations similar to those seen in stress responses [30]. Indeed, we observed that peripubertal caffeine exposure reduced serum corticosterone in both male and female rats regardless of cortical size (Figure 5A). The adrenal cortex underwent a developmental catch-up after birth in male rats exposed to caffeine prenatally, but corticosterone secretion remained low [31]. Thus, during puberty, adrenal cortical thickness may not reflect secretory function. These hormonal changes in the adrenal cortex may lead to malfunctioning of metabolism, which could adversely affect normal development in puberty and also affect subsequent mental and physical health [6,13]. In addition, caffeine markedly increases serum levels of ACTH and corticosterone in adult animals [32]. We also noted increased ACTH, but not corticosterone in caffeine-fed groups (Figure 5B). Previous studies reported a differential sensitivity of the adrenal to ACTH in adolescence [30]. Therefore, peripubertal caffeine exposure may interfere with cortical function by blunting the secretory response to ACTH. In addition, adolescent caffeine consumption may also change the circadian rhythm in corticosterone secretion, which could affect the adrenal growth during puberty; this needs to be further clarified. Considering that ACTH is the principal hormone responsible for the maintenance of adrenal structure and function [33], caffeine exposure may cause more adverse effects in this period than in adulthood when development has ceased.

5. Conclusions

In conclusion, we have shown that the harmful effects of caffeine on the adrenal glands of immature rats differ between females and males. Although, based on the changes in the microarchitecture of the adrenal glands, female rats seem to be more susceptible to damage, caffeine also affected corticosterone production in male rats. Therefore, caffeine may induce an endocrine imbalance that disturbs the establishment of the hypothalamo–pituitary adrenal axis during puberty, thereby leading to abnormal stress responses. Further studies are needed to identify the cellular/molecular mechanisms by which caffeine affects adrenal steroidogenesis.

Author Contributions: K.-Y.R. participated in the experiments, data collection, and analysis; J.R., contributed to the design of the study, data analysis, supervision, and development of the manuscript. J.R. takes responsibility for the integrity of the data analysis. All authors read and approved the final manuscript.

Funding: This research received no external funding.

Acknowledgments: We thank Jisook Kim (Department of Anatomical Pathology, Hanyang University Hospital, Seoul, Korea) for technical support.

Conflicts of Interest: The authors declare no conflict of interest.

References

1. Reissig, C.J.; Strain, E.C.; Griffiths, R.R. Caffeinated energy drinks—A growing problem. *Drug Alcohol Depend.* **2009**, *99*, 1–10. [CrossRef] [PubMed]
2. Seifert, S.M.; Schaechter, J.L.; Hershorin, E.R.; Lipshultz, S.E. Health effects of energy drinks on children, adolescents, and young adults. *Pediatrics* **2011**, *127*, 511–528. [CrossRef] [PubMed]

3. Jackson, D.A.; Cotter, B.V.; Merchant, R.C.; Babu, K.M.; Baird, J.R.; Nirenberg, T.; Linakis, J.G. Behavioral and physiologic adverse effects in adolescent and young adult emergency department patients reporting use of energy drinks and caffeine. *Clin. Toxicol.* **2013**, *51*, 557–565. [CrossRef] [PubMed]
4. Díaz-Aguila, Y.; Cuevas-Romero, E.; Castelán, F.; Martínez-Gómez, M.; Rodríguez-Antolín, J.; Nicolás-Toledo, L. Chronic stress and high sucrose intake cause distinctive morphometric effects in the adrenal glands of post-weaned rats. *Biotech. Histochem.* **2018**, *93*, 565–574. [CrossRef]
5. Ribelin, W.E. The effects of drugs and chemicals upon the structure of the adrenal gland. *Fundam. Appl. Toxicol.* **1984**, *4*, 105–119. [CrossRef]
6. O'Neill, C.E.; Newsom, R.J.; Stafford, J.; Scott, T.; Archuleta, S.; Levis, S.C.; Spencer, R.L.; Campeau, S.; Bachtell, R.K. Adolescent caffeine consumption increases adulthood anxiety-related behavior and modifies neuroendocrine signaling. *Psychoneuroendocrinology* **2016**, *67*, 40–50. [CrossRef] [PubMed]
7. Robertson, D.; Wade, D.; Workman, R.; Woosley, R.L.; Oates, J.A. Tolerance to the humoral and hemodynamic effects of caffeine in man. *J. Clin. Investig.* **1981**, *67*, 1111–1117. [CrossRef]
8. Wu, D.M.; He, Z.; Ma, L.P.; Wang, L.L.; Ping, J.; Wang, H. Increased DNA methylation of scavenger receptor class B type I contributes to inhibitory effects of prenatal caffeine ingestion on cholesterol uptake and steroidogenesis in fetal adrenals. *Toxicol. Appl. Pharmacol.* **2015**, *285*, 89–97. [CrossRef]
9. He, Z.; Zhu, C.; Huang, H.; Liu, L.; Wang, L.; Chen, L.; Magdalou, J.; Wang, H. Prenatal caffeine exposure-induced adrenal developmental abnormality in male offspring rats and its possible intrauterine programming mechanisms. *Toxicol. Res.* **2016**, *5*, 388–398. [CrossRef]
10. Xu, D.; Zhang, B.; Liang, G.; Ping, J.; Kou, H.; Li, X.; Xiong, J.; Hu, D.; Chen, L.; Magdalou, J.; et al. Caffeine-induced activated glucocorticoid metabolism in the hippocampus causes hypothalamic-pituitary-adrenal axis inhibition in fetal rats. *PLoS ONE* **2012**, *7*, e44497. [CrossRef]
11. Xing, Y.; Lerario, A.M.; Rainey, W.; Hammer, G.D. Development of adrenal cortex zonation. *Endocrinol. Metab. Clin. N. Am.* **2015**, *44*, 243–274. [CrossRef] [PubMed]
12. Walker, C.D.; Sapolsky, R.M.; Meaney, M.J.; Vale, W.W.; Rivier, C.L. Increased pituitary sensitivity to glucocorticoid feedback during the stress nonresponsive period in the neonatal rat. *Endocrinology* **1986**, *119*, 1816–1821. [CrossRef]
13. Anderson, N.L.; Hughes, R.N. Increased emotional reactivity in rats following exposure to caffeine during adolescence. *Neurotoxicol. Teratol.* **2008**, *30*, 195–201. [CrossRef] [PubMed]
14. Goldman, L.; Winget, C.; Hollingshead, G.W.; Levine, S. Postweaning development of negative feedback in the pituitary-adrenal system of the rat. *Neuroendocrinology* **1973**, *12*, 199–211. [CrossRef] [PubMed]
15. Oyola, M.G.; Handa, R.J. Hypothalamic-pituitary-adrenal and hypothalamic-pituitary-gonadal axes: Sex differences in regulation of stress responsivity. *Stress* **2017**, *20*, 476–494. [CrossRef] [PubMed]
16. Park, M.; Choi, Y.; Choi, H.; Yim, J.Y.; Roh, J. High doses of caffeine during the peripubertal period in the rat impair the growth and function of the testis. *Int. J. Endocrinol.* **2015**, *2015*, 368475. [CrossRef] [PubMed]
17. Kwak, Y.; Choi, H.; Bae, J.; Choi, Y.Y.; Roh, J. Peri-pubertal high caffeine exposure increases ovarian estradiol production in immature rats. *Reprod. Toxicol.* **2017**, *69*, 43–52. [CrossRef] [PubMed]
18. Vik, T.; Bakketeig, L.S.; Trygg, K.U.; Lund-Larsen, K.; Jacobsen, G. High caffeine consumption in the third trimester of pregnancy: Gender-specific effects on fetal growth. *Paediatr. Perinat. Epidemiol.* **2003**, *17*, 324–331. [CrossRef] [PubMed]
19. Ojeda, S.R.; Skinner, M.K. Puberty in the rat. In *Knobil and Neill's Physiology of Reproduction*; Elsevier: Amsterdam, The Netherlands, 2006; pp. 2061–2126.
20. Huang, T.H.; Yang, R.S.; Hsieh, S.S.; Liu, S.H. Effects of caffeine and exercise on the development of bone: A densitometric and histomorphometric study in young Wistar rats. *Bone* **2002**, *30*, 293–299. [CrossRef]
21. Pietrobelli, A.; Faith, M.S.; Wang, J.; Brambilla, P.; Chiumello, G.; Heymsfield, S.B. Association of lean tissue and fat mass with bone mineral content in children and adolescents. *Obes. Res.* **2002**, *10*, 56–60. [CrossRef]
22. Ishimoto, H.; Jaffe, R.B. Development and function of the human fetal adrenal cortex: A key component in the feto-placental unit. *Endocr. Rev.* **2011**, *32*, 317–355. [PubMed]
23. Mesiano, S.; Jaffe, R.B. Developmental and functional biology of the primate fetal adrenal cortex. *Endocr. Rev.* **1997**, *18*, 378–403. [PubMed]
24. Beach, E.F.; Turner, J.J. An enzymatic method for glucose determination in body fluids. *Clin. Chem.* **1958**, *4*, 462–475.
25. Novello, L.; Speiser, P.W. Premature adrenarche. *Pediatr. Ann.* **2018**, *47*, e7–e11. [CrossRef] [PubMed]

26. Belloni, A.S.; Rebuffat, P.; Malendowicz, L.K.; Mazzocchi, G.; Rocco, S.; Nussdorfer, G.G. Age-related changes in the morphology and function of the zona glomerulosa of the rat adrenal cortex. *Tissue Cell* **1992**, *24*, 835–842. [CrossRef]
27. Bailey, S.A.; Zidell, R.H.; Perry, R.W. Relationships between organ weight and body/brain weight in the rat: What is the best analytical endpoint? *Toxicol. Pathol.* **2004**, *32*, 448–466. [CrossRef] [PubMed]
28. Majchrzak, M.; Malendowicz, L.K. Sex differences in adrenocortical structure and function. XII. Stereologic studies of rat adrenal cortex in the course of maturation. *Cell Tissue Res.* **1983**, *232*, 457–469. [CrossRef]
29. Rosol, T.J.; Yarrington, J.T.; Latendresse, J.; Capen, C.C. Adrenal gland: Structure, function, and mechanisms of toxicity. *Toxicol. Pathol.* **2001**, *29*, 41–48. [CrossRef]
30. McCormick, C.M.; Mathews, I.Z. HPA function in adolescence: Role of sex hormones in its regulation and the enduring consequences of exposure to stressors. *Pharmacol. Biochem. Behav.* **2007**, *86*, 220–233. [CrossRef]
31. Chen, G.; Yuan, C.; Duan, F.; Liu, Y.; Zhang, J.; He, Z.; Huang, H.; He, C.; Wang, H. IGF1/MAPK/ERK signaling pathway-mediated programming alterations of adrenal cortex cell proliferation by prenatal caffeine exposure in male offspring rats. *Toxicol. Appl. Pharmacol.* **2018**, *341*, 64–76. [CrossRef]
32. Leblanc, J.; Richard, D.; Racotta, I.S. Metabolic and hormone-related responses to caffeine in rats. *Pharmacol. Res.* **1995**, *32*, 129–133. [CrossRef]
33. Patz, M.D.; Day, H.E.; Burow, A.; Campeau, S. Modulation of the hypothalamo-pituitary-adrenocortical axis by caffeine. *Psychoneuroendocrinology* **2006**, *31*, 493–500. [CrossRef] [PubMed]

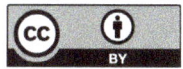

© 2019 by the authors. Licensee MDPI, Basel, Switzerland. This article is an open access article distributed under the terms and conditions of the Creative Commons Attribution (CC BY) license (http://creativecommons.org/licenses/by/4.0/).

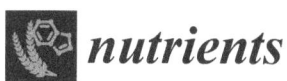

Discussion

Coffee Consumption and Risk of Colorectal Cancer: A Systematic Review and Meta-Analysis of Prospective Studies

Marina Sartini [1,*], Nicola Luigi Bragazzi [2], Anna Maria Spagnolo [1], Elisa Schinca [1], Gianluca Ottria [1], Chiara Dupont [1] and Maria Luisa Cristina [1]

1. Department of Health Sciences (DISSAL), University of Genoa, 16132 Genoa, Italy; am.spagnolo@unige.it (A.M.S.); elisa.schinca@unige.it (E.S.); gianluca.ottria@unige.it (G.O.); lioa@unige.it (C.D.); cristinaml@unige.it (M.L.C.)
2. Postgraduate School of Public Health, Department of Health Sciences (DISSAL), University of Genoa, 16132 Genoa, Italy; robertobragazzi@gmail.com
* Correspondence: sartini@unige.it

Received: 4 March 2019; Accepted: 19 March 2019; Published: 24 March 2019

Abstract: Coffee is a blend of compounds related to gastrointestinal physiology. Given its popularity and the epidemiology of colorectal cancer, the impact of this beverage on public health could be considerable. Our aim was to provide an updated synthesis of the relationship between coffee consumption and the risk of colorectal cancer. We conducted a systematic review and meta-analysis of 26 prospective studies. Regarding colorectal cancer, no significant relationship was detected. Stratifying for ethnicity, a protective effect emerged in US subjects. Concerning colon cancer, coffee proved to exert a protective effect in men and women combined and in men alone. Stratifying for ethnicity, a significant protective effect was noted in European men only and in Asian women only. Concerning rectal cancer, no association was found. Decaffeinated coffee exhibited a protective effect against colorectal cancer in men and women combined. Studies were appraised for their quality by means of the Newcastle-Ottawa Quality Assessment Scale for Cohort studies. Only one study proved to be of low quality. Ethnicity could explain the heterogeneity of the studies. However, little is known about the relationship between the genetic make-up and the risk of colorectal cancer associated with coffee. Further research is warranted.

Keywords: coffee/caffeine; systematic review and meta-analysis; prospective studies; epidemiology; cancer prevention; colorectal cancer

---

1. Introduction

Coffee is a complex blend of bioactive compounds. These are related to gastrointestinal physiology in various ways and may exert contrasting effects. On the one hand, coffee contains anti-oxidants and anti-mutagens, which could, as such, reduce exposure of the epithelial cells of the bowel to carcinogenic chemicals and compounds, and prevent and counteract the effect of potential promoters of intestinal carcinogenesis. Indeed, coffee seems to enhance bowel motility and functioning, reducing fecal transit times and increasing stool output. Furthermore, coffee contains lipidic compounds, such as cafestol and kahweol, which, by finely tuning cholesterol metabolism, reduce the synthesis and release of bile acids [1]. They act also as reactive oxygen species (ROS) scavengers, activating DNA repair enzymes [2] and phase-II enzymes involved in carcinogen detoxification. Furthermore, coffee modulates the microbiome of the gut. Caffeine has anti-apoptotic effects, inducing programmed cell death [3]. Caffeic acid is involved in several pathways related to inflammation, apoptosis and the cell cycle. Finally, chlorogenic acid seems to have antioxidant properties. On the other hand, coffee contains mutagens, such as glyoxal, methylglyoxal, ethylglyoxal, propylglyoxal, diacetyl, acetol and other dicarbonyls [4–7] or tannins [8], among others, which could counteract the protective effects of coffee.

Moreover, the quantity of these bioactive compounds varies according to the type of coffee. For example, unfiltered coffees, such as French press coffee or Turkish/Greek coffee, contain significant amounts of these compounds, unlike filtered blends, such as dip-brewed coffee. Moreover, filtered coffee also contains fewer phenols and polyphenols [2,9].

Being cheap and easy to prepare, coffee is a widespread beverage, its worldwide consumption of two billion cups per day being second only to that of water [2]. Given the popularity of coffee, its impact on public health could be considerable. Statistics on cancer reveal that colorectal cancer is the third most common cancer among men, after lung and prostate cancer, and the second most common cancer among women, after breast cancer; in terms of cancer-related death, it ranks fourth after lung, liver and stomach cancer [10]. We therefore aimed to provide an updated quantitative synthesis of the relationship between coffee consumption and the risk of colorectal cancer.

2. Materials and Methods

The Preferred Reporting Items for Systematic Reviews and Meta-analyses (PRISMA) guidelines [11] were used as a guide to ensure that the current standard for meta-analysis methodology were met (see also Supplementary Materials). We searched PubMed/MEDLINE and Scopus archives and databases for a combination of keywords such as "coffee" and "colorectal cancer", using Medical Subject Headings (MeSH) terms as vocabulary, according to the National Center for Biotechnology Information (NCBI) nomenclature and guidelines and, where appropriate, a wild-card option.

Inclusion criteria were: (1) articles with relevant quantitative details and information on the relationship between coffee consumption and the risk of developing colorectal cancer; (2) prospective studies. Exclusion criteria were: (1) items not directly pertinent to the query string; (2) articles not containing sufficient information on the relationship between coffee consumption and the risk of colorectal cancer; (3) articles not meeting the PICOS criteria (P: patients with colorectal cancer; I: consuming coffee; C: coffee consumption versus non-consumption, and/or comparison between different kinds of coffee: caffeinated or decaffeinated, etc.; O: risk ratio, RR, of colorectal cancer associated to coffee consumption; S: prospective study); all such articles were consequently discarded. No time filter or language filter was applied. For further details of the search strategy, see Table 1.

Table 1. Search strategy adopted in the present systematic review and meta-analysis.

Search Strategy	Details
Search string	(coffee OR caffeine) AND (tumor OR cancer OR neoplasm) AND (colon OR rectal OR colorectal)
Databases	PubMed/MEDLINE, Scopus
Inclusion criteria	P (patients/population): general population/patients suffering from colorectal cancer I (intervention/exposure): subjects consuming coffee C (comparisons/comparators): coffee consumers versus non-consumers; different kinds of coffee (caffeinated/decaffeinated) O (outcome): incidence of colorectal cancer S (study design): prospective study
Exclusion criteria	Experimental studies investigating in vitro or animal models Study design: editorial, commentaries, expert opinions, letters to editor, review articles, original non-prospective studies, articles with insufficient details
Time filter	None (from inception)
Language filter	None (any language)

Two of the authors independently screened the literature. Any case of disagreement was solved by discussion until consensus was reached. After the full text review, the papers included were retained for data extraction.

Data for the meta-analysis were extracted from the studies included by means of a standardized documentation form. The parameters extracted were: the surname of the first author, the year and country of publication, sample size, percentages of females and males, incidence of colorectal cancer (broken down by clinical site: colon and rectum), and the amount and type of coffee consumed.

RR of developing colorectal cancer on the basis of coffee consumed (i.e., RR of subjects with colorectal cancer who consumed the greatest amount of coffee versus subjects who did not consume coffee) were calculated as effect size estimates, with their 95% confidence intervals (CIs). Additional analyses were performed after stratification by type of coffee, study region, publication period and gender.

Study quality was appraised by two researchers, working independently, with respect to the appropriateness of the research questions tested and of the methods employed. For this purpose, the Newcastle-Ottawa Quality Assessment Scale for Cohort studies (NOS) was used; scores of ≥ 7 indicated high-quality and <7 indicated low-quality studies. Any disagreement was solved by consensus.

Statistical heterogeneity was also assessed in our meta-analysis by means of I^2 statistics and chi-square test, heterogeneity being deemed significant if the p value (χ^2) was <0.1. In detail, it was determined that the values of 25%, 50% and 75% in the I^2 test corresponded to low, moderate and high levels of heterogeneity, respectively. In the event of significant (moderate or high) heterogeneity among the studies, a random-effects model was used for the meta-analysis. The RR of the meta-analyses were deemed significant when the confidence intervals did not contain the value "1"; indeed, if the confidence interval contains the value "1", we cannot exclude the absence of an association between exposure and disease. A narrower CI than that of the individual studies indicates less imprecision.

Meta-analyses were carried out by means of the STATA SE14^R (StataCorp LP, College Station, TX, USA) software. To identify sources of variation, further stratification was performed with respect to study quality. In addition, in the sensitivity analyses, the stability of the pooled estimate with respect to each study was investigated by excluding individual studies from the analysis. Possible publication bias was visually inspected by means of a funnel plot. If asymmetry was detected by visual assessment, exploratory analyses using trim and/or fill analysis were performed in order to investigate and adjust the effect-size estimate. In addition, the probability of publication bias was tested by means of Egger's linear regression, a value of $p < 0.05$ being indicative of publication bias.

3. Results

Concerning the systematic review, our initial query resulted in 390 hits (specifically, 376 articles from PubMed/MEDLINE and Scopus, and 14 from other sources); after removal of duplicate items, the resulting list comprised of 270 non-redundant articles. Only 33 studies were retained in the qualitative synthesis, and 26 were finally considered in our systematic review and meta-analysis (186 articles were discarded as not being directly pertinent to the topic under investigation and 51 as not meeting the inclusion criteria). For further details, see Figure 1.

The full list of studies included [12–37] and their main characteristics are shown in Table 2.

The studies examined included 3,308,028 subjects. Eleven studies were performed in European countries, seven in Asian countries and seven in the USA. Nineteen studies were on colorectal cancer, 19 on colon cancer and 18 on rectal cancer.

With regard to colorectal cancer, from the pooled RR, no significant relationship between coffee consumption and the risk of developing cancer was detected (Table 3).

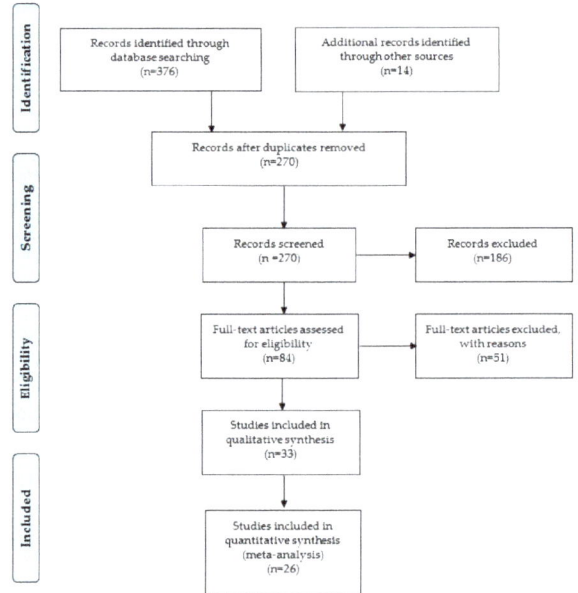

Figure 1. Flowchart of study selection, inclusion and synthesis.

Table 2. Characteristics of studies included.

First Authors (year)	Country	Study Subject	Coffee Consumption ("high" vs. "low")	No. Cases
Jacobsen (1986) [12]	Sweden	All (16,555) F (2891); M (13,664)	≥7 cups/d vs. ≤2 cups/d	97 CC—63 RC
Wu (1987) [13]	USA	All (11,632) F (7456); M (4163)	≥4 cups/d vs. ≤1 cup/d	NA (CRC)
Klatsky (1988) [14]	USA	All (10,572)	Continuous variable (cups/d)	203 CC—66 RC
Stensvold (1994) [15]	Sweden	F (21,238); M (21,735)	≥7 cups/d vs. ≤2 cups/d	F: 52 CC—38 RC; M: 78 CC—41 RC
Terry (2001) [16]	Sweden	F (61,463)	≥4 cups/d vs. <1 cup/d	291 CC—159 RC—460 CRC
Khan (2004) [17]	Japan	F (1634); M (1524)	Continuous variable (cups/d)	F: 14 CRC; M: 15 CRC
Michels (2005) [18]	USA	All (133,893) F (87,794); M (46,099)	>5 cups/d vs. none (caffeinated, decaffeinated)	Caffeinated: 1170 CC—260 RC—1431 CRC Decaffeinated: 913 CC—224 RC—1138 CRC
Larsson (2006) [19]	Sweden	All (106,739)	≥4 cups/d vs. <1 cup/d	843 CC—440 RC—1279 CRC
Mucci (2006) [20]	Sweden	F (61,467)	≥4 cups/d vs. ≤1 cup/d	504 CC—237 RC—741 CRC
Oba (2006) [21]	Japan	F (16,327); M (13,894)	≥1 cups/d vs. none	F: 102 CC; M: 111 CC
Lee (2007) [22]	Japan	F (50,139); M (46,023)	≥3 cups/d vs. none	F: 286 CC—151 RC—437 CRC M: 174 CC—102 RC—276 CRC
Naganuma (2007) [23]	Japan	All (47,605) F (24,769); M (22,836)	≥3 cups/d vs. none	ALL: 281 CC—180 RC—457 CRC F: 106 CC—68 RC—173 CRC M: 175 CC—112 RC—284 CRC

Table 2. *Cont.*

First Authors (year)	Country	Study Subject	Coffee Consumption ("high" vs. "low")	No. Cases
Bidel (2010) [24]	Finland	All (60,041) F (30,882); M (29,159)	≥10 cups/d vs. none	ALL: 333 CC—252 RC—538 CRC F: 167 CC—123 RC—271 CRC M: 166 CC—129 RC—267 CRC
Nilsson (2010) [25]	Sweden	All (64,603)	≥4 cups/d vs. <1 cup/d	321 CRC
Simons (2010) [26]	Netherlands	F (62,573) M (58,279)	>6 cups/d vs. ≤2 cups/d	F: 173 RC—939 CRC M: 322 RC—1260 CRC
Zhang (2010) [27]	Multi-center (conducted in USA and in Europe)	All (731,441)	High quintile vs. low quintile	5,604 CC
Sinha (2012) [28]	USA	All (489,706)	≥6 cups/d vs. none (all, caffeinated, decaffeinated)	5,072 CC—2863 Prox CC—1993 Distal CC—1874 RC—6946 CRC
Dominianni (2013) [29]	USA	All (57,398)	≥4 cups/d vs. none	681 CRC
Perrigue (2013) [30]	USA	All (67,912)	≥7 cups/d vs. <7 cups/d	409 CRC
Dik (2014) [31]	EPIC study (Europe)	All (521,448) F (365,014); M (156,434)	High quintile vs. low quintile (all, caffeinated, decaffeinated)	2691 CC—1242 Prox CC—1202 Distal CC—1543 RC—4234 CRC
Hartmann (2014) [32]	Finland	M (27,111)	>6 cups/d vs. ≤4 cups/d	106 CC—79 RC
Peterson (2014) [33]	Singapore	All (61,321)	≥2 cups/d vs. <1 cup/d	591 CC—370 RC
Yamada (2014) [34]	Japan	F (34,614) M (23,607)	≥4 cups/d vs. <1 cup/d	F: 332 CC—112 RC—444 CRC M: 355 CC—202 RC—557 CRC
Groessl (2016) [35]	USA	F (83,972)	≥4 cups/d vs. none	1,083 CC—160 RC—12,852 CRC
Lukic (2016) [36]	Norway	F (79,461)	>7 cups/d vs. ≤1 cup/d	1266 CRC
Kashino (2018) [37]	Japan	F (170,388) M (149,934)	≥3 cups/d vs. <1 cup/d	F: 1963 CC—770 RC—2689 CRC M: 2619 CC—1402 RC—4022 CRC

Abbreviations: CC (colon cancer); CRC (colorectal cancer); d (day); F (female); M (male); NA (not available); prox (proximal); RC (rectal cancer); vs. (versus).

Table 3. Risk ratio (RR) and 95% CI for all meta-analyses carried out. Values in bold are statistically significant.

Tumor and Geographic Provenience of the Studies		Men and Women RR [95%CI]; (N. Studies)	Men RR [95%CI]; (N. Studies)	Women RR [95%CI]; (N. Studies)
CRC	All	0.96 [0.88–1.03]; (8)	0.96 [0.88–1.04]; (9)	1.06 [0.97–1.14]; (13)
	EU studies only	1.07 [0.96–1.17]; (4)	0.93 [0.80–1.06]; (3)	1.10 [0.98–1.22]; (6)
	Asian studies only	NA	0.97 [0.87–1.08]; (5)	0.94 [0.78–1.09]; (5)
	USA studies only	**0.83 [0.72–0.95]; (3)**	NA	1.14 [0.92–1.36]; (2)
	Caffeinated coffee	0.96 [0.77–1.17]; (3)	NA	NA
	Decaffeinated coffee	**0.88 [0.78–0.97]; (3)**	NA	NA
CC	All	**0.91 [0.83–0.998]; (9)**	**0.94 [0.89–0.99]; (11)**	0.92 [0.80–1.03]; (13)
	EU studies only	0.96 [0.84–1.09]; (4)	**0.85 [0.72–0.99]; (4)**	1.05 [0.93–1.18]; (5)
	Asian studies only	0.91 [0.73–1.09]; (2)	0.94 [0.82–1.06]; (5)	**0.73 [0.58–0.88]; (5)**
	USA studies only	0.83 [0.66–1.01]; (7)	NA	0.90 [0.38–1.12]; (2)
	Caffeinated coffee	0.92 [0.68–1.15]; (3)	NA	NA
	Decaffeinated coffee	0.93 [0.81–1.05]; (3)	NA	NA
Distal CC	All	0.98 [0.95–1.02]; (5)	0.94 [0.87–1.01]; (5)	1.00 [0.96–1.04]; (6)
	EU studies only	NA	**0.77 [0.57–0.98]; (2)**	1.09 [0.82–1.36]; (3)
	Asian studies only	NA	0.83 [0.60–1.05]; (2)	0.91 [0.56–1.25]; (2)
	USA studies only	0.88 [0.65–1.12]; (2)	NA	NA
	Caffeinated coffee	0.99 [0.79–1.91]; (2)	NA	NA
	Decaffeinated coffee	1.05 [0.79–1.32]; (2)	NA	NA
Proximal CC	All	0.93 [0.73–1.15]; (5)	0.98 [0.92–1.04]; (5)	0.99 [0.96–1.03]; (6)
	EU studies only	NA	0.90 [0.66–1.14]; (2)	1.17 [0.90–1.44]; (3)
	Asian studies only	NA	1.08 [0.83–1.32]; (2)	0.85 [0.57–1.13]; (2)
	USA studies only	0.92 [0.23–1.60]; (2)	NA	NA
	Caffeinated coffee	0.85 [0.32–1.36]; (2)	NA	NA
	Decaffeinated coffee	0.86 [0.66–1.06]; (2)	NA	NA
RC	All	1.00 [0.89–1.11]; (9)	1.01 [0.87–1.14]; (9)	1.08 [0.94–1.23]; (11)
	EU studies only	1.17 [0.97–1.37]; (4)	0.96 [0.78–1.14]; (5)	1.04 [0.87–1.21]; (6)
	Asian studies only	1.04 [0.79–1.29]; (2)	1.07 [0.85–1.29]; (4)	1.28 [0.96–1.60]; (4)
	USA studies only	0.88 [0.72–1.04]; (3)	NA	NA
	Caffeinated coffee	1.18 [0.98–1.38]; (3)	NA	NA
	Decaffeinated coffee	0.71 [0.41–1.01]; (3)	NA	NA

Abbreviations: CC (colon cancer); CRC (colorectal cancer); EU (European countries); NA (not available); RC (rectal cancer).

Stratifying for ethnicity, a significant protective effect emerged among US subjects (men and women), with a RR of 0.83 (95% CI 0.72–0.95). While no statistical significance emerged for caffeinated coffee, decaffeinated coffee exhibited a protective effect on men and women combined (RR 0.88 (95% CI 0.78–0.97)).

Concerning colon cancer (Table 3), coffee consumption proved to exert a protective effect on men and women combined (RR 0.91 (95% CI 0.83–0.998)) (Figure 2), and on men only (RR 0.94 (95% CI 0.89–0.99)) (Figure 3).

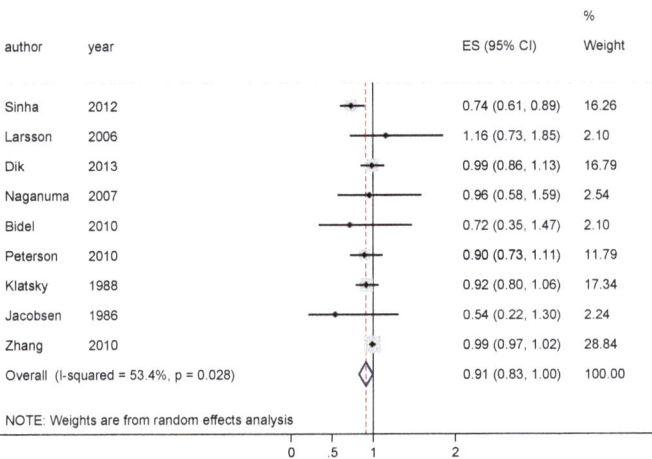

Figure 2. Forest plot of colon cancer in men and women combined.

Stratifying for ethnicity, a statistically significant protective effect was noted in European men only (RR 0.85 (95% CI 0.72–0.99)), and in Asian women only (RR 0.73 (95% CI 0.58–0.88)) (Figure 4A,B).

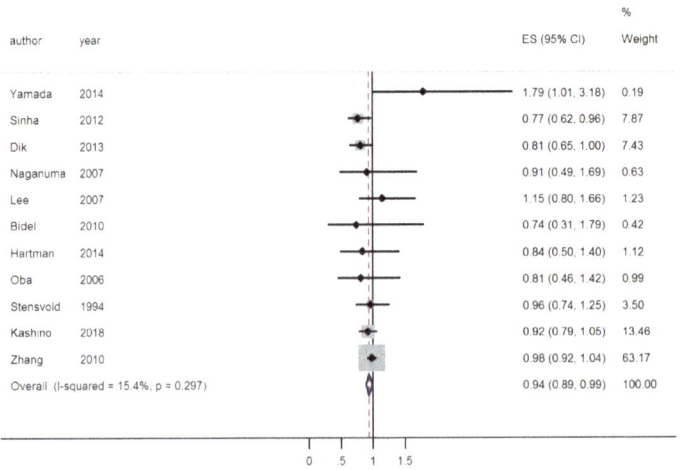

Figure 3. Forest plot of colon cancer in men.

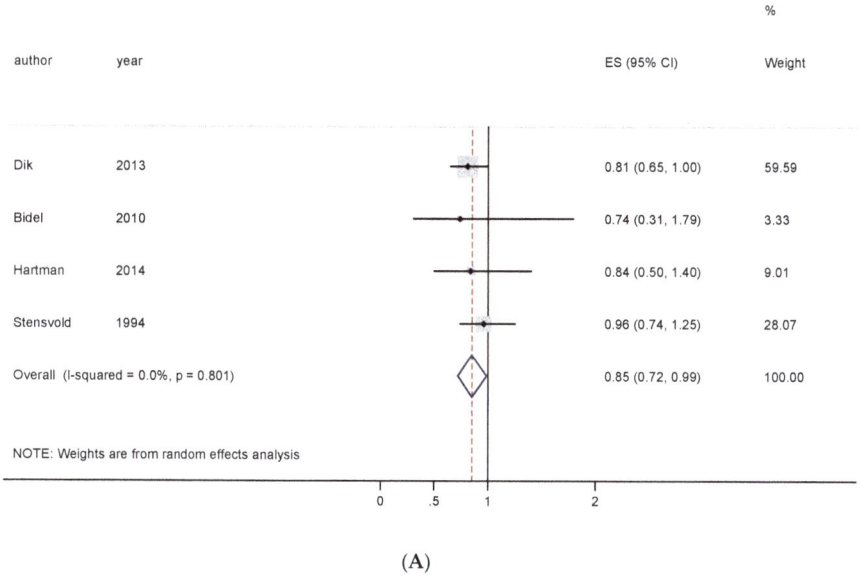

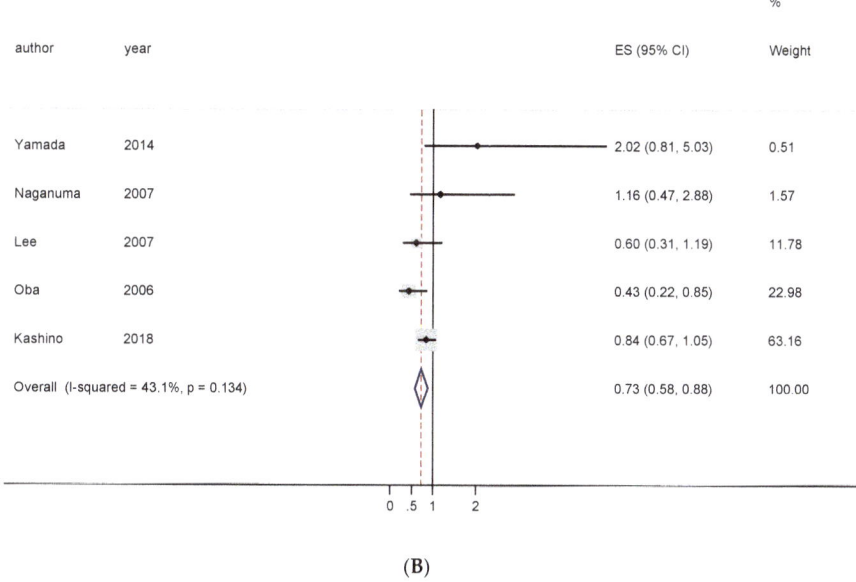

Figure 4. Forest plot of colon cancer in European men (**A**) and in Asian women (**B**).

Focusing on distal colon cancer (Table 3), coffee consumption proved protective in European men only (RR 0.77 (95% CI 0.57–0.98)). With regard to proximal colon cancer (Table 3), no significant association was found.

Concerning rectal cancer (Table 3), no significant association could be found.

No significant publication bias was detected. Finally, concerning the assessment of the risk of bias, no significant biases emerged. Only one study was deemed to be of low quality (Wu: NOS score = 5). Retaining or removing this study from the meta-analyses did not change the results.

4. Discussion

Performing the meta-analysis of prospective studies, we found a significantly high degree of heterogeneity.

With specific regard to rectal cancer, no evidence of an association between coffee consumption and the development of the disease could be found. For colorectal cancer, we found evidence of a protective effect only in US men and women together. Stratification by type of coffee—caffeinated or decaffeinated—did not reveal any differences linked to the presence of caffeine, since the types of coffee appeared to be protective in some studies and non-significant in others. Moreover, the quantity of caffeine in coffee also depends on the type of mixture used [38], a parameter that was not investigated in the studies considered. Instead, in the present systematic review and meta-analysis decaffeinated coffee consumption showed a protective role against colorectal cancer, despite the low number of investigations.

Regarding colon cancer, evidence of a protective effect of coffee consumption was found, both considering men and women together and considering men alone.

Stratifying for ethnicity, we found that the pooled RR was significant for European men and for Asian women. We can speculate that this might be due to the particular type of coffee consumed; for example, in Asia, coffee is rarely consumed boiled or decaffeinated [22]. Another possible explanation may lie in the biological make-up of the subjects; this might also explain why coffee drinking proved protective in a particular gender but not in the other. In this regard, Platt et al. found that cultural, dietary and lifestyle factors influenced the impact of coffee intake in terms of the risk of developing metabolic syndrome [39]. Similarly, Kumar et al. found a differential effect of caffeine intake on the onset of Parkinson's disease, the effect being mediated by genetic variants [40]. Other biological events or diseases have been found to be characterized by a complex gene–caffeine interaction, such as variability in the cardiovascular response to caffeine [41], coffee consumption and the risk of developing neurodegenerative disorders [42], epithelial ovarian cancer [43], breast cancer [44], or myocardial infarction [45], among others. These genes include cytochrome P450 1A2 (CYP1A2), adenosine A2a receptor (ADORA2A), and leucine-rich repeat kinase 2 or dardarin (LRRK2).

As potential mechanisms that may explain the inverse association between coffee consumption and the development of colon cancer, a review by Higdon [46] hypothesizes the presence of diterpenes as a factor of protection. Indeed, in vitro studies have reported that this molecule is able to reduce the formation of DNA adducts by several genotoxic carcinogens, including 2-amino-1-methyl-6-phenylimidazo[4,5-b]pyridine (PhIP), a heterocyclic amine implicated in colon carcinogenesis. Moreover, it would seem that diterpenes can promote the elimination of carcinogens and improve antioxidant status.

A major limitation of the present meta-analysis lies in the fact that most studies did not specify whether the coffee blend was caffeinated or decaffeinated, filtered or unfiltered, thus hindering the possibility of precisely stratifying the pooled RR according to the type of coffee consumed.

A major difficulty in interpreting epidemiological data is that studies often do not clearly indicate the quantity of coffee consumed (which is usually expressed as cups/day and not in mL); estimates are therefore "rough".

Moreover, the considerable variability in the composition of the beverage makes it difficult to accurately determine the potential quantity of bioactive substances involved in the process.

5. Conclusions

The development of colorectal carcinoma is a complex, multi-step process characterized by a series of both genetic and epigenetic changes, which involve different cellular cascades and pathways, including DNA repair, proliferation, apoptosis, intra- and extracellular signaling, and adhesion, among others [47]. Ethnicity seems to be an important variable in the relationship between coffee consumption and the risk of developing colorectal cancer. However, little is known about the relationship between genetic make-up and the risk of colorectal cancer associated with coffee consumption. Furthermore, given the above-mentioned limitations, further research in the field is warranted.

In conclusion, the available studies are not sufficient to define a protective role of coffee against colorectal cancer.

Supplementary Materials: The following are available online at http://www.mdpi.com/2072-6643/11/3/694/s1, PRISMA 2009 Checklist.

Author Contributions: Data curation, A.M.S., E.S. and G.O.; formal analysis, M.S. and N.L.B.; investigation, M.S.; methodology, M.S. and N.L.B.; project administration, M.S. and M.L.C.; software, E.S., G.O. and C.D.; writing—original draft, M.S., N.L.B. and M.L.C.; writing—review and editing, M.S., N.L.B., A.M.S., E.S., G.O., C.D. and M.L.C.

Conflicts of Interest: The authors declare no conflict of interest.

References

1. Rustan, A.C.; Halvorsen, B.; Huggett, A.C.; Ranheim, T.; Drevon, C.A. Effect of coffee lipids (cafestol and kahweol) on regulation of cholesterol metabolism in HepG2 cells. *Arterioscler. Thromb. Vasc. Biol.* **1997**, *17*, 2140–2149. [CrossRef]
2. Gaascht, F.; Dicato, M.; Diederich, M. Coffee provides a natural multitarget pharmacopeia against the hallmarks of cancer. *Genes Nutr.* **2015**, *10*, 51. [CrossRef]
3. Bode, A.M.; Dong, Z. The enigmatic effects of caffeine in cell cycle and cancer. *Cancer Lett.* **2007**, *247*, 26–39. [CrossRef]
4. Nagao, M.; Fujita, Y.; Sugimura, T.; Kosuge, T. Methylglyoxal in beverages and foods: Its mutagenicity and carcinogenicity. *IARC Sci. Publ.* **1986**, *70*, 283–291.
5. Nagao, M.; Fujita, Y.; Wakabayashi, K.; Nukaya, H.; Kosuge, T.; Sugimura, T. Mutagens in coffee and other beverages. *Environ. Health Perspect.* **1986**, *67*, 89–91. [CrossRef] [PubMed]
6. Nagao, M.; Wakabayashi, K.; Fujita, Y.; Tahira, T.; Ochiai, M.; Sugimura, T. Mutagenic compounds in soy sauce, Chinese cabbage, coffee and herbal teas. *Prog. Clin. Biol. Res.* **1986**, *206*, 55–62. [PubMed]
7. Pericleous, M.; Mandair, D.; Caplin, M.E. Diet and supplements and their impact on colorectal cancer. *J. Gastrointest. Oncol.* **2013**, *4*, 409–423.
8. Savolainen, H. Tannin content of tea and coffee. *J. Appl. Toxicol.* **1992**, *12*, 191–192. [CrossRef]
9. Niseteo, T.; Komes, D.; Belščak-Cvitanović, A.; Horžić, D.; Budec, M. Bioactive composition and antioxidant potential of different commonly consumed coffee brews affected by their preparation technique and milk addition. *Food Chem.* **2012**, *134*, 1870–1877. [CrossRef] [PubMed]
10. Valle, I.; Tramalloni, D.; Bragazzi, N.L. Cancer prevention: State of the art and future prospects. *J. Prev. Med. Hyg.* **2015**, *56*, E21–E27.
11. Moher, D.; Liberati, A.; Tetzlaff, J.; Altman, D.G. PRISMA Group. Preferred Reporting Items for Systematic Reviews and Meta-Analyses: The PRISMA Statement. *PLoS Med.* **2009**, *6*, e1000097. [CrossRef] [PubMed]
12. Jacobsen, B.K.; Bjelke, E.; Kvåle, G.; Heuch, I. Coffee drinking, mortality, and cancer incidence: Results from a Norwegian prospective study. *J. Natl. Cancer Inst.* **1986**, *76*, 823–831.
13. Wu, A.H.; Paganini-Hill, A.; Ross, R.K.; Henderson, B.E. Alcohol, physical activity and other risk factors for colorectal cancer: A prospective study. *Br. J. Cancer* **1987**, *55*, 687–694. [CrossRef]
14. Klatsky, A.L.; Armstrong, M.A.; Friedman, G.D.; Hiatt, R.A. The relations of alcoholic beverage use to colon and rectal cancer. *Am. J. Epidemiol.* **1988**, *128*, 1007–1015. [CrossRef]
15. Stensvold, I.; Jacobsen, B.K. Coffee and cancer: A prospective study of 43,000 Norwegian men and women. *Cancer Causes Control* **1994**, *5*, 401–408. [CrossRef]

16. Terry, P.; Bergkvist, L.; Holmberg, L.; Wolk, A. Coffee consumption and risk of colorectal cancer in a population based prospective cohort of Swedish women. *Gut* **2001**, *49*, 87–90. [CrossRef] [PubMed]
17. Khan, M.M.; Goto, R.; Kobayashi, K.; Suzumura, S.; Nagata, Y.; Sonoda, T.; Sakauchi, F.; Washio, M.; Mori, M. Dietary habits and cancer mortality among middle aged and older Japanese living in Hokkaido, Japan by cancer site and sex. *Asian Pac. J. Cancer Prev.* **2004**, *5*, 58–65. [PubMed]
18. Michels, K.B.; Willett, W.C.; Fuchs, C.S.; Giovannucci, E. Coffee, tea, and caffeine consumption and incidence of colon and rectal cancer. *J. Natl. Cancer Inst.* **2005**, *97*, 282–292. [CrossRef]
19. Larsson, S.C.; Bergkvist, L.; Giovannucci, E.; Wolk, A. Coffee consumption and incidence of colorectal cancer in two prospective cohort studies of Swedish women and men. *Am. J. Epidemiol.* **2006**, *163*, 638–644. [CrossRef]
20. Mucci, L.A.; Adami, H.O.; Wolk, A. Prospective study of dietary acrylamide and risk of colorectal cancer among women. *Int. J. Cancer* **2006**, *118*, 169–173. [CrossRef]
21. Oba, S.; Shimizu, N.; Nagata, C.; Shimizu, H.; Kametani, M.; Takeyama, N.; Ohnuma, T.; Matsushita, S. The relationship between the consumption of meat, fat, and coffee and the risk of colon cancer: A prospective study in Japan. *Cancer Lett.* **2006**, *244*, 260–267. [CrossRef]
22. Lee, K.J.; Inoue, M.; Otani, T.; Iwasaki, M.; Sasazuki, S.; Tsugane, S. JPHC Study Group. Coffee consumption and risk of colorectal cancer in a population-based prospective cohort of Japanese men and women. *Int. J. Cancer* **2007**, *121*, 1312–1318. [CrossRef]
23. Naganuma, T.; Kuriyama, S.; Akhter, M.; Kakizaki, M.; Nakaya, N.; Matsuda-Ohmori, K.; Shimazu, T.; Fukao, A.; Tsuji, I. Coffee consumption and the risk of colorectal cancer: A prospective cohort study in Japan. *Int. J. Cancer* **2007**, *120*, 1542–1547. [CrossRef]
24. Bidel, S.; Hu, G.; Jousilahti, P.; Antikainen, R.; Pukkala, E.; Hakulinen, T.; Tuomilehto, J. Coffee consumption and risk of colorectal cancer. *Eur. J. Clin. Nutr.* **2010**, *64*, 917–923. [CrossRef] [PubMed]
25. Nilsson, L.M.; Johansson, I.; Lenner, P.; Lindahl, B.; Van Guelpen, B. Consumption of filtered and boiled coffee and the risk of incident cancer: A prospective cohort study. *Cancer Causes Control* **2010**, *21*, 1533–1544. [CrossRef] [PubMed]
26. Simons, C.C.; Leurs, L.J.; Weijenberg, M.P.; Schouten, L.J.; Goldbohm, R.A.; van den Brandt, P.A. Fluid intake and colorectal cancer risk in the Netherlands Cohort Study. *Nutr. Cancer* **2010**, *62*, 307–321. [CrossRef] [PubMed]
27. Zhang, X.; Albanes, D.; Beeson, W.L.; van den Brandt, P.A.; Buring, J.E.; Flood, A.; Freudenheim, J.L.; Giovannucci, E.L.; Goldbohm, R.A.; Jaceldo-Siegl, K.; et al. Risk of colon cancer and coffee, tea, and sugar-sweetened soft drink intake: Pooled analysis of prospective cohort studies. *J. Natl. Cancer Inst.* **2010**, *102*, 771–783. [CrossRef]
28. Sinha, R.; Cross, A.J.; Daniel, C.R.; Graubard, B.I.; Wu, J.W.; Hollenbeck, A.R.; Gunter, M.J.; Park, Y.; Freedman, N.D. Caffeinated and decaffeinated coffee and tea intake and risk of colorectal cancer in a large prospective study. *Am. J. Clin. Nutr.* **2012**, *96*, 374–381. [CrossRef] [PubMed]
29. Dominianni, C.; Huang, W.Y.; Berndt, S.; Hayes, R.B.; Ahn, J. Prospective study of the relationship between coffee and tea with colorectal cancer risk: The PLCO Cancer Screening Trial. *Br. J. Cancer* **2013**, *109*, 1352–1359. [CrossRef]
30. Perrigue, M.M.; Kantor, E.D.; Hastert, T.A.; Patterson, R.; Potter, J.D.; Neuhouser, M.L.; White, E. Eating frequency and risk of colorectal cancer. *Cancer Causes Control* **2013**, *24*, 2107–2115. [CrossRef]
31. Dik, V.K.; Bueno-de-Mesquita, H.B.; Van Oijen, M.G.; Siersema, P.D.; Uiterwaal, C.S.; Van Gils, C.H.; Van Duijnhoven, F.J.; Cauchi, S.; Yengo, L.; Froguel, P.; et al. Coffee and tea consumption, genotype-based CYP1A2 and NAT2 activity and colorectal cancer risk-results from the EPIC cohort study. *Int. J. Cancer* **2014**, *135*, 401–412. [CrossRef] [PubMed]
32. Hartman, T.J.; Tangrea, J.A.; Pietinen, P.; Malila, N.; Virtanen, M.; Taylor, P.R.; Albanes, D. Tea and coffee consumption and risk of colon and rectal cancer in middle-aged Finnish men. *Nutr. Cancer* **1998**, *31*, 41–48. [CrossRef]
33. Peterson, S.; Yuan, J.M.; Koh, W.P.; Sun, C.L.; Wang, R.; Turesky, R.J.; Yu, M.C. Coffee intake and risk of colorectal cancer among Chinese in Singapore: The Singapore Chinese Health Study. *Nutr. Cancer* **2009**, *62*, 21–29. [CrossRef]

34. Yamada, H.; Kawado, M.; Aoyama, N.; Hashimoto, S.; Suzuki, K.; Wakai, K.; Suzuki, S.; Watanabe, Y.; Tamakoshi, A.; JACC Study Group. Coffee consumption and risk of colorectal cancer: The Japan Collaborative Cohort Study. *J. Epidemiol.* **2014**, *24*, 370–378. [CrossRef]
35. Groessl, E.J.; Allison, M.A.; Larson, J.C.; Ho, S.B.; Snetslaar, L.G.; Lane, D.S.; Tharp, K.M.; Stefanick, M.L. Coffee Consumption and the Incidence of Colorectal Cancer in Women. *J. Cancer Epidemiol.* **2016**, *2016*, 6918431. [CrossRef]
36. Lukic, M.; Licaj, I.; Lund, E.; Skeie, G.; Weiderpass, E.; Braaten, T. Coffee consumption and the risk of cancer in the Norwegian Women and Cancer (NOWAC) Study. *Eur. J. Epidemiol.* **2016**, *31*, 905–916. [CrossRef]
37. Kashino, I.; Akter, S.; Mizoue, T.; Sawada, N.; Kotemori, A.; Matsuo, K.; Oze, I.; Ito, H.; Naito, M.; Nakayama, T.; et al. Coffee drinking and colorectal cancer and its subsites: A pooled analysis of 8 cohort studies in Japan. *Int. J. Cancer* **2018**, *143*, 307–316. [CrossRef] [PubMed]
38. Ludwig, I.A.; Clifford, M.N.; Lean, M.E.; Ashihara, H.; Crozier, A. Coffee: Biochemistry and potential impact on health. *Food Funct.* **2014**, *5*, 1695–1717. [CrossRef] [PubMed]
39. Platt, D.E.; Ghassibe-Sabbagh, M.; Salameh, P.; Salloum, A.K.; Haber, M.; Mouzaya, F.; Gauguier, D.; Al-Sarraj, Y.; El-Shanti, H.; Zalloua, P.A.; et al. Caffeine Impact on Metabolic Syndrome Components Is Modulated by a CYP1A2 Variant. *Ann. Nutr. Metab.* **2016**, *68*, 1–11. [CrossRef] [PubMed]
40. Kumar, P.M.; Paing, S.S.; Li, H.; Pavanni, R.; Yuen, Y.; Zhao, Y.; Tan, E.K. Differential effect of caffeine intake in subjects with genetic susceptibility to Parkinson's Disease. *Sci. Rep.* **2015**, *5*, 15492. [CrossRef]
41. Renda, G.; Zimarino, M.; Antonucci, I.; Tatasciore, A.; Ruggieri, B.; Bucciarelli, T.; Prontera, T.; Stuppia, L.; De Caterina, R. Genetic determinants of blood pressure responses to caffeine drinking. *Am. J. Clin. Nutr.* **2012**, *95*, 241–248. [CrossRef] [PubMed]
42. Chuang, Y.H.; Lill, C.M.; Lee, P.C.; Hansen, J.; Lassen, C.F.; Bertram, L.; Greene, N.; Sinsheimer, J.S.; Ritz, B. Gene-Environment Interaction in Parkinson's Disease: Coffee, ADORA2A, and CYP1A2. *Neuroepidemiology* **2016**, *47*, 192–200. [CrossRef] [PubMed]
43. Kotsopoulos, J.; Vitonis, A.F.; Terry, K.L.; De Vivo, I.; Cramer, D.W.; Hankinson, S.E.; Tworoger, S.S. Coffee intake, variants in genes involved in caffeine metabolism, and the risk of epithelial ovarian cancer. *Cancer Causes Control* **2009**, *20*, 335–344. [CrossRef] [PubMed]
44. Kotsopoulos, J.; Ghadirian, P.; El-Sohemy, A.; Lynch, H.T.; Snyder, C.; Daly, M.; Domchek, S.; Randall, S.; Karlan, B.; Zhang, P.; et al. The CYP1A2 genotype modifies the association between coffee consumption and breast cancer risk among BRCA1 mutation carriers. *Cancer Epidemiol. Biomark. Prev.* **2007**, *16*, 912–916. [CrossRef]
45. Cornelis, M.C.; El-Sohemy, A.; Kabagambe, E.K.; Campos, H. Coffee, CYP1A2 genotype, and risk of myocardial infarction. *JAMA* **2006**, *295*, 1135–1141. [CrossRef] [PubMed]
46. Higdon, J.V.; Frei, B. Coffee and Health: A review of recent Human Research. *Crit. Rev. Food Sci. Nutr.* **2006**, *46*, 101–123. [CrossRef] [PubMed]
47. Marciniak, K.; Kiedrowski, M.; Gajewska, D.; Deptała, A.; Włodarek, D. Wpływ spożycia warzyw, owoców, herbaty oraz kawy na rozwój raka jelita grubego [The impact of the consumption of vegetables, fruits, coffee and tea on the development of colorectal carcinoma]. *Pol. Merkur. Lekarski.* **2016**, *41*, 205–208. (In Polish) [PubMed]

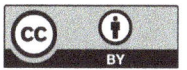

© 2019 by the authors. Licensee MDPI, Basel, Switzerland. This article is an open access article distributed under the terms and conditions of the Creative Commons Attribution (CC BY) license (http://creativecommons.org/licenses/by/4.0/).

MDPI
St. Alban-Anlage 66
4052 Basel
Switzerland
Tel. +41 61 683 77 34
Fax +41 61 302 89 18
www.mdpi.com

Nutrients Editorial Office
E-mail: nutrients@mdpi.com
www.mdpi.com/journal/nutrients

www.ingramcontent.com/pod-product-compliance
Lightning Source LLC
LaVergne TN
LVHW071939080526
838202LV00064B/6638